OXFORD MEDICAL PUBLICATIONS

AN INTRODUCTION TO ORTHODONTICS

An Introduction to Orthodontics

Second edition
LAURA MITCHELL

MDS, BDS, FDSRCPS (Glas), D. Orth RCS (Eng), M. Orth RCS (Eng)
Consultant Orthodontist, St. Luke's Hospital, Bradford
Honorary Clinical Lecturer, Leeds Dental Institute, Leeds

With contributions from
NIGEL E. CARTER

MSc, BDS, FDSRCS (Eng), D. Orth RCS (Eng), M. Orth RCS (Eng)
Consultant Orthodontist, Newcastle Dental Hospital and School, Newcastle

And
BRIDGET DOUBLEDAY

PhD, M. Med. Sci., BDS, FDSRCPS (Glas), M. Orth
Consultant Orthodontist, Leeds Dental Institute, Leeds

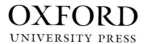

OXFORD
UNIVERSITY PRESS

OXFORD
UNIVERSITY PRESS

Great Clarendon Street, Oxford OX2 6DP
Oxford University Press is a department of the University of Oxford.
It furthers the University's objective of excellence in research, scholarship,
and education by publishing worldwide in

Oxford New York
Auckland Cape Town Dar es Salaam Hong Kong Karachi Kuala Lumpur
Madrid Melbourne Mexico City Nairobi New Delhi Taipei Toronto
Shanghai
With offices in
Argentina Austria Brazil Chile Czech Republic France Greece
Guatemala Hungary Italy Japan South Korea Poland Portugal
Singapore Switzerland Thailand Turkey Ukraine Vietnam

Oxford is a registered trade mark of Oxford University Press
in the UK and in certain other countries

Published in the United States
by Oxford University Press Inc., New York

First edition published 1996
Reprinted 1998, 2000
Second edition published 2001
Reprinted 2004, 2005

A catalogue record for this title is available from the British Library

Library of Congress Cataloging in Publication Data

Mitchell, Laura, 1958–
An introduction to orthodontics/Laura Mitchell, with contribution from
Nigel E. Carter and Bridget Doubleday – 2nd ed. (Oxford medical publications)
Includes index.
1. Orthodontics. I. Carter, Nigel E. II.Doubleday, Bridget. III. Title. IV. Series.
RK521.M58 2001   617.6'43–dc21   00–064993

ISBN 13: 978-0-19-263184–8
ISBN 10: 0-19-263184–5

5 7 9 10 8 6

Typeset by EXPO Holdings, Malaysia

Printed in Italy
by Lito Terrazzi s.r.l.

PREFACE FOR SECOND EDITION

I must admit I was delighted to be asked to produce a second edition of *An Introduction to Orthodontics*. Clinical practice changes so fast it is satisfying to have the chance to update this book for the 21st century.

Being an author is a very exposed position and therefore I would like to express my gratitude to all those who have made positive comments about the first edition of this book. In addition, I would like to thank my co-authors for kindly agreeing to revise some of the chapters and to the staff that have patiently worked with me to produce some of the clinical results seen in the illustrations.

I am greatly indebted to my husband, who not only has helped me with Chapters 20 and 21, but has also been very understanding when the 'the book' has taken priority over other areas of our life.

ACKNOWLEDGEMENTS

Firstly I would like to thank my co-author Nigel Carter not only for relieving me of the burden of two chapters, but also for his thoughtful help in setting the right level for the remainder of the book. Nigel's command of the English language is far in advance of mine and his patience in correcting my poor grammar was much appreciated. I should also mention Evelyn May who generously provided some of the illustrations that eluded me. Permission to use the Index of Orthodontic Treatment Need was kindly granted by VUMAN Limited (Skelton House, Manchester Science Park, Manchester, M15 6SH). I would like to thank the staff of Oxford University Press, who have been helpful and supportive throughout. Finally, I must pay tribute to the help provided by my long-suffering husband, David Mitchell, without whose forbearance and assistance this book would not have reached completion.

CONTENTS

1 The rationale for orthodontic treatment

1.1. DEFINITION

Orthodontics is that branch of dentistry concerned with facial growth, with development of the dentition and occlusion, and with the diagnosis, interception, and treatment of occlusal anomalies.

1.2. PREVALENCE OF MALOCCLUSION

Numerous surveys have been conducted to investigate the prevalence of malocclusion. It should be remembered that the figures for a particular occlusal feature or dental anomaly will depend upon the size and composition of the group studied (for example age and racial characteristics), the criteria used for

Table 1.1   UK Child Dental Health Survey 1993

In the 12-year-old age band:	
Crowding sufficient to impede/prevent eruption	18%
Overjet >5 mm	27%
At least one instanding incisor	8%

assessment, and the methods used by the examiners (for example whether radiographs were employed).

It has been estimated that approximately 66 per cent of 12-year-olds in the UK require some form of orthodontic intervention, and around 33 per cent need complex treatment. In addition, now that a greater proportion of the population are keeping their teeth for longer, orthodontic treatment has an increasing adjunctive role prior to restorative work.

1.3. NEED FOR TREATMENT

It is perhaps pertinent to begin this section by reminding the reader that malocclusion is one end of the spectrum of normal variation and is not a disease.

Ethically, no treatment should be embarked upon unless a demonstrable benefit to the patient is feasible. In addition, the potential advantages should be viewed in the light of possible risks and side-effects, including failure to achieve the aims of treatment. Appraisal of these factors is called risk–benefit analysis and, as in all branches of medicine and dentistry, needs to be considered before treatment is embarked upon for an individual patient. In parallel, financial constraints coupled with the increasing costs of health care have led to an an increased focus upon the cost–benefit ratio of treatment. Obviously the threshold for treatment and the amount of orthodontic intervention will differ between a system that is primarily funded by the state and one that is private or based on insurance schemes.

The decision to embark upon a course of treatment will be influenced by the perceived benefits to the patient in terms of improved function and aesthetics, balanced against the risks of appliance therapy and the prognosis for achieving the aims of treatment successfully. In this chapter we consider each of these areas in turn, starting with the results of research into the possible benefits of orthodontic treatment upon dental health and psychological well-being.

1.3.1. Dental health

Caries

Research has failed to demonstrate a significant association between malocclusion and caries, whereas diet and the use of fluoride toothpaste are correlated with caries experience. However, clinical experience suggests that in susceptible children with a poor diet, malalignment may reduce the potential for natural tooth-cleansing and increase the risk of decay.

Periodontal disease

The association between malocclusion and periodontal disease is weak, as research has shown that individual motivation has more impact than tooth alignment upon effective tooth brushing. Certainly, in the partially edentulous mouth the last remaining teeth are usually the lower incisors — an area which is commonly associated with crowding. Nevertheless, certain occlusal anomalies may prejudice periodontal support.

Crowding may lead to one or more teeth being squeezed buccally or lingually out of their investing bone, resulting in a reduction of periodontal support. This may also occur in a Class III malocclusion where the lower incisors in cross-bite are pushed labially, leading to gingival recession. Traumatic overbites can also lead to increased loss of periodontal suppport and therefore are another indication for orthodontic intervention.

Finally, an increased dental awareness has been noted in patients following orthodontic treatment, and this may be of long-term benefit to oral health.

Trauma to the anterior teeth

The risk of trauma to the upper incisors increases with the size of the overjet. The 1983 Child Dental Health Survey found that children with overjets in excess of 9 mm were twice as likely to experience trauma. Boys and patients with incompetent lips appear to be more at risk; however, the prevalence of trauma reduces with age, with the peak incidence occurring around 10 years.

Masticatory function

Patients with anterior open bites and those with markedly increased or reverse overjets often complain of difficulty with eating, particularly when incising food.

Speech

The soft tissues show remarkable adaptation to the changes that occur during the transition between the primary and mixed dentitions, and when the incisors have been lost owing to trauma or disease. In the main, speech is little affected by malocclusion, and correction of an occlusal anomaly has little effect upon abnormal speech. However, if a patient cannot attain contact between the incisors anteriorally, this may contribute to the production of a lisp (interdental sigmatism).

Tooth impaction

Unerupted teeth may rarely cause pathology. Unerupted impacted teeth, for example maxillary canines, may cause resorption of the roots of adjacent teeth. Dentigerous cyst formation can occur around unerupted third molars or canine teeth. Supernumerary teeth may also give rise to problems, most importantly where their presence prevents normal eruption of an associated permanent tooth or teeth.

Temporomandibular joint dysfunction syndrome

This topic is considered in more detail in Section 1.7, where the effects of both malocclusion and orthodontic treatment upon the temporomandibular joint and associated musculature are considered.

In summary, there are a number of dental traits which do appear to have an adverse effect upon the longevity of the dentition, indicating that their correction would benefit long-term dental health. These include the following:

- Increased overjet
- Increased traumatic overbites
- Anterior crossbites (causing a decrease in labial periodontal support of affected lower incisors)
- Unerupted impacted teeth (where there is a danger of pathology).
- Crossbites associated with mandibular displacement.

1.3.2. Psychosocial well-being

While it is accepted that dentofacial anomalies and severe malocclusion do have a negative effect on the pyschological well-being and self-esteem of the individual, the impact of more minor occlusal problems is more variable and is modified by social and cultural factors. Research has shown that an unattractive dentofacial appearance does have a negative effect on the expectations of teachers and employers. However, in this respect, background facial appearance would appear to have more impact than dental appearance.

A patient's perceptions of the impact of dental variation upon his or her self-image is subject to enormous diversity and is modified by cultural and racial influences. This results in some individuals being unaware of marked malocclusions, whilst others complain bitterly about very minor irregularities.

The dental health component of the Index of Orthodontic Treatment Need was developed to try and quantify the impact of a particular malocclusion upon long-term dental health. The index also comprises an aesthetic element which is an attempt to quantify the aesthetic handicap that a particular arrangement of the teeth poses for a patient. Both aspects of this index are discussed in more detail in Chapter 2.

1.4. DEMAND FOR TREATMENT

After working with the general public for a short period of time, it can readily be appreciated that demand for treatment does not necessarily reflect need for treatment. Some patients will complain bitterly about mild rotations of the upper incisors, whilst others are blithely unaware of markedly increased overjets. It has been demonstated that awareness of tooth alignment and malocclusion, and willingness to undergo orthodontic treatment, are greater in the following groups.

- females
- higher socio-economic families/groups
- in areas which have a smaller population to orthodontist ratio, presumably because appliances become more accepted.

One interesting example of the latter has been observed in countries where provision of orthodontic treatment is mainly privately funded, for example, the USA, as orthodontic appliances are now perceived as a 'status symbol'.

With the increasing dental awareness shown by the public and the increased acceptability of appliances, the demand for treatment is increasing rapidly, particularly among the adult population who may not have had ready access to orthodontic treatment as children. In addition, increased dental awareness also means that patients are seeking a higher standard of treatment result. These combined pressures place considerable strain upon the limited resources of state-funded systems of care. As it appears likely that the demand for treatment will contine to escalate, some form of rationing of state-funded treatment is inevitable and is already operating in some countries. In Sweden for example, the contribution made by the state towards the cost of treatment is based upon need for treatment as determined by the Swedish Health Board's Index.

1.5. THE DISADVANTAGES AND POTENTIAL RISKS OF ORTHODONTIC TREATMENT

Like any other branch of medicine or dentistry, orthodontic treatment is not without potential risks (see Table 1.2).

Table 1.2 Potential risks of orthodontic treatment

Problem	Avoidance/Management of risk
Decalcification	Dietary advice, improve oral hygiene, increase availablity of fluoride
	Abandon treatment
Periodontal attachment loss	Improve oral hygiene
Root resorption	Avoid treatment in patients with resorbed, blunted, or tapered roots
Loss of vitality	If history of previous trauma to incisors, counsel patient

1.5.1. Root resorption

It is now accepted that some root resorption is inevitable as a consequence of tooth movement. During the course of a conventional two-year fixed-appliance treatment around 1 mm of root length will be lost on average. However, this mean masks a wide range of individual variation, as some patients appear to be more susceptible and undergo more marked root resorption. Radiographic signs which indicate an increased susceptibility include shortened roots with evidence of previous root resorption, pipette-shaped or blunted roots, and teeth which have previously suffered an episode of trauma. In addition, more marked resorption is seen in cases where extensive movement of root apices has been undertaken.

1.5.2. Loss of periodontal support

As a result of reduced access for cleansing, an increase in gingival inflammation is commonly seen following the placement of fixed appliances. This normally reduces or resolves following removal of the appliance, but some apical migration of periodontal attachment and alveolar bony support is usual during a two-year course of orthodontic treatment. In most individuals this is minimal, but if oral hygiene is poor, more marked loss may occur.

Removable appliances may also be associated with gingival inflammation, particularly of the palatal tissues, in the presence of poor oral hygiene.

1.5.3. Decalcification

Caries or decalcification occurs when a cariogenic plaque occurs in association with a high-sugar diet. The presence of a fixed appliance predisposes to plaque accumulation as tooth cleaning around the components of the appliance is more difficult. Decalcification during treatment with fixed appliances is a real risk, with a reported prevalence of between 2 and 96 per cent (see Chapter 17, Section 17.7).

1.5.4. Soft tissue damage

Traumatic ulceration can occur during treatment with both fixed and removable appliances, although it is more commonly seen in association with the former as a removable appliance which is uncomfortable is usually removed. Over-enthusiastic apical movement, can lead to a reduction in blood supply to the pulp and even pulpal death. Teeth which have undergone a previous episode of trauma appear to be particularly susceptible, probably because the pulpal tissues are already compromised.

Temporomandibular joint dysfunction syndrome

This is discussed in Section 1.7.

1.6. THE EFFECTIVENESS OF TREATMENT

The decision to embark upon orthodontic treatment must also consider the effectiveness of appliance therapy in correcting the malocclusion of the individual concerned. This has several aspects.

● Are the tooth movements planned attainable? This is considered in more detail in the chapter on treatment planning but, in brief, tooth movement is only feasible within the constraints of the skeletal and growth patterns of the individual patient. The wrong treatment plan, or failure to anticipate adverse growth changes, will reduce the chances of success. In addition, the probable stability of the completed treatment needs to be considered. If a stable result is not possible, do the benefits conferred by proceeding justify prolonged retention, or the possibility of relapse?

- There is a wealth of evidence to show that orthodontic treatment is more likely to achieve a pleasing and successful result if fixed rather than removable appliances are used, and if the operator has had some post-graduate training in orthodontics.
- Patient co-operation.

The likelihood that orthodontic treatment will benefit a patient is increased if the malocclusion is severe and appliance therapy is planned and carried out by an experienced orthodontist. The likelihood of gain is reduced if the malocclusion is mild and treatment is undertaken by an inexperienced operator.

In essence, it may be better not to embark on treatment at all, rather than run the risk of failing to achieve a worthwhile improvement.

Table 1.3   Failure to achieve treatment objectives

Operator factors	Patient factors
Errors of diagnosis	Poor oral hygiene
Errors of treatment planning	Failure to wear appliances
Anchorage loss	Failed appointments
Technique errors	

1.7. THE TEMPOROMANDIBULAR JOINT AND ORTHODONTICS

The aetiology and management of temporomandibular pain dysfunction syndrome (TMPDS) have aroused considerable controversy in all branches of dentistry. The debate has been particularly heated regarding the role of orthodontics, with some authors claiming that orthodontic treatment can cause TMPDS, whilst at the same time others have advocated appliance therapy in the management of the condition.

There are a number of factors that have contributed to the confusion surrounding TMPDS. The objective view is that TMPDS is of multifactorial aetiology, with psychological, traumatic, and occlusal factors all being implicated. Of these, stress is probably the most important, with its effect being mediated by parafunctional activity, for example bruxism, which causes muscle pain and spasm. Success has been claimed for a wide assortment of treatment modalities, reflecting both the multifactorial aetiology and the self-limiting nature of the condition. Apart from internal derangement of the joint, the symptoms of TMPDS usually respond to any treatment which helps to reduce abnormal parafunctional muscle activity.

1.7.1. Orthodontic treatment as a contributory factor in TMPDS

A survey of the literature reveals that those articles claiming that orthodontic treatment (with or without extractions) can contribute to the development of TMPDS are predominantly of the viewpoint (based on the authors' opinion) and case report type. In contrast, controlled longitudinal studies have indicated a trend towards a lower incidence of the symptoms of TMPDS among post-orthodontic patients compared with matched groups of untreated patients.

The consensus view is that orthodontic treatment, either alone or in combination with extractions, does not 'cause' TMPDS.

1.7.2. The role of orthodontic treatment in the prevention and management of TMPDS

Some authors maintain that minor occlusal imperfections lead to abnormal paths of closure and/or bruxism, which then result in the development of TMPDS. If this were the case, then given the high incidence of malocclusion in the population (50–75 per cent), one would expect a higher prevalence of TMPDS than the reported 5–30 per cent. A number of carefully controlled longitudinal studies have been carried out in the USA, and these have found no relationship between the signs and symptoms of TMPDS and the presence of non-functional occlusal contacts or mandibular displacements. However, other studies have found a small but statistically significant association between TMPDS and crossbites, anterior open bite and Class III malocclusions. It is important to remember the multifactorial nature of TMPDS — perhaps, the presence of a displacing contact in susceptible individuals contact may act as the focus of a parafunctional habit mediated by stress.

PRINCIPAL SOURCES AND FURTHER READING

American Journal of Orthodontics and Dentofacial Orthopedics, **101** (1) (1992).
● This is a special issue dedicated to the results of several studies set up by the American Association of Orthodontists to investigate the link between orthodontic treatment and the temporomandibular joint. It is essential reading for all those involved in dentistry.
Harris, M., Feinmann, C., Wise, M., and Treasure, F. (1993). Temporomandibular joint and orofacial pain: clinical and medicolegal management problems. *British Dental Journal*, **174**, 129–36.
● Discusses the role of psychogenic factors in the aetiology of TMPDS.
Holmes, A. (1992). The subjective need and demand for orthodontic treatment. *British Journal of Orthodontics*, **19**, 287–97.
Luther, F. (1998). Orthodontics and the TMJ: Where are we now? *Angle Orthodontist*, **68**, 295–318.
● An authoritative review of the literature on this subject.
Murray, A. M. (1989). Discontinuation of orthodontic treatment: a study of the contributing factors. *British Journal of Orthodontics*, **16**, 1–7.
Office of Population Censuses and Surveys (1994). *Children's dental health in the United Kingdom 1993*. HMSO, London.
Richmond, S. (1993). The provision of orthodontic care in the general dental services of England and Wales: extraction patterns, treatment duration, appliance types and standards. *British Journal of Orthodontics*, **20**, 345–50.
Salonen, L., Mohlin, B., Götzlinger, B., and Helldén, L. (1992). Need and demand for orthodontic treatment in an adult Swedish population. *European Journal of Orthodontics*, **14**, 359–68.
Shaw, W. C., O'Brien, K. D., Richmond, S. and Brook, P. (1991). Quality control in orthodontics: risk/benefit considerations. *British Dental Journal*, **170**, 33–7.
● A rather pessimistic view of orthodontics.
Tang, E. L. K. and Wei, S. H. Y. (1990) Assessing treatment effectiveness of removable and fixed orthodontic appliances with the occlusal index. *American Journal of Orthodontics and Dentofacial Orthopedics*, **99**, 550–6.
● The authors concluded that the effectiveness of fixed appliances (as measured with the occlusal index) is much greater than that of removable appliances.
Turbill, E. A., Richmond, S., and Wright, J. L. (1999). A closer look at GDS orthodontics in England and Wales 1: Factors influencing effectiveness. *British Dental Journal*, **187**, 211–16.
Wassell, R. W. (1989) Do occlusal factors play a part in temporomandibular dysfunction? *Journal of Dentistry*, **17**, 101–10.
● The restorative viewpoint.

Wheeler, T. T. McGorray, S. P., Yurkiewicz, L., Keeling, S. D., and King, G. J. (1994) Orthodontic treatment demand and need in third and fourth grade schoolchildren. *American Journal of Orthodontics and Dentofacial Orthopedics*, **106**, 22–33.
● Contains a good discussion on the need and demand for treatment.

2 The aetiology and classification of malocclusion

2.1. THE AETIOLOGY OF MALOCCLUSION

The aetiology of malocclusion is a fascinating subject about which there is still much to elucidate and understand. At a basic level, malocclusion can occur as a result of genetically determined factors, which are inherited, or environmental factors, or more commonly a combination of both inherited and environmental factors acting together. For example, failure of eruption of an upper central incisor may arise as a result of dilaceration following an episode of trauma during the deciduous dentition which led to intrusion of the primary predecessor — an example of environmental aetiology. Failure of eruption of an upper central incisor can also occur as a result of the presence of a supernumerary tooth — a scenario which questioning may reveal also affected the patient's parent, suggesting an inherited problem. However, if in the latter example caries (an environmental factor) has led to early loss of many of the deciduous teeth, then forward drift of the first permanent molar teeth may also lead to superimposition of the additional problem of crowding.

While it is relatively straightforward to trace the inheritance of syndromes such as cleft lip and palate (see Chapter 21), it is more difficult to determine the aetiology of features which are in essence part of normal variation, and the picture is further complicated by the compensatory mechanisms that exist. Evidence for the role of inherited factors in the aetiology of malocclusion has come from studies of families and twins. The facial similarity of members of a family, for example the prognathic mandible of the Hapsburg royal family, is easily appreciated. However, more direct testimony is provided in studies of twins and triplets, which indicate that skeletal pattern and tooth size and number are largely genetically determined.

Examples of environmental influences include digit-sucking habits and premature loss of teeth as a result of either caries or trauma. Soft tissue pressures acting upon the teeth for more than 6 hours per day can also influence tooth position. However, because the soft tissues including the lips are by necessity attached to the underlying skeletal framework, their effect is also mediated by the skeletal pattern.

Crowding is extremely common in Caucasians, affecting approximately two-thirds of the population. As was mentioned above, the size of the jaws and teeth are mainly genetically determined; however, environmental factors, for example premature deciduous tooth loss, can precipitate or exacerbate crowding. In evolutionary terms both jaw size and tooth size appear to be reducing. However, crowding is much more prevalent in modern populations than it was in prehistoric times. It has been postulated that this is due to the introduction of a less abrasive diet, so that less interproximal tooth wear occurs during the lifetime of an individual. However, this is not the whole story, as a change from a rural to an urban life-style can also apparently lead to an increase in crowding after about two generations.

Although this discussion may at first seem rather theoretical, the aetiology of malocclusion is a vigorously debated subject. This is because if one believes that the basis of malocclusion is genetically determined, then it follows that orthodontics is limited in what it can achieve. However, the opposite viewpoint is that every individual has the potential for ideal occlusion and that orthodontic intervention is required to eliminate those environmental factors that have led to a particular malocclusion. Research suggests that for the majority of malocclusions the aetiology is multifactorial, and orthodontic treatment can effect only limited skeletal change. Therefore, as a patient's skeletal and growth pattern is largely genetically determined, if orthodontic treatment is to be successful clinicians must recognize and work within those parameters.

Of necessity, the above is a brief summary, but it can be appreciated that the aetiology of malocclusion is a complex subject, much of which is still not fully understood. The reader seeking more information is advised to consult the publications listed in the section on further reading.

2.2. CLASSIFYING MALOCCLUSION

The categorization of a malocclusion by its salient features is helpful for describing and documenting a patient's occlusion. In addition, classifications and indices allow the prevalence of a malocclusion within a population to be recorded, and also aid in the assessment of need, difficulty, and success of orthodontic treatment.

Malocclusion can be recorded qualitatively and quantitatively. However, the large number of classifications and indices which have been devised, are testimony to the problems inherent in both these approaches. All have their limitations, and these should be borne in mind when they are applied.

Two terms are often mentioned in relation to indices:

- **Validity** — Can the index measure what it was designed to measure?
- **Reproducibility** — Does the index give the same result when recorded on two different occasions, and by different examiners?

2.2.1. Qualitative assessment of malocclusion

Essentially, a qualitative assessment is descriptive and therefore this category includes the diagnostic classifications of maloccusion. The main drawback to a qualitative approach is that malocclusion is a continuous variable so that clear cut-off points between different categories do not always exist. This can lead to problems when classifying borderline malocclusions. In addition, although a qualitative classification is a helpful shorthand method of describing the salient features of a malocclusion, it does not provide any indication of the difficulty of treatment.

Qualitative evaluation of malocclusion was attempted historically before quantative analysis. One of the better known classifications was devised by Angle in 1899, but other classifications are now more widely used, for example the British Standards Institute (1983) classification of incisor relationship.

2.2.2. Quantitative assessment of malocclusion

In quantitative indices two differing approaches can be used:

- Each feature of a malocclusion is given a score and the summed total is then recorded (e.g. the PAR Index).
- The worst feature of a malocclusion is recorded (e.g. the Index of Orthodontic Treatment Need).

2.3. COMMONLY USED CLASSIFICATIONS AND INDICES

2.3.1. Angle's classification

Angle's classification was based upon the premise that the first permanent molars erupted into a constant position within the facial skeleton, which could be used to assess the anteroposterior relationship of the arches. In addition to the fact that Angle's classification was based upon an incorrect assumption, the problems experienced in categorizing cases with forward drift or loss of the first permanent molars have resulted in this particular approach being superseded by other classifications. However, Angle's classification is still used to describe molar relationship, and the terms used to describe incisor relationship have been adapted into incisor classification.

Angle described three groups (Fig. 2.1):

- *Class I or neutrocclusion* — the mesiobuccal cusp of the upper first molar occludes with the mesiobuccal groove of the lower first molar. In practice discrepancies of up to half a cusp width either way were also included in this category.
- *Class II or distocclusion* — the mesiobuccal cusp of the lower first molar occludes distal to the Class I position. This is also known as a postnormal relationship.
- *Class III or mesiocclusion* — the mesiobuccal cusp of the lower first molar occludes mesial to the Class I position. This is also known as a prenormal relationship.

2.3.2. British Standards Institute classification

This is based upon incisor relationship and is the most widely used descriptive classification. The terms used are similar to those of Angle's classification, which can be a little confusing as no regard is taken of molar relationship. The categories defined by British Standard 4492 are as follows:

- *Class I* — the lower incisor edges occlude with or lie immediately below the cingulum plateau of the upper central incisors (Fig. 2.2).
- *Class II* — the lower incisor edges lie posterior to the cingulum plateau of the upper incisors. There are two subdivisions of this category:

    Division 1 — the upper central incisors are proclined or of average inclination and there is an increase in overjet (Fig. 2.3).

    Division 2 — The upper central incisors are retroclined. The overjet is usually minimal or may be increased (Fig. 2.4).

- *Class III* — The lower incisor edges lie anterior to the cingulum plateau of the upper incisors. The overjet is reduced or reversed (Fig. 2.5).

As with any descriptive analysis it is difficult to classify borderline cases. Some workers have suggested introducing a Class II intermediate category for those cases where the upper incisors are upright and the overjet increased between 4 and 6 mm. However, this suggestion has not gained widespread acceptance.

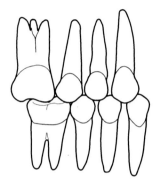

Class I

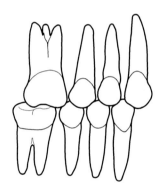

Class II

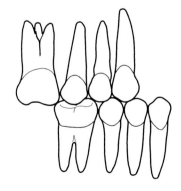

Class III

Fig. 2.1. Angle's classification.

2.3.3. Summers occlusal index

This index was developed by Summers, in the USA, during the 1960s. It is popular in the USA, particularly for research purposes. Good reproducibility has been reported and it has also been employed to determine the success of treatment with acceptable results. The index scores nine defined parameters including molar relationship, overbite, overjet, posterior crossbite, posterior open bite, tooth displacement, midline relation, maxillary median diastema, and absent upper incisors. Allowance is made for different stages of development by varying the weighting applied to certain parameters in the deciduous, mixed, and permanent dentition.

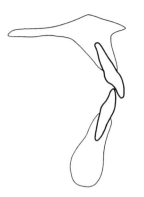

Fig. 2.2. Incisor classification — Class I.

2.3.4. Index of Orthodontic Treatment Need (IOTN)

The Index of Orthodontic Treatment Need was developed as a result of a government initiative. The purpose of the index was to help determine the likely impact of a malocclusion on an individual's dental health and psychosocial well-being. It comprises two elements.

Dental health component

This was developed from an index used by the Dental Board in Sweden designed to reflect those occlusal traits, which could affect the function and longevity of the dentition. The single worst feature of a malocclusion is noted (the index is not cumulative) and categorized into one of five grades reflecting need for treatment (Table 2.1):

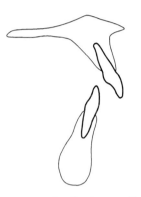

Fig. 2.3. Incisor classification — Class II division 1.

- *Grade 1* — no need
- *Grade 2* — little need
- *Grade 3* — moderate need
- *Grade 4* — great need
- *Grade 5* — very great need.

A ruler has been developed to help with assessment of the dental health component (Fig. 2.6), and these are available commercially.

Aesthetic component

This aspect of the index was developed in an attempt to assess the aesthetic handicap posed by a malocclusion and thus the likely psychosocial impact upon the patient — a task fraught with potential pitfalls (see Chapter 1). The aesthetic component comprises a set of ten standard photographs (Fig. 2.7), which are also graded from score 1, the most aesthetically pleasing, to score 10, the least aesthetically pleasing. Colour photographs are available for use with a patient in the clinical situation and black-and-white photographs for scoring from study

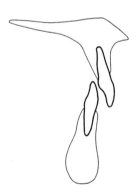

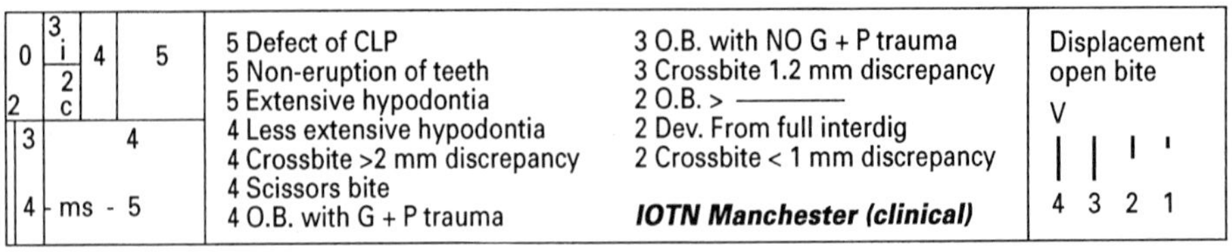

Fig. 2.4. Incisor classification — Class II division 2.

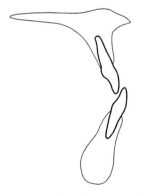

Fig. 2.5. Incisor classification — Class III.

0	3 i 2 c	4	5	5 Defect of CLP 5 Non-eruption of teeth 5 Extensive hypodontia 4 Less extensive hypodontia 4 Crossbite >2 mm discrepancy 4 Scissors bite 4 O.B. with G + P trauma	3 O.B. with NO G + P trauma 3 Crossbite 1.2 mm discrepancy 2 O.B. >⸺ 2 Dev. From full interdig 2 Crossbite < 1 mm discrepancy ***IOTN Manchester (clinical)***	Displacement open bite V | | ʲ ' 4 3 2 1
2	3		4			
4	ms - 5					

Fig. 2.6. IOTN ruler.

Table 2.1 The Index of Orthodontic Treatment Need

Grade 1 (None)

1   Extremely minor malocclusions including displacements less than 1 mm

Grade 2 (Little)

2a   Increased overjet 3.6–6 mm with competent lips
2b   Reverse overjet 0.1–1 mm
2c   Anterior or posterior crossbite with up to 1 mm discrepancy between retruded contact position and intercuspal position
2d   Displacement of teeth 1.1–2 mm
2e   Anterior or posterior open bite 1.1–2 mm
2f   Increased overbite 3.5 mm or more, without gingival contact
2g   Prenormal or postnormal occlusions with no other anomalies; includes up to half a unit discrepancy.

Grade 3 (Moderate)

3a   Increased overjet 3.6–6 mm with incompetent lips
3b   Reverse overjet 1.1–3.5 mm
3c   Anterior or posterior crossbites with 1.1–2 mm discrepancy
3d   Displacement of teeth 2.1–4 mm
3e   Lateral or anterior open bite 2.1–4 mm
3f   Increased and complete overbite without gingival trauma

Grade 4 (Great)

4a   Increased overjet 6.1–9 mm
4b   Reversed overjet greater than 3.5 mm with no masticatory or speech difficulties
4c   Anterior or posterior crossbites with greater than 2 mm discrepancy between retruded contact position and intercuspal position.
4d   Severe displacement of teeth, greater than 4 mm.
4e   Extreme lateral or anterior open bites, greater than 4 mm.
4f   Increased and complete overbite with gingival or palatal trauma.
4h   Less extensive hypodontia requiring pre-restorative orthodontic space closure to obviate the need for a prosthesis
4l   Posterior lingual crossbite with no functional occlusal contact in one or both buccal segments
4m   Reverse overjet 1.1–3.5 mm with recorded masticatory and speech difficulties
4t   Partially erupted teeth, tipped and impacted against adjacent teeth
4x   Supplemental teeth

Grade 5 (Very Great)

5a   Increased overjet greater than 9 mm
5h   Extensive hypodontia with restorative implications (more than one tooth missing in any quadrant) requiring pre-restorative orthodontics
5i   Impeded eruption of teeth (with the exception of third molars) due to crowding, displacement, the presence of supernumerary teeth, retained deciduous teeth, and any pathological cause
5m   Reverse overjet greater than 3.5 mm with reported masticatory and speech difficulties
5p   Defects of cleft lip and palate
5s   Submerged deciduous teeth

Reproduced with the kind permission of Vuman Ltd.

Fig. 2.7. Aesthetic component of IOTN.

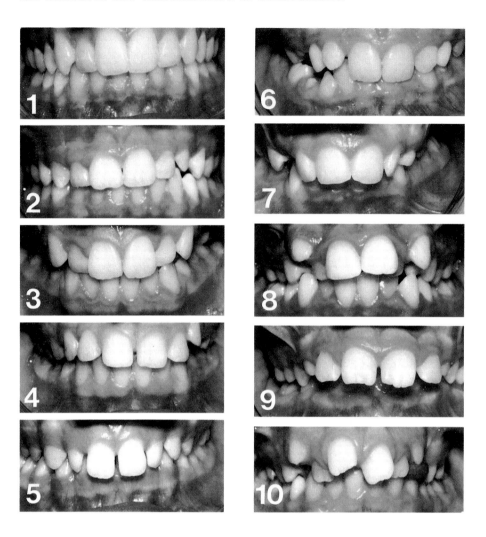

models alone. The patient's teeth (or study models), in occlusion, are viewed from the anterior aspect and the appropriate score determined by choosing the photograph that is thought to pose an equivalent aesthetic handicap. The scores are categorized acccording to need for treatment as follows:

- score 1 or 2 — none
- score 3 or 4 — slight
- score 5, 6, or 7 — moderate/borderline
- score 8, 9, or 10 — definite

An average score can be taken from the two components, but the dental health component alone is more widely used. The aesthetic component has been criticized for being subjective, and particular difficulty is experienced in accurately assessing Class III malocclusions or anterior open bites, as the photographs are composed of Class I and Class II cases.

2.3.5. Peer Assessment Rating (PAR)

The PAR index was developed primarily to measure the success (or otherwise) of treatment. Scores are recorded for a number of parameters (listed below), before and at the end of treatment, using study models. Unlike IOTN, the scores are cumulative; however, a weighting is accorded to each component to reflect current opinion in the UK as to their relative importance. The features recorded are listed below, with the current weightings in parenthesis:

- crowding — by contact point displacement (×1)
- buccal segment relationship — in the anteroposterior, vertical, and transverse planes (×1)
- overjet (×6)
- overbite (×2)
- centrelines (×4).

The difference between the PAR scores at the start and on completion of treatment can be calculated, and from this the percentage change in PAR score, which is a reflection of the success of treatment, is derived. A high standard of treatment is indicated by a mean percentage reduction of greater than 70 per cent. A change of 30 per cent or less indicates that no appreciable improvement has been achieved. The size of the PAR score at the beginning of treatment gives an indication of the severity of a malocclusion. Obviously it is difficult to achieve an significant reduction in PAR in cases with a low pretreatment score.

2.3.6 Index of Complexity Outcome and Need (ICON)

This new index incorporates features of both the Index of Orthodontic Need (IOTN) and the Peer Assessment Rating (PAR). The aesthetic component of IOTN is included along with scores for upper arch crowding/spacing; presence of crossbite; overbite/open bite, and buccal segment relationship. As in the PAR, weightings are added to reflect current orthodontic opinion. The sum of the scores and their weightings gives a pretreatment score, which is said to reflect the need for, and likely complexity of, the treatment required. Following treatment the index is scored again to give an improvement grade (pretreatment score minus 4 × post-treatment score) and thus the outcome of treatment. This ambitious index is currently undergoing evaluation.

PRINCIPAL SOURCES AND FURTHER READING

Angle, E. H. (1899). Classification of malocclusion. *Dental Cosmos*, **41**, 248–64.

Markovic, M. (1992). At the crossroads of oral facial genetics. *European Journal of Orthodontics*, **14**, 469–81.

- A fascinating study of twins and triplets with Class II/2 malocclusions.

Mossey, P. A. (1999). The heritability of malocclusion. *British Journal of Orthodontics*, **26**, 103–13, 195–203.

Richmond, S., Shaw, W. C., O'Brien, K. D., Buchanan, I. B., Jones, R., Stephens, C. D., *et al.* (1992). The development of the PAR index (Peer Assessment Rating): reliability and validity. *European Journal of Orthodontics*, **14**, 125–39.

- The PAR index, part 1.

Richmond, S., Shaw, W. C., Roberts, C. T., and Andrews, M. (1992). The PAR index (Peer Assessment Rating): methods to determine the outcome of orthodontic treatment in terms of improvements and standards. *European Journal of Orthodontics*, **14**, 180–7.

- The PAR index, part 2.

Summers, C. J. (1971). A system for identifying and scoring occlusal disorders. *American Journal of Orthodontics*, **59**, 552–67.

- For readers requiring further information on Summers' occlusal index.

Shaw, W. C., O'Brien, K. D., and Richmond, S. (1991). Quality control in orthodontics: indices of treatment need and treatment standards. *British Dental Journal*, **170**, 107–12.

- An interesting paper on the role of indices, with good explanations of the IOTN and the PAR index.

Tang, E. L. K. and Wei, S. H. Y. (1993). Recording and measuring malocclusion: a review of the literature. *American Journal of Orthodontics and Dentofacial Orthopedics*, **103**, 344–51.
- Useful for those researching the subject.

3 Management of the developing dentition

Many dental practitioners find it difficult to judge when to intervene in a developing malocclusion and when to let nature take its course. This is because experience is only gained over years of careful observation, and decisions to intercede are often made in response to pressure exerted by the parents 'to do something'. It is hoped that this chapter will help impart some of the former, so that the reader is better able to resist the latter.

3.1. NORMAL DENTAL DEVELOPMENT

It is important to realize that 'normal' in this context means average, rather than ideal. An appreciation of what constitutes the range of normal development is essential. One area in which this is particularly pertinent is eruption times (Table 3.1).

3.1.1. Calcification and eruption times

Knowledge of the calcification times of the permanent dentition is invaluable if one wishes to impress patients and colleagues. It is also helpful for assessing dental as opposed to chronological age, for determining whether a developing tooth not present on radiographic examination can be considered absent, and for estimating the timing of any possible causes of localized hypocalcification or hypoplasia (chronological hypoplasia).

3.1.2. The transition from primary to mixed dentition

The eruption of a baby's first tooth is heralded by the proud parents as a major landmark in their child's development. This milestone is described in many baby-care books as occurring at 6 months of age, which can lead to unnecessary concern as it is normal for the mandibular incisors to erupt at any time in the first year. Dental textbooks often dismiss 'teething', ascribing the symptoms that occur at this time to the diminution of maternal antibodies. Any parent will be able to correct this fallacy!

Eruption of the primary dentition (Fig. 3.1) is usually completed around 3 years of age. The deciduous incisors erupt upright and spaced — a lack of spacing strongly suggests that the permanent successors will be crowded. Overbite reduces throughout the primary dentition until the incisors are edge to edge, which can contribute to marked attrition.

The mixed dentition phase is usually heralded by the eruption of either the first permanent molars or the lower central incisors. The lower labial segment teeth erupt before their counterparts in the upper arch and develop lingual to their

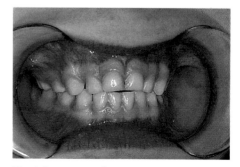

Fig. 3.1. Primary dentition.

Table 3.1 Average calcification and eruption times

	Calcification commences (weeks *in utero*)	Eruption (months)
Primary dentition		
Central incisors	12–16	6–7
Lateral incisors	13–16	7–8
Canines	15–18	18–20
First molars	14–17	12–15
Second molars	16–23	24–36

Root calcification complete $1-1\frac{1}{2}$ years after eruption

	Calcification commences (months)	Eruption (years)
Permanent dentition		
Mand. central incisors	3–4	6–7
Mand. lateral incisors	3–4	7–8
Mand. canines	4–5	9–10
Mand. first premolars	21–24	10–12
Mand. second premolars	27–30	11–12
Mand. first molars	Around birth	5–6
Mand. second molars	30–36	12–13
Mand. third molars	96–120	17–25
Max. central incisors	3–4	7–8
Max. lateral incisors	10–12	8–9
Max. canines	4–5	11–12
Max. first premolars	18–21	10–11
Max. second premolars	24–27	10–12
Max. first molars	Around birth	5–6
Max. second molars	30–36	12–13
Max. third molars	84–108	17–25

Root calcification complete 2–3 years after eruption

predecessors. It is usual for there to be some crowding of the permanent lower incisors as they emerge into the mouth, which reduces with intercanine growth. As a result the lower incisors often erupt slightly lingually placed and/or rotated (Fig. 3.2), but will usually align spontaneously if space becomes available. If the arch is inherently crowded, this space shortage will not resolve with intercanine growth.

The upper permanent incisors also develop lingual to their predecessors. Additional space is gained to accommodate their greater width because they erupt onto a wider arc and are more proclined than the primary incisors. If the arch is intrinsically crowded, the lateral incisors will not be able to move labially following eruption of the central incisors and therefore may erupt palatal to the arch. Pressure from the developing lateral incisor often gives rise to spacing between the central incisors which resolves as the laterals erupt. They in turn are tilted distally by the canines lying on the distal aspect of their root. This latter stage of development used to be described as the 'ugly duckling' stage of development (Fig. 3.3), although it is probably diplomatic to describe it as normal dental development to concerned parents. As the canines erupt, the lateral incisors usually upright themselves and the spaces close. The upper canines

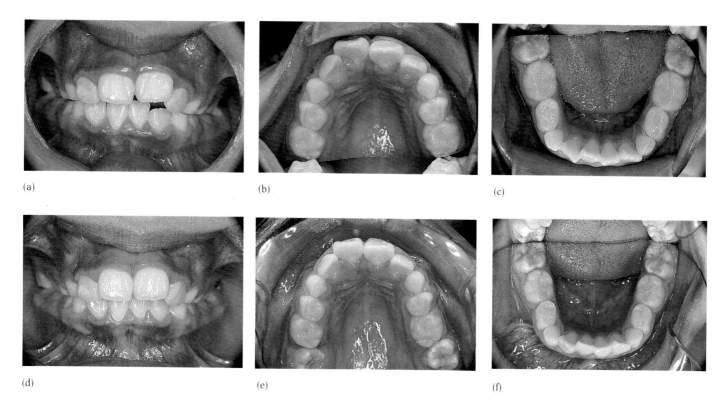

(a)

(b)

(c)

(d)

(e)

(f)

develop palatally, but migrate labially to come to lie slightly labial and distal to the root apex of the lateral incisors. In normal development they can be palpated buccally from as young as 8 years of age.

The combined width of the deciduous canine, first molar, and second molar is greater than that of their permanent successors, particularly in the lower arch. This difference in widths is called the leeway space (Fig. 3.4) and in general is of the order of 1–1.5 mm in the maxilla and 2–2.5 mm in the mandible (in Caucasians). This means that if the deciduous buccal segment teeth are retained until their normal exfoliation time, there will be sufficient space for the permanent canine and premolars.

The deciduous second molars usually erupt with their distal surfaces flush anteroposteriorly. The transition to the stepped Class I molar relationship occurs

Fig. 3.2. Crowding of the labial segment reducing with growth in intercanine width: (a), (b), (c) age 8 years; (d), (e), (f) age 9 years.

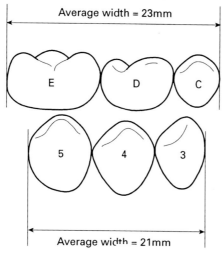

Fig. 3.4. Leeway space.

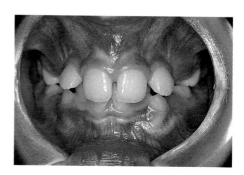

Fig. 3.3. 'Ugly duckling' stage.

during the mixed dentition as a result of differential mandibular growth and/or the leeway space.

3.1.3. Development of the dental arches

Intercanine width is measured across the cusps of the deciduous/permanent canines, and during the primary dentition an increase of around 1–2 mm is seen. In the mixed dentition an increase of about 3 mm occurs, but this growth is largely completed around a developmental stage of 9 years with some minimal increase up to age 13. After this time a gradual decrease is the norm.

Arch width is measured across the arch between the lingual cusps of the second deciduous molars or second premolars. Between the ages of 3 and 18 years an increase of 2–3 mm occurs; however, for clinical purposes arch width is largely established in the mixed dentition.

Arch circumference is determined by measuring around the buccal cusps and incisal edges of the teeth to the distal aspect of the second deciduous molars or second premolars. On average, there is little change with age in the maxilla; however, in the mandible arch circumference decreases by about 4 mm because of the leeway space. In individuals with crowded mouths a greater reduction may be seen.

In summary, on the whole there is little change in the size of the arch anteriorly after the establishment of the primary dentition, except for an increase in intercanine width which results in a modification of arch shape. Growth posteriorly provides space for the permanent molars, and considerable appositional vertical growth occurs to maintain the relationship of the arches during vertical facial growth.

3.2. ABNORMALITIES OF ERUPTION AND EXFOLIATION

3.2.1. Screening

Early detection of any abnormalities in tooth development and eruption is essential to give the opportunity for interceptive action to be taken. This requires careful observation of the developing dentition for evidence of any problems, for example deviations from the normal sequence of eruption. If an abnormality is suspected then further investigation including radiographs is indicated. Around 9 to 10 years of age it is important to palpate the buccal sulcus for the permanent maxillary canines in order to detect any abnormalities in the eruption path of this tooth.

3.2.2. Natal teeth

A tooth, which is present at birth, or erupts soon after, is described as a natal tooth. These most commonly arise anteriorly in the mandible and are typically a lower primary incisor, which has erupted prematurely (Fig. 3.5). Because root formation is not complete at this stage, natal teeth can be quite mobile, but they usually become firmer relatively quickly. If the tooth (or teeth) interferes with breast feeding or is so mobile that there is a danger of inhalation, removal is indicated and this can usually be accomplished with topical anaesthesia. If the tooth is symptomless, it can be left *in situ*.

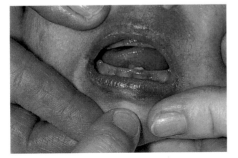

Fig. 3.5. Natal tooth present at birth.

3.2.3. Eruption cyst

An eruption cyst is caused by an accumulation of fluid or blood in the follicular space overlying the crown of an erupting tooth (Fig. 3.6). They usually rupture spontaneously, but very occasionally marsupialization may be necessary.

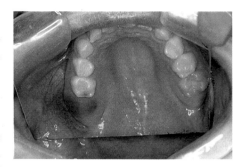

Fig. 3.6. Eruption cyst.

3.2.4. Failure of/delayed eruption

There is a wide individual variation in eruption times, which is illustrated by the patients in Fig. 3.7. Where there is a generalized tardiness in tooth eruption in an otherwise fit child, a period of observation is indicated. However, the following may be indicators of some abnormality and therefore warrant further investigation (Fig. 3.8):

- A disruption in the normal sequence of eruption.
- An asymmetry in eruption pattern between contralateral teeth. If a tooth on one side of the arch has erupted and 6 months later there is still no sign of its equivalent on the other side, radiographic examination is indicated.

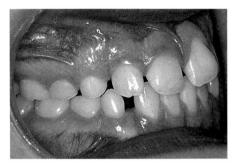

(a)

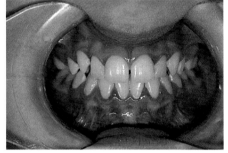

(b)

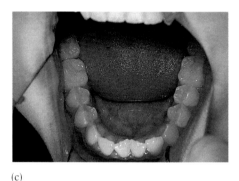

(c)

Fig. 3.7. Normal variation in eruption times: (a) patient aged 12.5 years with deciduous canines and molars still present; (b), (c) patient aged nine years with all permanent teeth to the second molars erupted.

Table 3.2 Causes of delayed eruption

Generalized causes
Hereditary gingival fibromatosis
Down syndrome
Cleidocranial dysostosis
Cleft lip and palate
Ricketts

Localized causes
Congenital absence
Crowding
Delayed exfoliation of primary predecessor
Supernumerary tooth (see below)
Dilaceration
Abnormal position of crypt
Primary failure of eruption

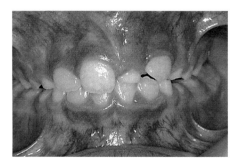

Fig. 3.8. Disruption of normal eruption sequence as 21/2 erupted, but /1 unerupted.

3.3. MIXED DENTITION PROBLEMS

3.3.1. Premature loss of deciduous teeth

Balancing extraction is the removal of the contralateral tooth. **Compensating extraction** is the removal of the equivalent opposing tooth.

The major effect of early loss of a primary tooth, whether due to caries, premature exfoliation, or planned extraction, is localization of pre-existing crowding. In an uncrowded mouth this will not occur. However, where some crowding exists and a primary tooth is extracted, the adjacent teeth will drift or tilt around into the space provided. The extent to which this occurs depends upon the degree of crowding, the patient's age, and the site. Obviously, as the degree of crowding increases so does the pressure for the remaining teeth to move into the extraction space. The younger the child is when the primary tooth is extracted, the greater is the potential for drifting to ensue. The effect of the site of tooth loss is best considered by tooth type, but it is important to bear in mind the increased potential for mesial drift in the maxilla.

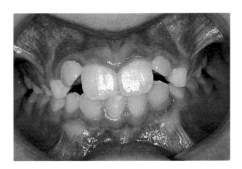

Fig. 3.9. Centre-line shift to patient's left owing to early unbalanced loss of lower left deciduous canine.

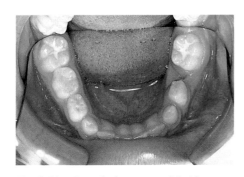

Fig. 3.10. Loss of a lower second deciduous molar leading to forward drift of first permanent molar.

- **Deciduous incisor:** premature loss of a deciduous incisor has little impact, mainly because they are shed relatively early in the mixed dentition.

- **Deciduous canine:** unilateral loss of a primary canine in a crowded mouth will lead to a centreline shift (Fig. 3.9). As this is a difficult problem to treat, often requiring fixed appliances, prevention is preferable and therefore premature loss of a deciduous canine should be balanced in any patient with even the mildest crowding.

- **Deciduous first molar:** unilateral loss of this tooth may result in a centreline shift. In most cases an automatic balancing extraction is not necessary, but the centreline should be kept under observation and, if indicated, a tooth on the opposite side of the arch removed.

- **Deciduous second molar:** if a second primary molar is extracted the first permanent molar will drift forwards (Fig. 3.10). This is particularly marked if loss occurs before the eruption of the permanent tooth and for this reason it is better, if at all possible, to try to preserve the second deciduous molar at least until the first permanent molar has appeared. In most cases balancing or compensating extractions of other sound second primary molars is not necessary. However, where extraction of a carious upper deciduous molar alone would change the molar relationship from a half-unit Class II to a full Class II, it may be advisable to consider balancing with the extraction of the lower second deciduous molar.

It should be emphasized that the above are suggestions, not rules, and at all times a degree of common sense and forward planning should be applied. For example, if extraction of a carious first primary molar is required and the contralateral tooth is also doubtful, then it might be preferable in the long term to extract both. Also, in children with an absent permanent tooth (or teeth) early extraction of the primary buccal segment teeth may be advantageous to encourage forward movement of the first permanent molars if space closure (rather then space opening) is planned.

The effect of early extraction of a primary tooth on the eruption of its successor is variable and will not necessarily result in a hastening of eruption.

3.3.2. Retained deciduous teeth

A difference of more than 6 months between the shedding of contralateral teeth should be regarded with suspicion. Provided that the permanent successor is present, retained primary teeth should be extracted, particularly if they are causing deflection of the permanent tooth (Fig. 3.11).

3.3.3. Infra-occluded (submerged) primary molars

Infra-occlusion is now the preferred term for describing the process where a tooth fails to achieve or maintain its occlusal relationship with adjacent or opposing teeth. Most infra-occluded deciduous teeth erupt into occlusion, but subsequently become 'submerged' because bony growth and development of the adjacent teeth continues (Fig. 3.12). Estimates vary, but this anomaly would appear to occur in around 1–9 per cent of children.

Resorption of the primary teeth is not a continuous process. In fact, resorption is interchanged with periods of repair, although in most cases the former prevails. If a temporary predominance of repair occurs this can result in ankylosis and infra-occlusion of the affected primary molar.

The results of recent epidemiological studies have suggested a genetic tendency to this phenomenon and also an association with other dental anomalies including ectopic eruption of first permanent molars, palatal displacement of maxillary canines, and congenital absence of premolar teeth. Therefore, it is advisable to be vigilant in patients exhibiting any of these features.

Where a permanent successor exists the phenomenon is usually temporary, and studies have shown no difference in the age at exfoliation of a submerged primary molar compared with an unaffected contralateral tooth. Therefore extraction of a submerged primary tooth is only necessary under the following conditions:

● There is a danger of the tooth disappearing below gingival level (Fig. 3.13).

● Root formation of the permanent tooth is nearing completion (as eruptive force reduces markedly after this event).

● The permanent successor is missing, as in this situation the submergence may be progressive.

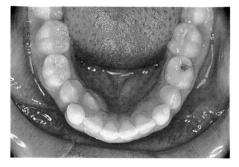

Fig. 3.11. Retained primary tooth contributing to deflection of the permanent successor.

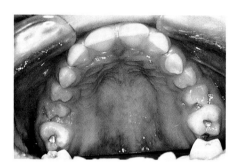

Fig. 3.12. Ankylosed primary molars.

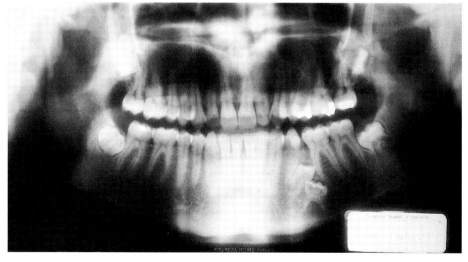

Fig. 3.13. Marked submergence of deciduous molar (with second premolar affected).

3.3.4. Impacted first permanent molars

Impaction of a first permanent molar tooth against the second deciduous molar occurs in approximately 2–6 per cent of children and is indicative of crowding. It

Fig. 3.14. Impacted bilateral upper first permanent molars.

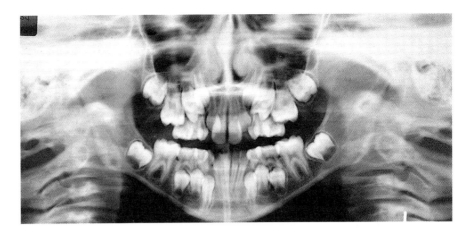

most commonly occurs in the upper arch (Fig. 3.14). Spontaneous disimpaction may occur, but this is rare after 8 years of age. Mild cases can sometimes be managed by tightening a brass separating wire around the contact point between the two teeth over a period of about 2 months. This can have the effect of pushing the permanent molar distally, thus letting it jump free. In more severe cases the impaction can be kept under observation, although extraction of the deciduous tooth may be indicated if it becomes abscessed or the permanent tooth becomes carious and restoration precluded by poor access. The resultant space loss can be dealt with in the permanent dentition.

3.3.5. Dilaceration

Dilaceration is a distortion or bend in the root of a tooth.

Aetiology

There appear to be two distinct aetiologies:

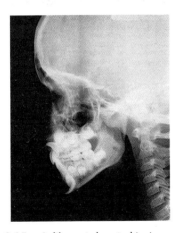

Fig. 3.15. A dilacerated central incisor.

- Developmental — this anomaly usually affects an isolated central incisor and occurs in females more often than males. The crown of the affected tooth is turned upward and labially and no disturbance of enamel and dentine is seen (Fig. 3.15).
- Trauma — intrusion of a deciduous incisor leads to displacement of the underlying developing permanent tooth germ. Characteristically, this causes the developing permanent tooth crown to be deflected palatally, and the enamel and dentine forming at the time of the injury are disturbed, giving rise to hypoplasia. The sexes are equally affected and more than one tooth may be involved depending upon the extent of the trauma.

Management

Dilaceration usually causes failure of eruption. Where the dilaceration is severe there is often no alternative but to remove the affected tooth. In milder cases it may be possible to expose the crown surgically and apply traction to align the tooth, provided that the root apex will be sited within cancellous bone at the completion of crown alignment.

3.3.6. Supernumerary teeth

A supernumerary tooth is one that is additional to the normal series. This anomaly occurs in the permanent dentition in approximately 2 per cent of the population and in the primary dentition in less than 1 per cent, though a supernumerary in the deciduous dentition is often followed by a supernumerary in the permanent dentition. The aetiology is not completely understood, but suggestions include an offshoot of the dental lamina of the permanent dentition or a tertiary dentition. This anomaly occurs more commonly in males than females. Supernumerary teeth are also commonly found in the region of the cleft in individuals with a cleft of the alveolus.

Supernumerary teeth can be described according to their morphology or position in the arch.

Morphology

- **Supplemental**: this type resembles a tooth and occurs at the end of a tooth series, for example an additional lateral incisor, second premolar, or fourth molar (Fig. 3.16).
- **Conical**: the conical or peg-shaped supernumerary most often occurs between the upper central incisors (Fig. 3.17). It is said to be more commonly associated with displacement of the adjacent teeth, but can also cause failure of eruption or have no effect at all.
- **Tuberculate**: this type is described as being barrel-shaped, but usually any supernumerary which does not fall into the conical or supplemental categories is included. Classically, this type is associated with failure of eruption (Fig. 3.18).
- **Odontome**: This variant is rare. Both compound and complex forms have been described.

Position

Supernumerary teeth can occur within the arch, but when they develop between the central incisors they are often described as a mesiodens. A supernumerary tooth distal to the arch is called a distomolar, and one adjacent to the molars is known as a paramolar.

Effects of supernumerary teeth and their management

Failure of eruption

The presence of a supernumerary tooth is the most common reason for the non-appearance of a maxillary central incisor. However, failure of eruption of any tooth in either arch can be caused by a supernumerary.

Management of this problem involves removing the supernumerary tooth and ensuring that there is sufficient space to accommodate the unerupted tooth in the arch. If the tooth does not erupt spontaneously within 1 year, then a second operation to expose it and apply orthodontic traction may be required. Management of a patient with this problem is illustrated in Fig. 3.19.

Displacement

The presence of a supernumerary tooth can be associated with displacement or rotation of an erupted permanent tooth (Fig. 3.20). Management involves firstly removal of the supernumerary, usually followed by fixed appliances to align the affected tooth or teeth. It is said that this type of displacement has a high tendency to relapse following treatment, but this may be a reflection of the fact that the malposition is usually in the form of a rotation or an apical displacement which are particularly liable to relapse.

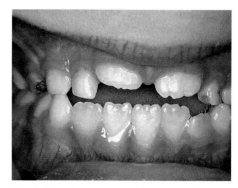

Fig. 3.16. A supplemental lower lateral incisor.

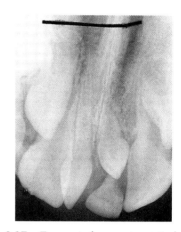

Fig. 3.17. Two conical supernumeraries lying between 1/1 with /A retained.

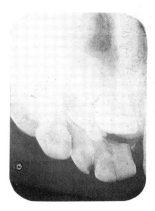

Fig. 3.18. A tuberculate supernumerary lying occlusal to 2/.

Fig. 3.19. Management of a patient with failure of eruption of the upper central incisors owing to the presence of two supernumerary teeth: (a) patient on presentation aged 10 years; (b) radiograph showing unerupted central incisors and associated conical supernumerary teeth; (c) following removal of the supernumerary teeth a URA was fitted to open space for the central incisors, until 1/ erupted 10 months later; (d) 7 months later /1 erupted and a second URA with a buccal spring was used to align /1; (e) occlusion 3 years after initial presentation.

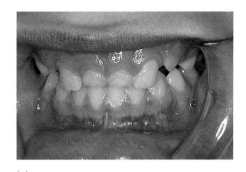

(a)

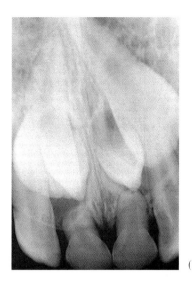

(b)

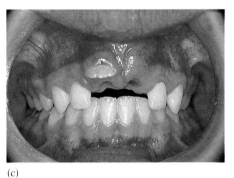

(c)

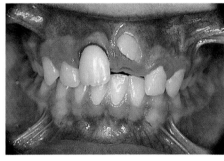

(d)

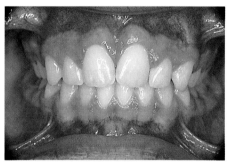

(e)

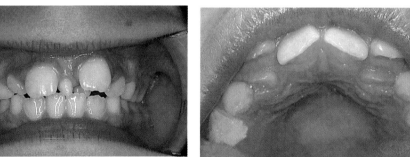

Fig. 3.20. Displacement of 1/1 caused by two erupted conical supernumerary teeth.

Fig. 3.21. Crowding due to the presence of two supplemental upper lateral incisors.

Crowding

This is caused by the supplemental type and is treated by removing the most poorly formed or more displaced tooth (Fig. 3.21).

No effect

Occasionally a supernumerary tooth (usually of the conical type) is detected as a chance finding on a radiograph of the upper incisor region (Fig. 3.22). Provided that the extra tooth will not interfere with any planned movement of the upper incisors, it can be left *in situ* under radiographic observation. In practice these teeth usually remain symptomless and do not give rise to any problems.

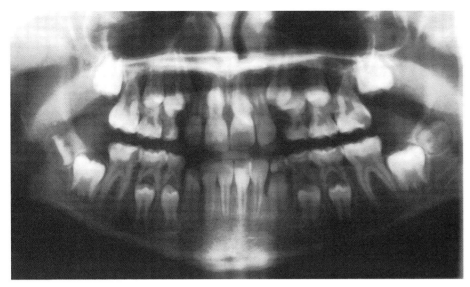

(a)

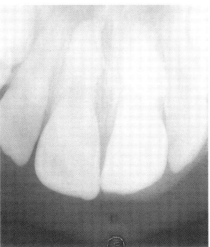

(b)

Fig. 3.22. Chance finding of a supernumerary on routine radiographic examination.

3.3.7. Habits

The effect of a habit will depend upon the frequency and intensity of indulgence. This problem is discussed in greater detail in Chapter 9, Section 9.1.4.

3.3.8. First permanent molars of poor long-term prognosis

Treatment planning for a child with poor-quality first permanent molars is always difficult because several competing factors have to be considered before a decision can be reached for a particular individual. First permanent molars are never the first tooth of choice for extraction as their position within the arch means that little space is provided anteriorly for relief of crowding or correction of the incisor relationship unless appliances are used. Removal of maxillary first molars often compromises anchorage in the upper arch, and a good spontaneous result in the lower arch following extraction of the first molars is rare. However, patients for whom enforced extraction of the first molars is required are often the least able to support complicated treatment. Finally, it has to be remembered that, unless the caries rate is reduced, the premolars may be similarly affected a few years later. Nevertheless, if a two-surface restoration is present or required in the first permanent molar of a child, the prognosis for that tooth and the remain-

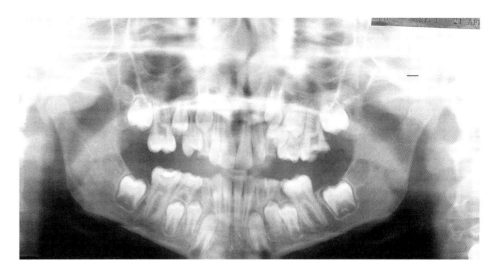

Fig. 3.23. All four first permanent molars were extracted in this patient because of the poor long-term prognosis for 6⌐ and ⌐6.

ing first molars should be considered as the planned extraction of first permanent molars of poor quality may be preferable to their enforced extraction later on (Fig. 3.23).

Factors to consider when assessing first permanent molars of poor long-term prognosis

It is impossible to produce hard and fast rules regarding the extraction of first permanent molars, and therefore the following should only be considered a starting point:

- Check for the presence of all permanent teeth. If any are absent, extraction of the first permanent molar in that quadrant should be avoided.
- If the dentition is uncrowded, extraction of first permanent molars should be avoided as space closure will be difficult.
- Remember that in the maxilla there is a greater tendency for mesial drift and so the timing of the extraction of upper first permanent molars is less critical.
- In the lower arch a good spontaneous result is more likely if:
  (a) the lower second permanent molar has developed as far as its bifurcation;
  (b) the angle between the long axis of the crypt of the lower second permanent molar and the first permanent molar is between 15° and 30°;
  (c) the crypt of the second molar overlaps the root of the first molar (a space between the two reduces the likelihood of good space closure).
- Extraction of the first molars will relieve buccal segment crowding, but will have little effect on a crowded labial segment.
- If space is needed anteriorly for the relief of labial segment crowding or for retraction of incisors (i.e. the upper arch in Class II cases or the lower arch in Class III cases), then it may be prudent to delay extraction of the first molar, if possible, until the second permanent molar has erupted in that arch. The space can then be utilized for correction of the labial segment.
- Serious consideration should be given to extracting the opposing upper first permanent molar, should extraction of a lower molar be necessary. If the upper molar is not extracted it will over-erupt and prevent forward drift of the lower second molar (Fig. 3.24).
- A compensating extraction in the lower arch (when extraction of an upper first permanent molar is necessary) should be avoided where possible as a good spontaneous result in the mandibular arch is less likely.

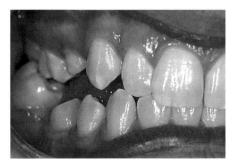

Fig. 3.24. Over-eruption of 6⌐ preventing forward movement of the lower right second permanent molar.

- Impaction of the third permanent molars is less likely, but not impossible, following extraction of the first molar.

3.3.9. Median diastema

Prevalence

Median diastema occurs in 98 per cent of 6-year-olds, 49 per cent of 11-year-olds, and 7 per cent of 12–18-year-olds.

Aetiology

Factors, which have been considered to lead to a median diastema include the following:

- physiological (normal dental development)
- small teeth in large jaws (a spaced dentition)
- missing teeth
- midline supernumerary tooth/teeth
- proclination of the upper labial segment
- prominent fraenum.

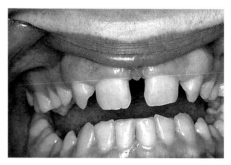

Fig. 3.25. Patient with missing 2/2 and a median diastema with a low fraenal attachment.

A median diastema is normally present between the maxillary permanent central incisors when they first erupt. As the lateral incisors and then the canines emerge the diastema usually closes. Therefore a midline diastema is a normal feature of the developing dentition; however, if it persists after eruption of the canines, it is unlikely that it will close spontaneously.

In the deciduous dentition the upper midline fraenum runs between the central incisors and attaches into the incisive papilla area. However, as the central incisors move together with eruption of the lateral incisors, it tends to migrate round onto the labial aspect. In a spaced upper arch, or where the upper lateral incisors are missing (Fig. 3.25), this recession of the fraenal attachment is less likely to occur and in such cases it is obviously not appropriate to attribute the persistence of a diastema to the fraenum itself. However, in a small proportion of cases the upper midline fraenum can contribute to the persistence of a diastema. Factors, which may indicate that this is the case include the following:

- When the fraenum is placed under tension there is blanching of the incisive papilla.
- Radiographically, a notch can be seen at the crest of the interdental bone between the upper central incisors (Fig. 3.26).
- The anterior teeth may be crowded.

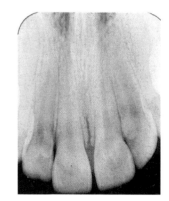

Fig. 3.26. Notch in interdental bone between 1/1 associated with a fraenal insertion running between 1/1 into the incisive papilla.

Management

It is advisable to take a periapical radiograph to exclude the presence of a midline supernumerary tooth prior to planning treatment for a midline diastema.

In the developing dentition a diastema of less than 3 mm rarely warrants intervention; in particular, extraction of the deciduous canines should be avoided as this will tend to make the diastema worse. However, if the diastema is greater than 3 mm and the lateral incisors are present, it may be necessary to consider appliance treatment to approximate the central incisors to provide space for the laterals and canines to erupt. However, care should be taken to ensure that the roots of the teeth being moved are not pressed against any unerupted crowns as this can lead to root resorption. If the crowns of the teeth are tilted distally, an upper removable appliance (URA) can be used to approximate the teeth, but fixed appliances are required for bodily movement. Closure of a diastema has a notable tendency to relapse, therefore long-term retention is required. This is most readily accomplished by placement of a bonded retainer.

3.4. SERIAL EXTRACTION

Serial extraction was first advocated in 1948 by Kjellgren, a Swedish orthodontist, as a solution to a shortage of orthodontists. Kjellgren hoped that his scheme would facilitate the treatment of patients with straightforward crowding by their own dentists, thus minimizing demands upon the orthodontic service. He suggested the employment of a planned sequence of extractions designed to allow crowded incisor segments to align spontaneously during the mixed dentition by shifting labial segment crowding to the buccal segments where it could be dealt with by premolar extractions.

3.4.1. Classical technique

- Extraction of the deciduous canines, as the lateral incisors were are erupting. This step was designed to allow the incisors to align.
- Extraction of the first deciduous molars when their roots were approximately half resorbed. The purpose of this was is to hasten the eruption of the first premolars.
- Extraction of the first premolars on eruption.

3.4.2. Pitfalls and disadvantages

- This approach involves putting the child through several sequences of extractions.
- As intercanine growth continues up to around 13 years of age, it is difficult to assess accurately how crowded a child's teeth will actually be at the stage when serial extraction is usually embarked upon.
- Extraction of the deciduous canines and first molars will allow forward drift of the buccal segment teeth and an effective increase in anterior crowding. This may be unhelpful in a child with severe crowding.
- Extraction of lower deciduous canines may result in the lower incisors tilting lingually, causing an increase in overbite. Therefore serial extraction should be avoided in Class II division 2 cases.
- Appliance therapy may still be required.

3.4.3. Conclusion

The technique of serial extraction can produce a nice result in carefully selected cases, namely Class I with moderate crowding and all permanent teeth present in a good position, but often this type of case also responds well to extraction of the first premolars upon eruption. Omitting the deciduous extractions removes some of the potential pitfalls and diminishes the guesswork involved, and, most importantly, reduces the number of extractions required.

3.4.4. Indications for the extraction of deciduous canines

Nevertheless there are a number of occasions where the timely extraction of the deciduous canines may avoid more complicated treatment later:

- In a crowded upper arch the erupting lateral incisors may be forced palatally. In a Class I malocclusion this will result in a crossbite and in addition the apex of an affected tooth will be palatally positioned, making later correction more difficult. Extraction of the deciduous canines whilst the lateral incisors are erupting often results in their being able to escape spontaneously into a better position.

- In a crowded lower labial segment one incisor may be pushed through the labial plate of bone, resulting in a compromised labial periodontal attachment. Relief of crowding by extraction of the lower deciduous canines usually results in the lower incisor moving back into the arch and improves periodontal support (Fig. 3.27).

- Extraction of the lower deciduous canines in a Class III malocclusion can be advantageous (Fig. 3.28).

- To provide space for appliance therapy in the upper arch, for example correction of an instanding lateral incisor, or to facilitate eruption of a incisor prevented from erupting by a supernumerary tooth.

- To improve the position of a displaced permanent canine (see Chapter 14).

PRINCIPAL SOURCES AND FURTHER READING

Bishara, S. E. (1997). Arch width changes from 6 weeks to 45 years of age. *American Journal of Orthodontics and Dentofacial Orthopedics*, **111**, 401–9.

Foster, T. D. and Grundy, M. C. (1986). Occlusal changes from primary to permanent dentitions. *British Journal of Orthodontics*, **13**, 187–93.

Gorlin, R. J., Cohen, M. M., and Levin, L. S. (1990). *Syndromes of the head and neck* (3rd edn). Oxford University Press, Oxford.

- Source of calcification and eruption dates (and a vast ammount of additional information not directly related to this chapter).

Kjellgren, B. (1948). Serial extraction as a corrective procedure in dental orthopaedic therapy. *Acta Odontologica Scandinavica*, **8**, 17–43.

Kurol, J. and Bjerklin, K. (1986). Ectopic eruption of maxillary first permanent molars: a review. *Journal of Dentistry for Children*, **53**, 209–15.

- All you need to know about impacted first permanent molars.

Kurol, J. and Koch, G. (1985). The effect of extraction of infraoccluded deciduous molars: a longitudinal study. *American Journal of Orthodontics*, **87**, 46–55.

Larsson, E. (1988). Treatment of children with a prolonged dummy or finger sucking habit. *European Journal of Orthodontics*, **10**, 244–8.

Mackie, I. C., Blinkhorn, A. S., and Davies, P. H. J. (1989). The extraction of permanent molars during the mixed-dentition period — a guide to treatment planning. *Journal of Paediatric Dentistry*, **5**, 85–92.

Peck, S. M., Peck, L., and Kataja, M. (1994). The palatally displaced canine as a dental anomaly of genetic origin. *Angle Orthodontist*, **64**, 249–256.

Stewart, D. J. (1978). Dilacerate unerupted maxillary incisors. *British Dental Journal*, **145**, 229–33.

Welbury, R. R. (ed.). (1996). *Paediatric Dentistry*. Oxford University Press, Oxford.

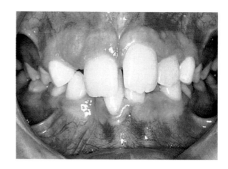

(a)

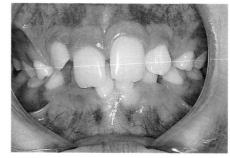

(b)

Fig. 3.27. (a) In this patient all four deciduous canines were extracted to relieve the labial segment crowding; (b) note how the periodontal condition of the lower right central incisor has improved six months later

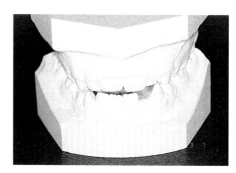

(a)

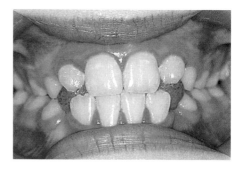

(b)

Fig. 3.28. (a) Class III prior to extraction of the lower deciduous canines; (b) same patient 13 months later.

4   Facial growth (N. E. Carter)

4.1. INTRODUCTION

Orthodontic treatment is usually carried out on children at a time when the face is growing. The clinician must be aware of the impact of growth upon the progress and outcome of treatment, and of how growth may hinder or help treatment. Orthodontic treatment itself may have some effect upon the growth of the face, and a basic knowledge of the processes of facial growth is essential for the practising clinical orthodontist.

The face is a very complex structure, and its growth and development are the result of many interacting processes. The purpose of this brief account is to highlight just a few aspects of facial growth which are relevant to clinical orthodontic practice, particularly the later stages of growth which very often coincide with orthodontic treatment. Of course, facial appearance is the result of growth of both hard and soft tissues, but the teeth are hard tissue structures and the main focus of study has been on growth of the bony facial skeleton.

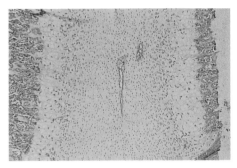

Fig. 4.1. Synchondrosis: ossification is taking place on both sides of the primary growth cartilage (Photo: D. J. Reid).

4.2. MECHANISMS OF BONE GROWTH

Bone is laid down in two ways: by replacing cartilage and by membrane activity. Bone does not grow interstitially, i.e. it does not expand by cell division within its mass; rather, it grows by activity at the margins of the bone tissue.

4.2.1. Endochondral ossification

At cartilaginous growth centres, chondroblasts lay down a matrix of cartilage within which ossification occurs. At primary growth centres, these cells are aligned in columns along the direction of growth, in which there are recognizable zones of cell division, cell hypertrophy, and calcification (Fig. 4.1). This process is seen in both the epiphyseal plates of long bones and the synchondroses of the cranial base. Growth at these primary centres causes expansion despite any opposing compressive forces such as the weight of the body on the long bones, and thus the bones on either side of the spheno-occipital synchondrosis are moved apart as it grows. Condylar cartilage also lays down bone, and for a long time this was thought to be a similar mechanism to epiphyseal growth, but developmentally it is a secondary cartilage and its structure is different Proliferating condylar cartilage cells do not show the ordered columnar arrangement seen in epiphyseal cartilage, and the articular surface is covered by a layer of dense fibrous connective tissue (Fig. 4.2). The role of the condylar cartilage during growth is not yet fully understood, but it is clear that it is different from that of the primary cartilages and its growth seems to be a reactive process in response to the growth of other structures in the face.

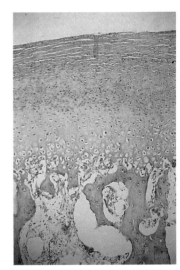

Fig. 4.2. Condylar cartilage of young adult (Photo: D. J. Reid).

4.2.2. Intramembranous ossification

Bone is both laid down and resorbed by the investing periosteum and by the endosteum within the bone. These processes of deposition and resorption together constitute **remodelling** (Fig. 4.3). Growth does not consist simply of enlargement of a bone by deposition on its surface: periosteal (surface) remodelling is also needed to maintain the overall shape of the bone as it grows. Thus, as well as having areas where new bone is being laid down, a growing bone always undergoes resorption of some parts of its surface. At the same time, endosteal remodelling maintains the internal architecture of cortical plates and trabeculae, but of course it cannot cause the bone to enlarge. Remodelling is a very important mechanism of facial growth, and the complex patterns of surface remodelling brought about by the periosteum which invests the facial skeleton have been studied extensively.

The bones of the face and skull articulate together mostly at **sutures**, and growth at sutures can be regarded as a special kind of periosteal remodelling — an infilling of bone in response to tensional growth forces separating the bones on either side (Fig. 4.4).

Growth which causes the mass of a bone to be moved relative to its neighbours is known as **displacement** of the bone; an example is forward and downward translation of the maxillary complex (Fig. 4.5). The change in position of a bony

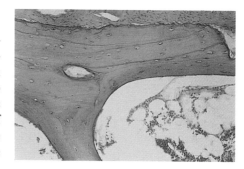

Fig. 4.3. Periosteal remodelling, showing reversal lines where bone resorption has been followed by deposition (Photo: D. J. Reid).

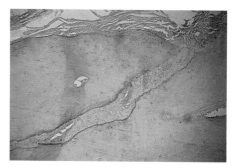

Fig. 4.4. Cranial suture (Photo: D. J. Reid).

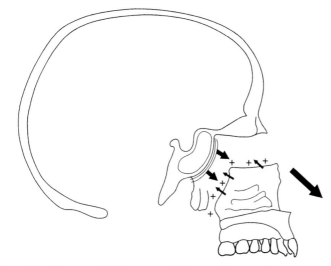

Fig. 4.5. Forward and downward displacement of the maxillary complex associated with deposition of bone at sutures. (After Enlow, D. H.: Facial Growth, W. B. Saunders Co., Philadelphia, 1990.)

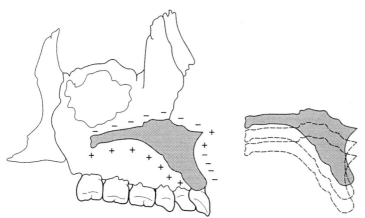

Fig. 4.6. Downwards migration of the hard palate due to drift. (From Enlow, D. H.: Facial Growth, W. B. Saunders Co., Philadelphia, 1990.)

structure owing to remodelling of that structure is called **drift**, and Fig. 4.6 shows an example of this where the palate moves downwards during growth as a result of bone being laid down on its inferior surface and resorbed on its superior surface.

4.3. GROWTH PATTERNS

It is not intended to describe in any detail here the processes by which the face grows, rather to give a picture of the patterns of facial growth. Early cephalometric growth studies gave the impression that, overall, as the face enlarges it grows downwards and forwards away from the cranial base (Fig. 4.7). However, it is now known that growth of the face is much more complex than this, involving many growth processes in the mandible, mid-face, cranial base, and so on. All of these are going on at the same time, and the overall pattern of growth results from the interplay between them. They must all harmonize with each other if a normal facial pattern is to result, and small deviations from a harmonious facial growth pattern will cause discrepancies of major significance to the orthodontist.

Different systems have different growth patterns in terms of rate and timing, and four main types are recognized: neural, somatic, genital, and lymphoid (Fig. 4.8). The first two are most relevant here.

Neural growth is essentially that which is determined by growth of the brain, and the calvarium follows this pattern of growth — in other words the bones grow in response to the growth of another structure. There is rapid growth in the early years of life, but this slows until by about the age of 8 years growth is almost complete. The orbits also follow a neural growth pattern.

Somatic growth is that followed by most structures. It is seen in the long bones, amongst others, and is the pattern followed by increase in body height. Unlike neural growth, somatic bone growth seems to be more an intrinsic property of the bones and under fairly tight genetic control. Growth is fairly rapid in

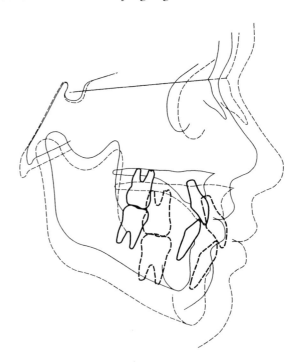

Fig. 4.7. Superimpositions on the cranial base showing overall downwards and forwards direction of facial growth. Solid line 8 years, broken line 18 years of age.

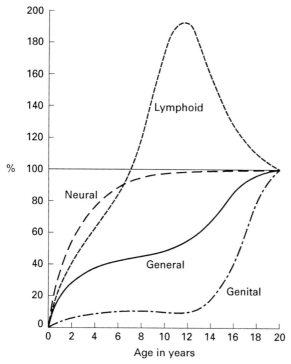

Fig. 4.8. Postnatal growth patterns shown as percentages of total increase (From Scammon, R. E.: The Measurement of Man, University of Minnesota Press, 1930.)

the early years, but slows in the prepubertal period. The pubertal growth spurt is a time of very rapid growth, which is followed by further slower growth. The pubertal growth spurt occurs on average at 12 years in girls, but in boys it is later at about 14 years. Although the timing of facial growth has been studied less extensively than the timing of growth in stature, growth of the facial skeleton follows approximately a somatic growth pattern.

Thus different parts of the skull follow different growth patterns, with much of the growth of the face occurring later than the growth of the cranial vault. As a result the proportions of the face to the cranium change during growth, and the face of the child represents a much smaller proportion of the skull than the face of the adult (Fig. 4.9).

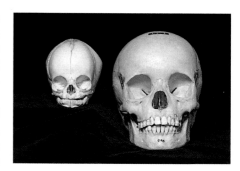

Fig. 4.9. The face in the neonate represents a much smaller proportion of the skull than the face of the adolescent (Photo: B. Hill).

4.4. CALVARIUM

The calvarium is that part of the skull which develops from the membrane bones surrounding the brain and therefore it follows the neural growth pattern. It comprises the frontal bones, the parietal bones, and the squamous parts of the temporal and occipital bones. These bones articulate with each other at sutures, which at birth are not yet united. Six fontanelles are also present at birth which close by 18 months. By the age of 6 years the calvarium has developed inner and outer cortical tables which enclose the diploë. Its growth consists of a combination of drift and displacement. Drift occurs because the intracranial aspects of the bones are resorbed while bone is laid down on the external surfaces. There is displacement as the bones are separated by the growing brain, with fill-in bone growth occurring at the sutures to maintain continuity of the cranial vault.

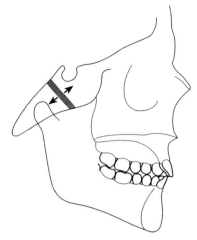

Fig. 4.10. Antero-posterior growth at the spheno-occipital synchondrosis affects the anteroposterior relationship of the jaws.

4.5. CRANIAL BASE

Growth of the cranial base is influenced by both neural and somatic growth patterns. As in the calvarium, there is both remodelling and sutural infilling as the brain enlarges, but there are also primary cartilaginous growth sites in this region — the synchondroses. Of these, the spheno-occipital synchondrosis is of special interest as it makes an important contribution to growth of the cranial base during childhood, continuing to grow until about 15 years of age, and fusing at approximately 20 years. Thus the middle cranial fossa enlarges both by anteroposterior growth at the spheno-occipital synchondrosis and by remodelling. The anterior cranial fossa enlarges and increases in anteroposterior length by remodelling, with resorption intracranially and corresponding extracranial deposition.

The spheno-occipital synchondrosis is anterior to the temporomandibular joints but posterior to the anterior cranial fossa, and therefore its growth is significant clinically as it influences the overall facial skeletal pattern (Fig. 4.10). Growth at the spheno-occipital synchondrosis increases the length of the cranial base, and since the maxillary complex lies beneath the anterior cranial fossa while the mandible articulates with the skull at the temporomandibular joints which lie beneath the middle cranial fossa, the cranial base plays an important part in determining how the mandible and maxilla relate to each other. For example, a Class II skeletal facial pattern is often associated with the presence of a long cranial base which causes the mandible to be set back relative to the maxilla.

In the same way, the overall shape of the cranial base affects the jaw relationship, with a smaller cranial base angle tending to cause a Class III skeletal pattern, and a larger cranial base angle being more likely to be associated with a Class II skeletal pattern (Fig. 4.11).

The anterior part of the cranial base is used in cephalometric analysis as a reference structure from which measurements can be taken, remote from the face itself and thus unaffected by orthodontic treatment. It is often represented by the Sella–Nasion line (see Chapter 6).

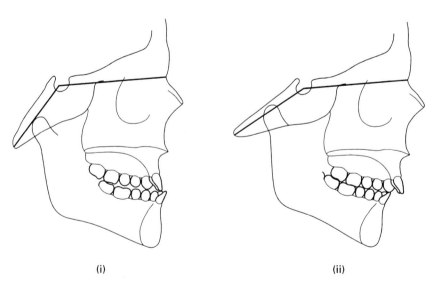

(i)   (ii)

Fig. 4.11. View (i) Low cranial base angle associated with Class III skeletal pattern.
View (ii) Large cranial base angle associated with a Class II skeletal pattern.

4.6. MAXILLARY COMPLEX

The maxilla derives from the maxillary processes of the first pharyngeal arch and from the frontal process. Ossification is intramembranous, beginning laterally to the cartilaginous nasal capsule.

Clinical orthodontic practice is primarily concerned with the dentition and its supporting alveolar bone which is part of the maxilla and premaxilla. However, the middle third of the facial skeleton is a complex structure and also includes, among others, the palatal, zygomatic, ethmoid, vomer, and nasal bones. These articulate with each other and with the anterior cranial base at sutures. Growth of the maxillary complex occurs in part by displacement with fill-in growth at sutures and in part by drift and periosteal remodelling.

The maxilla enlarges anteroposteriorly by deposition of bone posteriorly at the tuberosities, which of course also lengthens the dental arch. Forward growth of the maxilla is thus anterior displacement as bone is laid down on its posterior aspect (see Fig. 4.5). The zygomatic bones are also carried forwards, necessitating infilling at sutures, and at the same time they enlarge and remodel. In the upper part of the face, the ethmoids and nasal bones grow forwards by deposition on their anterior surfaces, with corresponding remodelling further back, including in the air sinuses, to maintain their anatomical form.

Downward growth occurs by vertical development of the alveolar process and eruption of the teeth, and also by inferior drift of the hard palate, i.e. the palate remodels downwards by deposition of bone on its inferior surface (the palatal vault) and resorption on its superior surface (the floor of the nose and maxillary sinuses) (see Fig. 4.6). These changes are also associated with some downward displacement of the bones as they enlarge, again necessitating infilling at sutures. Lateral growth in the mid-face occurs by displacement apart of the two halves of the maxilla, with deposition of bone at the midline suture. Internal remodelling leads to enlargement of the air sinuses and nasal cavity as the bones of the mid-face increase in size.

Thus there are complex patterns of surface remodelling on the anterior and lateral surfaces of the maxilla which maintain the overall shape of the bone as it enlarges. Despite being translated anteriorly, much of the anterior surface of the maxilla is in fact resorptive in order to maintain the concave contours beneath the pyriform fossa and zygomatic buttresses.

Maxillary growth ceases on average at about 15 years in girls and rather later, at about 17 years, in boys.

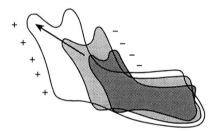

Fig. 4.12. Growth at the condylar cartilage elongates the mandible, causing anterior displacement, while its shape is maintained by remodelling, including posterior drift of the ramus. (After Enlow, D. H. 1990 *Facial growth*, Saunders, Philadelphia, 1990.).

4.7. MANDIBLE

The mandible derives from the first pharyngeal arch and is a membrane bone, ossifying laterally to Meckel's cartilage. Secondary cartilages appear, including the condylar cartilage, but the role of the condylar cartilage in the growth of the mandible is not yet entirely clear. It seems probable that, since it is a secondary cartilage, it is not a primary growth centre in its own right, but rather it grows in response to some other controlling factors. However, what is clear is that normal growth at the condylar cartilage is required for normal mandibular growth to take place.

However, most mandibular growth occurs as a result of periosteal activity. Muscular processes develop at the angles of the mandible and the coronoids, and the alveolar processes develop vertically to keep pace with the eruption of the teeth. As the mandible elongates with growth at the condylar cartilage, so its anterior part is displaced forwards, while at the same time periosteal remodelling

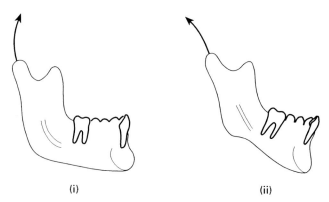

Fig. 4.13. Direction of condylar growth and mandibular growth rotations:
View (i) Forward rotation
View (ii) Backward rotation

maintains its shape (Fig. 4.12). Bone is laid down on the posterior margin of the vertical ramus and resorbed on the anterior margin, and this posterior drift of the ramus allows lengthening of the dental arch posteriorly. At the same time the vertical ramus becomes taller to accommodate the increase in height of the alveolar processes. Remodelling also brings about an increase in the width of the mandible, particularly posteriorly. Lengthening of the mandible and anterior remodelling together cause the chin to become more prominent, an obvious feature of facial maturation especially in males. Indeed, just as in the maxilla, the whole surface of the mandible undergoes many complex patterns of remodelling as it grows in order to maintain its proper anatomical form.

Mandibular growth ceases rather later than maxillary growth, on average at about 17 years in girls and 19 years in boys, although it may continue for longer.

4.8. GROWTH ROTATIONS

Early studies of facial growth indicated that during childhood the face enlarges progressively and consistently, growing downwards and forwards away from the cranial base (see Fig. 4.7). These studies looked only at average trends and failed to demonstrate the huge variation which exists between the growth patterns of individual children. Later work by Björk has shown that the direction of facial growth is curved, giving a rotational effect (Fig. 4.13). The growth rotations

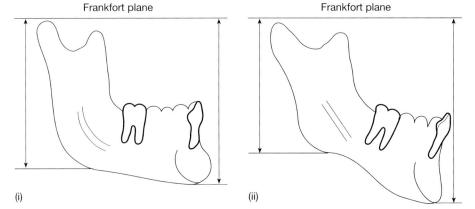

Fig. 4.14. Mandibular growth rotations reflect the ratio between the anterior and posterior face heights, here shown relative to the Frankfort horizontal plane: (i) forward rotation, (ii) backward rotation.

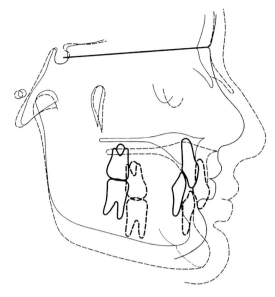

Fig. 4.15. Forward growth rotation. Solid line 11 years, broken line 18 years of age.

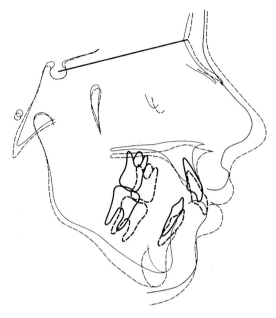

Fig. 4.16. Backward growth rotation. Solid line 12 years, broken line 19 years of age.

were demonstrated by placing small titanium implants into the surface of the facial bones, and subsequently taking cephalometric radiographs at intervals during growth. Since bone does not grow interstitially, the implants could be used as fixed reference points on the serial radiographs from which to measure the growth changes.

Growth rotations are most obvious and have their greatest impact on the mandible; their effects on the maxilla are small and are almost completely masked by surface remodelling. In the mandible, however, their effect is significant, particularly in the vertical dimension. Mandibular growth rotations result from the interplay of the growth of a number of structures which together determine the ratio of posterior to anterior facial heights (Fig. 4.14). The posterior face height is determined by factors including the direction of the growth at the condyles and vertical growth at the spheno-occipital synchondrosis. The anterior facial height is affected by the eruption of teeth and vertical growth of the soft tissues, including the masticatory musculature and the suprahyoid musculature and fasciae, which are in turn influenced by growth of the spinal column. The overall direction of growth rotation is thus the result of the growth of many structures.

Forward growth rotations are more common than backward rotations, with the average being a mild forward rotation which produces a well-balanced facial appearance. A marked forward growth rotation tends to result in reduced anterior vertical facial proportions and an increased overbite (Fig. 4.15), and the more severe the forward rotation the more difficult it will be to reduce the overbite. Similarly, a more backward rotation will tend to produce increased anterior vertical facial proportions and a reduced overbite or anterior open bite (Fig. 4.16).

Not only is the vertical dimension affected, but there are also important antero-posterior effects. For example, correction of a Class II malocclusion will be helped by a forward growth rotation but made more difficult by a backward rotation. Growth rotations may also have an effect on the position of the lower labial segment. A forward growth rotation tends to cause retroclination of the lower labial segment which is often associated with shortening of the dental arch anteriorly and crowding of the lower incisors. A possible explanation for this is that, as the lower arch is carried forwards with mandibular growth, forward movement of the lower incisor crowns is limited by contact with the upper incisors, causing them to crowd. This is common in the very late stages of growth when mandibular growth continues after maxillary growth has finished, although facial growth is only one of a number of possible aetiological factors in late lower incisor crowding.

Thus growth rotations play an important part in the aetiology of certain malocclusions and must be taken into account in planning orthodontic treatment. It is necessary to try to assess the direction of mandibular growth rotation clinically. This is not entirely straightforward since the effect of growth rotation upon the mandible is masked to some extent by surface remodelling, particularly along the lower border of the mandible and at the angle. However, it is possible to make a useful assessment of a patient's facial growth pattern by examining the anterior facial proportions and mandibular plane angle as described in Chapter 5. Increased facial proportions and a steep mandibular plane indicate that the direction of mandibular growth has a substantial downward component, while reduced facial proportions and a horizontal mandibular plane suggest that the direction of growth is more forwards. It is also helpful to examine the shape of the lower border of the mandible. A concave lower border with a marked antegonial notch is associated with a backward rotation, while a convex lower border is associated with a forward growth rotation (see Figs 4.15 and 4.16).

4.9. GROWTH OF THE SOFT TISSUES

The importance of the oral musculature in orthodontic practice is that it influences significantly the form of the dental arches, since the teeth lie in a position of equilibrium between the lingual and bucco-labial musculature. Therefore they are important factors in the aetiology of malocclusion, and greatly affect the stability of the result after orthodontic treatment.

The facial musculature is well developed at birth, considerably in advance of the limbs, because of the need for the baby to suckle and maintain the airway. Other functions soon develop: mastication as teeth erupt, facial expressions, a mature swallowing pattern (as opposed to suckling), and speech.

The lips, tongue, and cheeks guide the erupting teeth towards each other to achieve a functional occlusion. This serves as a compensatory mechanism for a discrepancy in the skeletal pattern; for example, in a Class III subject the lower incisors may become retroclined and the upper incisors proclined to obtain incisor contact. Sometimes this compensatory mechanism fails, either because the skeletal problem is too severe or the soft tissue behaviour is abnormal. An example of this is where lower lip function worsens a Class II division 1 malocclusion by acting behind the upper incisors rather than anteriorly to them. In the late stages of growth the lips lengthen as they mature, tending to become more competent.

Muscle growth must be coordinated with the growth of the associated bones, with the muscles lengthening as their bony attachments separate. Neuromuscular activity regulates the positions of the jaws, and it has been suggested that the whole process of facial skeletal growth is determined by the soft tissues which surround the bones.

4.10. CONTROL OF FACIAL GROWTH

The mechanisms that control facial growth are poorly understood but are the subject of considerable interest and research. As with all growth and development, there is an interaction between genetic and environmental factors, but if environmental factors can make a significant impact on facial growth then the possibility exists for clinicians to alter facial growth with appliances.

It is often difficult to distinguish the effects of heredity and environment, but it is helpful to consider how tightly the growth and development of a structure or tissue are under genetic control. Two simple examples illustrate this: gender is genetically determined and does not change no matter how extreme the environmental conditions, while obesity is very strongly affected by the nature and amount of food consumed. Most structures, including the facial skeleton and soft tissues, are influenced by both genetic and environmental factors, and the effect that the latter can have depends upon how tightly growth is under genetic control.

Genetic control is undoubtedly significant in facial growth, as is clearly shown by facial similarities in members of a family. The extent to which the facial skeleton itself is under genetic control has been debated at length in recent decades, with the development of two opposing schools of thought. Growth at the primary cartilages is regarded as being under tight genetic control, with the cartilage itself containing the necessary genetic programming. Therefore those who view growth of the whole facial skeleton as being directly and tightly genetically controlled have looked for primary cartilaginous growth centres in the facial bones. The condylar cartilages seemed to fulfil this role in the mandible, while the nasal septal cartilage was thought to serve a similar function in the maxilla. However, the structure and behaviour of these cartilages is different from primary growth cartilages, and at present it is thought that, while their presence is necessary for normal growth to take place, they are probably not primary growth centres in their own right.

The other school of thought proposed that bone growth itself is only under loose genetic control and takes place in response to growth of the surrounding soft tissues — the **functional matrix** which invests the bone. This idea looks to the example of the neural growth pattern of the calvarium and orbits, which develop intramembranously and enlarge in response to growth of the brain and eyes. However, the functional matrix theory ran into difficulty with regard to facial growth as there are no similarly expanding structures within the middle and lower face. It has attracted a lot of attention as, if taken to its logical conclusion, it implies that orthodontic appliances can be used to alter facial growth.

There is much yet to be understood about how growth of the face is controlled. As to whether appliances influence facial growth, the truth appears to lie somewhere between the two extremes of opinion, but research in this field faces considerable problems, some of which are discussed in Chapter 18 in relation to functional appliances. At present, the evidence is that the impact of current orthodontic treatment methods on facial growth is on average quite small, but there is considerable variation in the response of individual patients.

4.11. GROWTH PREDICTION

It would be extremely useful if we could predict the future growth of a child's face, particularly in cases which are at the limits of what orthodontic treatment can achieve. For growth prediction to be useful clinically it would need to be able to predict the amount, direction, and timing of growth of the various parts of the facial skeleton to a high level of accuracy.

At present there are no known predictors which can be measured, either clinically on the patient or from radiographs, which will enable future growth to be predicted with the necessary precision. Much work has been done to try to find measurements which can be taken from cephalometric radiographs which will predict future facial growth to a useful level of precision, but so far with limited success. Assessment of stature (height) and secondary sex characteristics help to indicate whether the patient has entered the pubertal growth spurt, an important observation when functional appliances are being considered. Since growth of the jaws follows a somatic growth pattern, the possibility has been investigated that observation of the developmental stage of other parts of the skeleton would give an indication of the stage of facial development. The stage of maturation of the metacarpal bones and the phalanges as seen on a hand–wrist radiograph is used as a measure of skeletal development, but the correlation of this with jaw growth has been found to be too poor to give clinically useful information.

The best which can be done is to add average growth increments to the patient's existing facial pattern, but this has only limited value. This can be done manually using a grid superimposed on the patient's lateral cephalometric tracing, and average annual growth increments are read off to predict the change in position of the various cephalometric landmarks. Computer programs can be used for the same purpose, after the points and outlines from the lateral skull radiograph have been digitized. These programs can refine the prediction process further but they still have to make some assumptions about the rate and direction of facial growth. Unfortunately, the assumption that a patient's future growth pattern will be average is least appropriate in those individuals whose facial growth differs significantly from the average, and who are the very subjects where accurate prediction would be most useful. As growth proceeds, the rate and direction of growth in an individual vary enough that study of the past pattern of a patient's facial growth does not allow prediction of future growth to the level of precision required for it to be clinically useful. However, many clinicians find it helpful to assess the direction of mandibular growth rotation (see Section 4.8) on the assumption that this pattern is likely to continue.

Clinical experience has shown that for most patients, whose growth patterns are close to the average, it can be assumed for treatment-planning purposes that their growth will continue to be average.

PRINCIPAL SOURCES AND FURTHER READING

Björk, A. and Skieller, V. (1983). Normal and abnormal growth of the mandible. A synthesis of longitudinal cephalometric implant studies over a period of 25 years. *European Journal of Orthodontics*, **5**, 1–46.
● A summary of the implant work on mandibular growth rotations.
Enlow, D. H. and Hans M. G. (1996). *Essentials of facial growth*. Saunders, Philadelphia.
● The Bible of facial growth.
Houston, W. J. B. (1979). The current status of facial growth prediction: a review. *British Journal of Orthodontics*, **6**, 11–17.
● An authoritative assessment of the value of growth prediction.
Houston, W. J. B. (1988). Mandibular growth rotations — their mechanism and importance. *European Journal of Orthodontics*, **10**, 369–73.
● A concise review of the aetiology and clinical importance of growth rotations.
Mills, J. R. E. (1983). A clinician looks at facial growth. *British Journal of Orthodontics*, **10**, 57–72.
● A clear description of the facial growth processes from a clinical orthodontic viewpoint.

5   Orthodontic assessment

A brief examination of the developing occlusion should be carried out around 7 to 8 years of age to check upon the presence and position of the permanent incisor teeth and to help detect at an early stage any incipient problems which may hinder the normal eruption sequence (see Chapter 3). Radiographic examination is indicated at this stage if an abnormality is suspected. In general dental practice, a child's dental and occlusal development should be checked yearly, and from around 10 years of age the routine dental examination should be extended to include palpation for unerupted maxillary permanent canines in the buccal sulcus.

5.1. PURPOSE AND AIMS OF AN ORTHODONTIC ASSESSMENT

Prior to the commencement of orthodontic treatment a full examination (including radiographs) and assessment of the occlusion needs to be carried out, which for most children is not before the eruption of the permanent dentition. However, for those with a skeletal discrepancy where treatment may need to be timed to coincide with the pubertal growth spurt, it may be prudent to carry out a full assessment earlier.

The purpose of an orthodontic assessment is to evaluate and record the features of a malocclusion in preparation for planning treatment, if indicated. The following approach is suggested because it has been successfully used by the author and others, but the exact sequence of the examination is unimportant. However, a consistent logical approach is essential to avoid omissions.

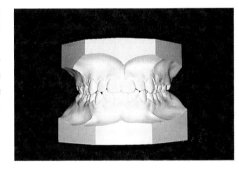

(a)

5.2. EQUIPMENT

5.2.1. Instruments

A mirror, probe, and stainless steel orthodontic (or engineer's) rule are required.

5.2.2. Study models

The assistance provided by a set of study models during assessment and treatment planning cannot be over-emphasized. In addition, they are essential as a pretreatment record if any appliance therapy is to be carried out. To be of value the study models should include all erupted teeth, the palate, and the full sulcus depth. They should at least be trimmed so that the upper and lower bases are parallel with the occlusal plane; however, traditionally orthodontic study models are trimmed so that the heels and sides are flush (Fig. 5.1), allowing the models to be placed down in any position and remain in occlusion.

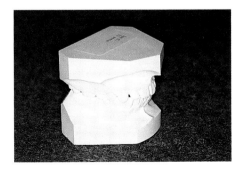

(b)

Fig. 5.1.   Trimmed orthodontic models.

5.2.3. Radiographs

See Section 5.8.

5.3. PRESENTING COMPLAINT

It is extremely important to determine the patient's opinion regarding the position and alignment of their teeth. It is not uncommon for an orthodontic opinion to be sought at the instigation of a anxious parent when the child concerned is quite happy with their occlusion and certainly not prepared to entertain the idea of wearing appliances. No matter how enthusiastic a patient's parents may be for their offspring to undergo orthodontic treatment, if the child itself is not willing, then a successful outcome is less likely. Adult patients are usually keen and cooperative once they have decided to go ahead with appliance treatment.

It is also important to ascertain exactly which features of the occlusion concern the patient. A child may be more concerned about the mild rotation of an upper central incisor than increased overjet, particularly if other members of the family have Class II division 1 malocclusions. Naturally they will not be content if, at the completion of treatment for their increased overjet the rotation is still present.

It is often helpful to determine the types of appliance that the patient is willing to accept — examples of the different appliances or good colour pictures are invaluable at this stage.

5.4. DENTAL HISTORY

Regular dental care and good oral health are an essential prerequisite to orthodontic treatment. The patient's past dental history should include details of any previous appliance therapy. If permanent teeth have been extracted, the timing of these extractions and the reason for removal should be ascertained if possible.

5.5. MEDICAL HISTORY

A thorough medical history should be taken. Conditions which might affect orthodontic treatment include the following:

- Rheumatic fever. If a patient is suspected of being at risk of infective endocarditis it is advisable to seek medical advice, preferably from a cardiologist. If the risk is confirmed then orthodontic treatment can be considered provided the patient is able to maintain good gingival health and accepts the risk involved. Invasive procedures, for example, extractions and band placement and removal (however, some authorities suggest bonds should be used in preference for bands in susceptible patients), should be covered with the recommended antibiotic cover regime. A chlorhexidine rinse prior to adjustment of a fixed appliance is a useful adjunct, although daily long-term use of chlorhexidine may lead to bacterial resistance. If the patient's oral hygiene deteriorates during treatment it may be advisable to discontinue appliance treatment.

- Epilepsy. Because of the risk of damage to the mouth caused by a broken appliance during an epileptic attack, it is prudent to delay treatment in this group of patients until the condition is well controlled.

- Recurrent apthous ulceration (RAU). This condition of (much) debated aetiology is known to be exacerbated by trauma to the mucosa. Cribs or springs on a removable appliance, or the components of a fixed appliance, may be sufficient to set off an attack in a susceptible individual. In patients with a history of RAU, it may be prudent to carry out a thorough investigation first, including referral for blood tests if indicated, and to determine the effect of appliances before any irreversible steps, for example extractions, are taken.

● Hay fever. Atopic children may experience problems with a functional appliance during the summer months.

Of course, there are many more esoteric conditions that will modify treatment in affected individuals. However, there is only space here to comment that when in doubt a specialist opinion should be sought.

5.6. EXTRA-ORAL EXAMINATION

The position of the teeth is determined largely by a patient's underlying skeletal pattern and the soft tissue environment. The purpose of this aspect of the examination is to evaluate their relative influence in the aetiology of a particular malocclusion and also the degree to which they can be modified or corrected by treatment.

5.6.1. Skeletal pattern

The patient should be comfortably seated upright. Tilting of the head upwards increases the prominence of the chin, and conversely tilting the head downwards has the opposite effect. Therefore it is important to ensure that the patient is positioned so that his or her Frankfort plane (uppermost aspect of the external auditory canal to the lowermost aspect of the orbital margin) is horizontal. The teeth should be together in maximum interdigitation — it is wise to check this, as often a patient will posture the mandible forwards with only the incisors in contact.

The skeletal pattern should be asesssed in all three planes of space.

Anteroposterior

The patient should be viewed from the side and the relative position of the maxilla and mandible assessed (Fig. 5.2). It is important to look at the region of the dental base rather than the lips, as their position will be influenced by proclination or retroclination of the incisors. The following classification of skeletal pattern is universally recognized:

● Class I — the mandible is 2–3 mm posterior to maxilla.
● Class II — the mandible is retruded relative to the maxilla.
● Class III — the mandible is protruded relative to the maxilla.

It is important to note that this classification only gives the position of the mandible and the maxilla relative to each other and does not indicate where the discrepancy lies. A lateral cephalometric radiograph is required for further assessment of the aetiology of the skeletal pattern. If a skeletal discrepancy is present, an assessment of its severity should be made.

Vertical

Again, the patient is viewed from the side. The vertical assessment comprises two separate evaluations:

Fig. 5.2. Assessment of anteroposterior skeletal pattern: (a) Class I; (b) Class II; (c) Class III.

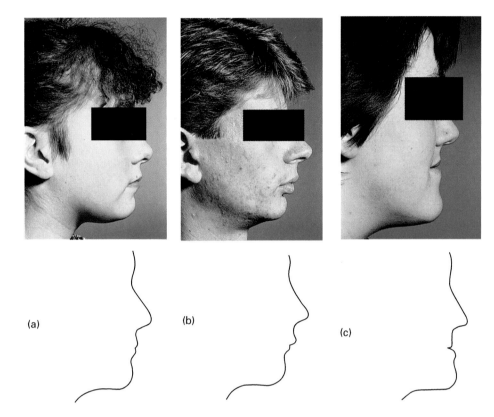

(a)　　　　(b)　　　　(c)

- Lower facial height (Fig. 5.3): the distance from the eyebrow to the base of the nose should equal the distance from the base of the nose to the lowermost point on the chin. If the latter distance is increased, the lower facial height is described as being increased, and vice versa.
- Frankfort mandibular planes angle (FMPA) (Fig. 5.4): assessment of the FMPA clinically by eye comes with experience, but the neophyte orthodontist may find it helpful to assess this angle by placing one hand level with the Frankfort plane (external auditory meatus to the lower border of the orbital margin) and the other hand level with the lower border of the mandible. Then in the 'mind's eye' extrapolate the planes and assess where they would cross. If the angle between these two planes is around the average of 28°, then the lines would intersect approximately at the back of the head. If the FMPA is increased the lines would meet before the back of the head, and if it is reduced they would cross beyond.

Transverse

It is important to remember that all faces are asymmetric to a small degree. However, any marked discrepancies should be noted. For this assessment the patient should be viewed anteriorly and, if an asymmetry is noted, also examined by looking down on the face from above. The extent of the asymmetry and whether only the lower facial third or the maxilla or orbits are involved should be recorded. Whether the occlusal plane follows the asymmetry and 'runs' down to one side should be established by asking the patient to bite onto a tongue spatula (Fig. 5.5).

5.6.2. Soft tissues

Assessment of the soft tissues should commence as soon as the patient enters the surgery and continue during the preliminary stages of the assessment in order to be able to observe normal function.

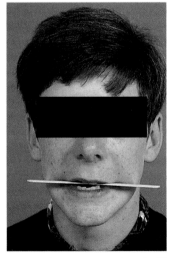

Fig. 5.5. Use of a tongue spatula to highlight a 'run' in the occlusal plane in addition to a small degree of facial asymmetry.

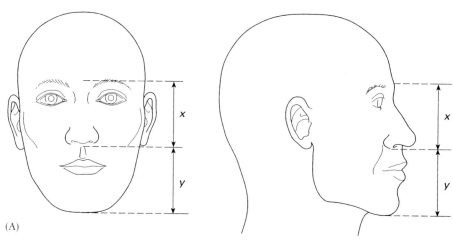

(A)

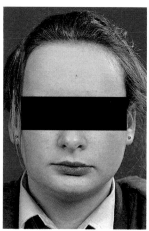

(b)

Fig. 5.3. (a) Assessment of lower facial height: in an averagely proportioned face the distance x from a point between the eyebrows to the base of the nose is equivalent to the distance y from the base of the nose to the chin. (b) A patient with a reduced lower facial height.

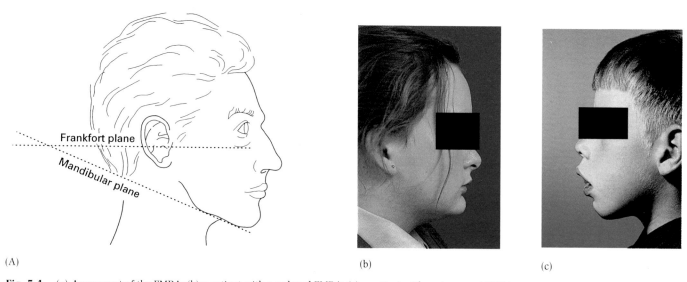

(A)   (b)   (c)

Fig. 5.4. (a) Assessment of the FMPA; (b) a patient with a reduced FMPA; (c) a patient with an increased FMPA.

Lips

The following should be considered:

- The form, tonicity, and fullness of the lips (Fig. 5.6). For example, are they full or thin, hyperactive, or with little tone?

- Lip competence. Competent lips meet together at rest without any muscular activity (Fig. 5.7). If a patient's lips are incompetent, the method by which they achieve an anterior oral seal should be evaluated. This is usually either by tongue to lower lip contact, with the lower lip being drawn up behind the upper incisors, or by the patient bringing the lips together. An assessment should also be made as to whether the lips are potentially competent (Fig. 5.8). This is most relevant in Class II division 1 malocclusions where it is important to assess whether the lower lip will act in front of the upper incisors to retain their corrected position following overjet reduction (see Chapter 9).

Fig. 5.6. (a) Full lips with little muscle tone; (b) thin lips with obvious muscular tone.

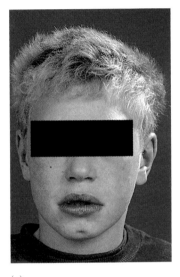
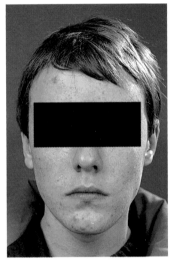

(a)   (b)

Fig. 5.7. (a) Competent lips which meet together at rest; (b) incompetent lips as they require muscular effort to achieve contact.

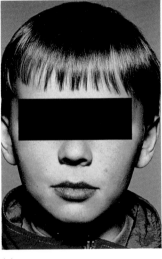
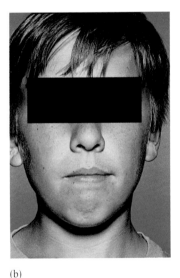

(a)   (b)

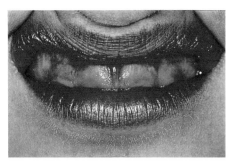 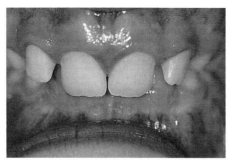

Fig. 5.9. High lower lip line relative to the upper central incisors which has resulted in their retroclination. The shorter lateral incisors have not been affected by the lip.

- Lower lip position relative to the upper incisors. A high lower lip line (Fig. 5.9) is often one of the aetiological factors in Class II division 2 malocclusions.
- The length of the upper lip and amount of upper incisor shown. The normal upper incisor show, at rest, is 2–3 mm in females and less in males (Fig. 5.10).

Tongue

Tongue thrusts are usually adaptive, i.e. the tongue is placed forward between the teeth to help achieve an anterior oral seal during swallowing. Rarely, patients are encountered who appear to have a habit of pushing their tongue between the upper and lower incisors when swallowing; this is described as an endogenous or primary tongue thrust. The significant difference between the two is that an adaptive tongue thrust will cease following treatment when a lip-to-lip contact can be achieved, whereas an endogenous tongue thrust will not and this often leads to relapse (this is discussed in greater detail in Chapter 12, Section 12.2.2).

5.6.3. Temporomandibular joints

Before any examination of the temporomandibular joints is carried out the patient should be asked about symptoms. The joints should be palpated simultaneously by placing the middle finger over the condylar head whilst the patient is instructed to open and close and to move laterally. Any clicks, crepitus, and locking should be recorded. It is probably prudent to record any negative findings

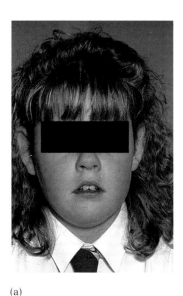 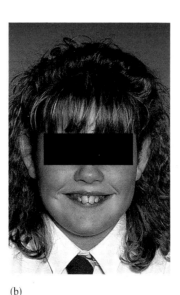

(a)   (b)

Fig. 5.8. Potentially competent lips.

Fig. 5.10. Excessive amount of upper incisor show (a) at rest and (b) when smiling.

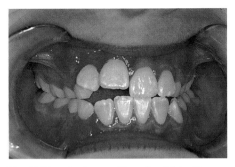

Fig. 5.11. Incisor position of a child with a persistent thumb-sucking habit.

as well. If definitive symptoms exist, the muscles of mastication should also be examined for areas of tenderness.

5.6.4. Habits

Enquire about any habits, whilst observing the patient's hands for any signs of digit sucking or nail-biting (the latter has been associated with a increased incidence of root resorption).

With a little experience it can be easy to spot the occlusal features of a finger- or thumb-sucking habit (Fig. 5.11). Some patients develop a lip-sucking habit, which can lead to a eczematous appearance of the skin below the lower lip in addition to retroclination of the lower labial segment.

The effects of any habit upon the dentition should be brought to the attention of the child and their parents.

5.7. INTRA-ORAL EXAMINATION

5.7.1. Dental examination

This should include the following:

- Charting all the erupted teeth.
- Noting any permanent teeth of poor prognosis, untreated caries, and the patient's caries rate.
- Oral hygiene and gingival condition. Any gingival recession, and any areas with a reduced width of attached gingiva, should also be noted.
- Any teeth with an abnormal morphology or size.
- Anterior teeth which have suffered trauma.

5.7.2. Path of closure

The patient's position of maximum interdigitation (intercuspal or centric position) should be examined together with their path of closure from the rest position. This can often be difficult at an initial consultation when the patient is a little apprehensive, and is occasionally impossible in the younger child. Therefore care is required to ensure that the patient's true intercuspal position is recorded, particularly in Class II division 1 malocclusions where the patient may tend to posture forwards. Asking the subject to curl the tongue up to touch the back of the palate, whilst closing the teeth together, can be helpful.

Displacement on closure

A premature contact encountered on closure from the rest position is uncomfortable and the patient soon learns to displace the mandible forwards or laterally to avoid the offending tooth or teeth (Fig. 5.12). This displaced position quickly becomes learned and so can be difficult to detect. It is advisable to assume that any unilateral crossbite is associated with a displacement until proved otherwise, and to examine carefully the path of closure and centrelines. Where a displacement exists, the occlusion should be assessed in maximum interdigitation and the direction and amount of displacement recorded.

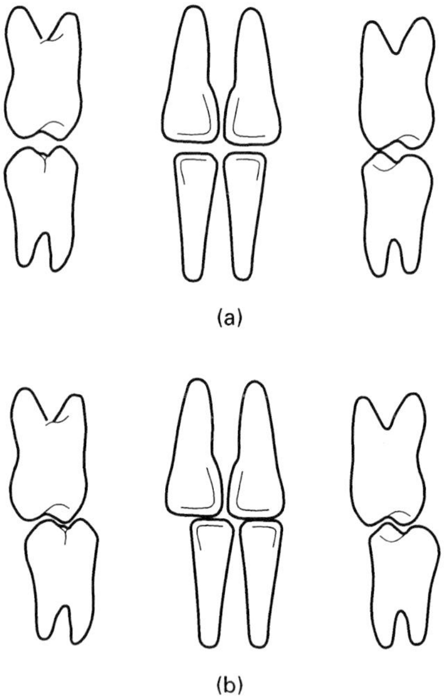

Fig. 5.12. Diagram to illustrate the displacement of the mandible laterally into a unilateral cross bite: (a) initial contact on hinge axis closure; (b) displacement into maximum interdigitation (note shift of lower centre line relative to upper arch).

Deviation on closure

This is most commonly seen in association with Class II division 1 malocclusions where the patient has a tendency to hold the mandible forward to mask the underlying problem. This used to be rather aptly described as a 'Sunday bite'. On closure from the rest into the intercuspal position, the mandible can be seen to translate backwards and upwards.

5.7.3. Labial segments

Labial segment alignment

First the lower and then the upper labial segment should be examined in turn and the following recorded:

- Angulation relative to mandibular/maxillary base.
- General alignment and the presence of crowding and spacing.
- Any rotated teeth and those displaced from the line of the arch.
- The inclination of the canines if they are erupted or, if not, whether they can be palpated buccally in a favourable position.

Labial segment relationship

The patient should be guided into maximum interdigitation and the following recorded:

- Incisor relationship (see Chapter 2, Section 2.3.2).
- Overjet — from the mesial aspect of the upper central incisors to the lower incisors in millimetres (Fig. 5.13).
- Overbite — in terms of overlap of the lower incisors by the upper incisors (Fig. 5.13). Normal overbite is a half to a third of the lower incisor crown height. However, it is usually sufficient to record overbite as increased, reduced, or normal. Whether the overbite is incomplete or complete onto tooth or the palate should also be noted, and if an anterior open bite is present, its extent should be recorded in millimetres. A traumatic overbite is said to be present if obvious ulceration is evident where the lower incisors make contact with the palatal tissues (Fig. 5.14).
- Presence of any anterior crossbites.
- Check whether the centrelines of each arch are coincident with the centre of the face and with each other. Measure and record any discrepancies in millimetres.

5.7.4. Buccal segments

Buccal segment alignment

Again, first the lower and then the upper buccal segments should be examined in turn and the following recorded:

- General alignment and the presence of crowding or spacing.
- Any rotated teeth and those displaced from the line of the arch.
- Angulation relative to their respective bases (Fig. 5.15). This is of most relevance where a posterior crossbite exists.

Buccal segment relationship

The patient should be guided into maximum interdigitation and the following recorded:

- Molar relationship (if a corresponding molar is present in each arch).
- Canine relationship (Fig. 5.16).
- Presence of any crossbites.

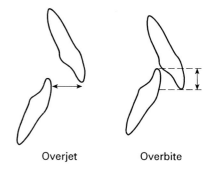

Overjet   Overbite

Fig. 5.13. Measurement of overjet and overbite.

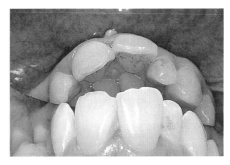

Fig. 5.14. A traumatic overbite.

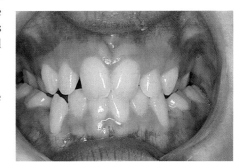

Fig. 5.15. Note how the upper buccal segment teeth are tilted palatally in this photograph.

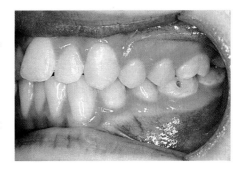

Fig. 5.16. Class I canine and molar relationship.

5.8. RADIOGRAPHIC EXAMINATION

Before radiographs can be prescribed a thorough examination of the patient should be carried out so that the views indicated on clinical grounds can be taken at the same visit. The commonly used views include the following:

- A panoramic view — an orthopantomographic (DPT) radiograph, or left and right lateral obliques.

- A lateral cephalometric radiograph — indicated for skeletal discrepancies and/or where anteroposterior movement of the incisors is required (see Chapter 6).

- A view of the upper incisors — either a periapical or an upper anterior occlusal. There has been some controversy as to the efficacy of this aspect of the radiographic examination in the light of radiographic dosage. It has been argued that only rarely does this view reveal a unexpected abnormal finding that is not indicated on the panoramic view (Fig. 5.17). Obviously where there is reason to suspect pathology (for example failure of eruption or a history of trauma) an intra-oral radiograph of this area is indicated. Also a panoramic view may need to be supplemented with an intra-oral view to

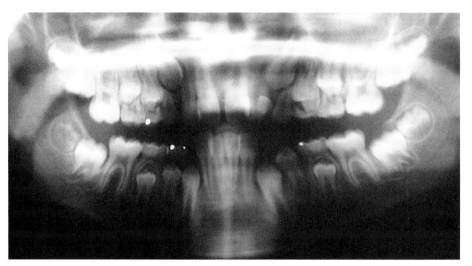

(a)

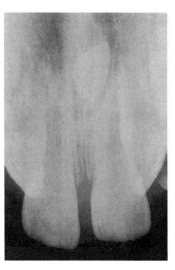

(b)

Fig. 5.17. (a) DPT and (b) peri-apical radiographs of the same patient. The intra-oral radiograph revealed a supernumerary tooth which was not evident on the OPG radiograph.

check the upper incisors radiographically prior to starting treatment to check for evidence of root resorption, root fracture, or supernumerary teeth.

The radiographs taken should be examined as follows:

- Check the clinical charting and to record the presence of any unerupted teeth. Any missing teeth (congenitally absent or previously extracted) should be noted.
- Assess the position and degree of development of any unerupted teeth which should also be studied for any abnormalities.
- Note any teeth with large restorations or untreated caries.
- Look for evidence of root resorption and apical pathology.
- Cephalometric tracing described in Chapter 6.

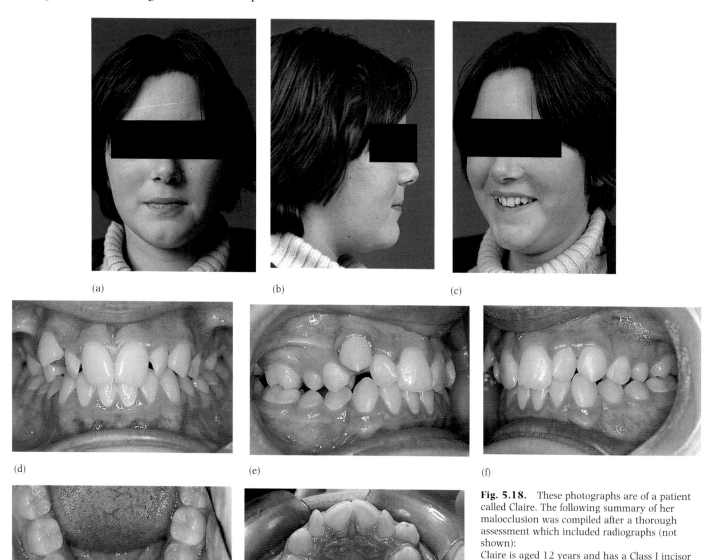

(a) (b) (c)

(d) (e) (f)

(g) (h)

Fig. 5.18. These photographs are of a patient called Claire. The following summary of her malocclusion was compiled after a thorough assessment which included radiographs (not shown):

Claire is aged 12 years and has a Class I incisor relationship on a mild Class III skeletal pattern with slightly increased vertical proportions. She has a mildly crowded lower arch and a moderately crowded upper arch with rotated upper lateral incisors and a buccally displaced 3/.

5.9. SUMMARY

Following a thorough orthodontic examination a summary of the salient features of the malocclusion should be recorded. This usually involves the following:

- The patient's name and age.
- A description of the incisor relationship, by classifying as Class I, Class II division 1, Class II division 2, or Class III (see Section 2.3.2) where possible. However, if there is any doubt it is often better to describe the overjet and overbite in words.
- Skeletal pattern.
- The presence of crowding or spacing.
- Any other features of note, for example absent teeth, displaced teeth, crossbites, or displacement on closure.

An example is given in Fig. 5.18. This approach helps to highlight the important features of a malocclusion and provides a problem list, thus facilitating treatment planning (Chapter 7).

PRINCIPAL SOURCES AND FURTHER READING

British Orthodontic Society Development and Standards Committee. (1999). *Orthodontic records: collection and management.*

Isaacson, K. G. and Jones, M. L. (ed.) (1994). *Orthodontic radiography: guidelines.* British Orthodontic Society, 291 Grays Inn Road London.

- This pamphlet gives the recommendations of the British Orthodontic Standards Working Party on which radiographs to take and their timing to achieve maximum diagnostic information with minimum X-ray dosage.

Khurana, M. and Martin, M. V. (1999). Orthodontics and Infective endocarditis. *British Journal of Orthodontics,* **26**, 295–8.

McDonald, F. and Ireland, A. J. (1998). *Diagnosis of the orthodontic patient.* Oxford University Press, Oxford.

Stephens, C. D., and Isaacson, K. (1990). *Practical orthodontic assessment.* Heinemann Medical Books, Oxford.

- This excellent book contains a very good résumé of diagnosis and treatment planning, but consists mainly of clinical cases for the reader to practise upon and learn from.

Taylor, N. G. and Jones, A. G. (1995). Are anterior occlusal radiographs indicated to supplement panoramic radiography during an orthodontic assessment? *British Dental Journal,* **179**, 377–81.

6 Cephalometrics

Cephalometry is the analysis and interpretation of standardized radiographs of the facial bones. In practice, cephalometrics has come to be associated with a true lateral view (Fig. 6.1). An anteroposterior radiograph can also be taken in the cephalostat, but this view is difficult to interpret and is usually only employed in cases with a skeletal asymmetry.

6.1. THE CEPHALOSTAT

In order to be able to compare the cephalometric radiographs of one patient taken on different occasions, or those of different individuals, some standardization is necessary. To achieve this aim the cephalostat was developed by B. Holly Broadbent in the period after the First World War (Fig. 6.2). The cephalostat consists of an X-ray machine which is at a fixed distance from a set of ear posts designed to fit into the patient's external auditory meatus. Thus the central beam of the machine is directed towards the ear posts, which also serve to stabilize the patient's head. The position of the head in the vertical axis is standardized by ensuring that the patient's Frankfort plane (for definition see below) is horizontal. This can be done by manually positioning the subject or, alternatively, by placing a mirror some distance away level with the patient's head and asking him or her to look into their own eyes. This is termed the natural head position, and some orthodontists claim that it is more consistent than a manual approach. It is normal practice to cone down the area exposed so that the skull vault is not routinely included in the X-ray beam.

Unfortunately, attempts to standardize the distances from the tube to the patient (usually between 5 and 6 feet (1.5 to 1.8 m)) and from the patient to the film (usually around 1 foot (around 30 cm)) have not been entirely successful as the values in parenthesis would suggest. Some magnification, usually of the order of 7–8 per cent, is inevitable with a lateral cephalometric film. In order to be able to check the magnification and thus the comparability of different films, it is helpful if a scale is included in the view (see Fig. 6.1).

To give a better definition of the soft tissue outline of the face, either a thin layer of barium paste can be placed down the central axis of the face or an aluminium wedge positioned so as to attenuate the beam in that area.

6.2. INDICATIONS FOR CEPHALOMETRIC EVALUATION

An increasing awareness of the risks associated with X-rays has led clinicians to re-evaluate the indications for taking a cephalometric radiograph. The following are considered valid.

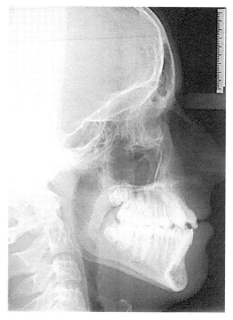

Fig. 6.1. A lateral cephalometric radiograph. Note the scale on the upper right-hand side.

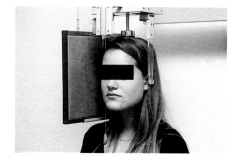

Fig. 6.2. A cephalostat.

6.2.1. An aid to diagnosis

It is possible to carry out successful orthodontic treatment without taking a cephalometric radiograph, particularly in Class I malocclusions. However, the information that cephalometric analysis yields is helpful in assessing the probable aetiology of a malocclusion and in planning treatment. The benefit to the patient in terms of the additional information gained must be weighed against the X-ray dosage. Therefore a lateral cephalometric radiograph is best limited to patients with a skeletal discrepancy and/or where anteroposterior movement of the incisors is planned. In a small proportion of patients it may be helpful to monitor growth to aid the planning and timing of treatment by taking serial cephalometric radiographs, although again the dosage to the patient must be justifiable.

In addition, a lateral view is often helpful in the accurate localization of unerupted displaced teeth and other pathology.

6.2.2. A pretreatment record

A lateral cephalometric radiograph is useful in providing a baseline record prior to the placement of appliances, particularly where movement of the upper and lower incisors is planned.

6.2.3. Monitoring the progress of treatment

In the management of severe malocclusions, where tooth movement is occurring in all three planes of space (for example treatments involving functional appliances, or upper and lower fixed appliances), it is common practice to take a lateral cephalometric radiograph during treatment to monitor anchorage requirements and incisor inclinations. A lateral cephalometric radiograph may also be useful in monitoring the movement of unerupted teeth and is the most accurate view for assessing upper incisor root resorption if this occurs during treatment.

6.2.4. Research purposes

A great deal of information has been obtained about growth and development by longitudinal studies which involved taking serial cephalometric radiographs from birth to the late teens or beyond. While the data provided by previous investigations are still used for reference purposes, it is no longer ethically possible to repeat this type of study. However, those views taken routinely during the course of orthodontic diagnosis and treatment can be used to study the effects of growth and treatment.

6.3. TRACING A CEPHALOMETRIC RADIOGRAPH

Before starting a tracing it is important to examine the radiograph for any abnormalities or pathology. For example, a pituitary tumour could result in an increase in the size of the sella turcica. Shortening of the roots of the incisors is often seen more clearly on a lateral cephalometric radiograph. This view is also helpful in assessing the patency of the airway, as enlarged adenoids can be easily seen.

In order to be able to derive meaningful information from a lateral cephalometric tracing, an accurate and systematic approach is required which also involves selecting the right conditions and equipment for the task.

- The tracing should be carried out in a darkened room on a light viewing box. All but the area being traced should be shielded to block out any extraneous light.

- Although it is possible to use tracing paper, proprietary acetate sheets are more transparent and give a more professional result.

- A sharp pencil should be used. The author recommends a 0.3 mm leaded propelling pencil (as this saves hours searching for pencil sharpeners). Some orthodontists with very steady hands use a fine ink stylus, but this is not advocated for the novice.

- The tracing paper or acetate sheet should be secured onto the film with masking tape, which does not leave a sticky residue when removed. The tracing should be oriented in the same position as the patient was when the radiograph was taken, i.e. with the Frankfort plane horizontal.

- Some orthodontists use stencils to obtain a neat outline of the incisor and molar teeth. However, too much artistic licence can lead to inaccuracies, particularly if the crown root angle of a tooth is not 'average'.

- For landmarks which are bilateral (unless they are directly superimposed) an average of the two should be taken.

- With a careful technique tracing errors should be of the order of + 0.5 mm for linear measurements and + 0.5° for angular measurements.

- It is a valuable 'learning experience' to trace the same radiograph on two separate occasions and compare the tracings. This helps to reduce the temptation to place undue emphasis upon small variations from normal cephalometric values.

An example of a tracing is shown in Fig. 6.3 (see also Fig. 6.4). Definitions of the various points and reference planes are given in Section 6.5.

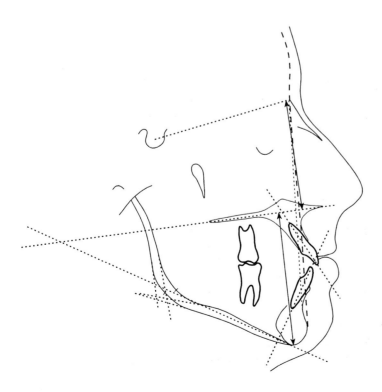

Fig. 6.3. A cephalometric tracing: patient LH (male) aged 14 years.

	LH	**Mean**
SNA	78.5°	81° ± 3°
SNB	77°	78° ± 3°
ANB	1.5°	3° ± 2°
UInc-MxPl	117.5°	109° ± 6°
LInc- MnPl	91.5°	93° ± 6°
MMPA	31°	27° ± 4°
LInc to APog	+4 mm	+1 mm ± 2 mm
FP	55%	55% ± 2%

6.3.1. Digitizers

A digitizer comprises an illuminated radiographic viewing screen which is connected to a computer. Information from a lateral cephalometric radiograph is entered into the computer by means of a cursor which records the horizontal and vertical (x, y) co-ordinates of cephalometric points or bony or soft tissue outlines. Specialized software can then be employed to utilize the information entered to produce a tracing and/or the analysis of choice. Studies have shown digitizers to be as accurate as tracing a radiograph by hand. Certainly, this approach is particularly useful for research as any number of radiographs can be entered, superimposed, and/or compared statistically.

6.4. CEPHALOMETRIC ANALYSIS — GENERAL POINTS

The orthodontic literature is replete with different cephalometric analyses, which in itself suggests that no single method is sufficient for all purposes and that all have their drawbacks. In a book of this size it is more appropriate to consider one analysis in depth. Therefore one of the approaches used commonly in the UK will be considered (Table 6.1). For details of other analyses the reader is referred to the publications cited in the section on further reading.

Table 6.1 Cephalometric norms for Caucasians (Eastman Standard).

Measurement	Mean value	Standard Deviation
SNA	81°	3°
SNB	78°	3°
ANB	3°	2°
UInc to MxPl	109°	6°
LInc to MnPl	93°*	6°
Inter-incisal angle	135°	10°
MMPA	27°	4°
Facial Proportion	55%	2%
LInc to APog line	+1 mm	2 mm
SN to MxPl	8°	3°

For definitions see Section 6.5.
*Or 120° — MMPA (see Section 6.8).

Cephalometric analyses are often based upon comparing the values obtained for certain measurements for a particular individual (or group of individuals) with the average values for their population (e.g. Caucasians). An indication of the significance of any difference between the actual measurement for an individual and the 'average' value can be obtained from the standard deviation. The range given by one standard deviation around the mean will include 66 per cent of the population and two standard deviations will include 97 per cent.

Cephalometric analysis is also of value in identifying the component parts of a malocclusion and probable aetiological factors — it is useful when a tracing is finished to reflect why that individual has that particular malocclusion. However, it is important not to fall into the trap of giving more credence to cephalometric analysis than it actually merits; it should always be remembered that it is an adjunctive tool to clinical diagnosis, and differences of cephalometric values from the average are not in themselves an indication for treatment, particularly as variations from normal in a specific value may be compensated for elsewhere in the facial skeleton or cranial base. In addition, cephalometric errors can occur owing to incorrect positioning of the patient and incorrect identification of landmarks.

A lateral cephalometric radiograph is a slightly magnified, two-dimensional representation of a three-dimensional object (the patient). For this reason angular measurements are generally to be preferred to linear measurements as the element of magnification is less important.

6.5. COMMONLY USED CEPHALOMETRIC POINTS AND REFERENCE LINES

The points and reference lines are shown in Fig. 6.4.

A point (A) — this is the point of deepest concavity on the anterior profile of the maxilla. It is also called subspinale. This point is taken to represent the anterior limit of the maxilla and is often tricky to locate accurately. However, tracing the outline of the root of the upper central incisor first and shielding all extraneous light often aids identification. The A point is located on alveolar bone and is liable to changes in position with tooth movement and growth.

Anterior nasal spine (ANS) — this is the tip of the anterior process of the maxilla and is situated at the lower margin of the nasal aperture.

B point (B) — the point of deepest concavity on the anterior surface of the mandibular symphysis. The B point is also sited on alveolar bone and can alter with tooth movement and growth.

Gonion (Go) — the most posterior inferior point on the angle of the symphysis. This point can be 'guesstimated', or determined more accurately by bisecting the angle formed by the tangents from the posterior border of the ramus and the inferior border of the mandible (Fig. 6.5).

Menton (Me) — the lowest point on the mandibular symphysis.

Nasion (N) — the most anterior point on the frontonasal suture. When difficulty is experienced locating nasion, the point of deepest concavity at the intersection of the frontal and nasal bones can be used instead.

Orbitale (Or) — the most inferior anterior point on the margin of the orbit. By definition, the left orbital margin should be used to locate this point. However,

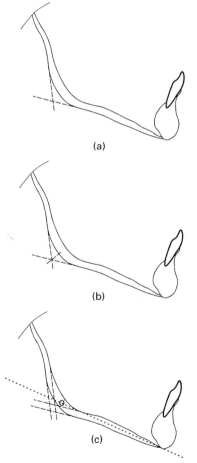

(a)

(b)

(c)

Fig. 6.5. Construction of Gonion (Go): (a) draw tangents to posterior and inferior borders; (b) bisect the angle formed by the tangents and mark where it crosses the angle of the mandible; (c) repeat for the other outline (if one is visible). Go is located midway between the two points.

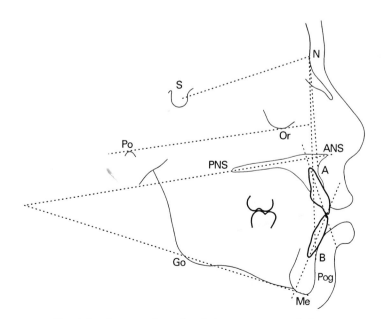

Fig. 6.4. Commmonly used cephalometric points and planes.

this can be a little tricky to determine radiographically, and so an average of the two images of left and right is usually taken.

Pogonion (Pog) — the most anterior point on the mandibular symphysis.

Porion (Po) — the uppermost outermost point on the bony external auditory meatus. This landmark can be obscured by the ear posts of the cephalostat, and some advocate tracing these instead. However, this is not recommended as they do not approximate to the position of the external auditory meatus. The uppermost surface of the condylar head is at the same level, and this can be used as a guide where difficulty is experienced in determining porion.

Posterior nasal spine (PNS) — this is the tip of the posterior nasal spine of the maxilla. This point is often obscured by the developing third molars, but lies directly below the pterygomaxillary fissure.

Sella (S) — the midpoint of the sella turcica.

SN line — this line, connecting the midpoint of sella turcica with nasion, is taken to represent the cranial base.

Frankfort plane — this is the line joining porion and orbitale. This plane is difficult to define accurately because of the problems inherent in determining orbitale and porion.

Mandibular plane — The line joining gonion and menton. This is only one of several definitions of the mandibular plane, but is probably the most widely used. Other definitions can be found in the publications listed in the section on further reading.

Maxillary plane — the line joining anterior nasal spine with posterior nasal spine. Where it is difficult to determine ANS and PNS accurately, a line parallel to the nasal floor can be used instead.

Functional occlusal plane — a line drawn between the cusp tips of the permanent molars and premolars (or deciduous molars in mixed dentition). It can be difficult to decide where to draw this line, particularly if there is an increased curve of Spee, or only the first permanent molars are in occlusion during the transition from mixed to permanent dentition. The functional plane can change orientation with growth and/or treatment, and so is not particularly reliable for longitudinal comparisons.

6.6. ANTEROPOSTERIOR SKELETAL PATTERN

6.6.1. Angle ANB (Fig. 6.6)

In order to be able to compare the position of the maxilla and mandible, it is necessary to have a fixed point or plane. The skeletal pattern is often determined cephalometrically by comparing the relationship of the maxilla and mandible with the cranial base by means of angles SNA and SNB. The difference between these two measurements, angle ANB, is classified broadly as follows:

ANB < 2°	Class III
2° ≤ ANB ≤ 4°	Class I
ANB > 4°	Class II

However, this approach assumes (incorrectly in some cases) that the cranial base, as indicated by the line SN, is a reliable basis for comparison and that points A and B are indicative of maxillary and mandibular basal bone. Variations in the position of nasion can also affect angles SNA and SNB and thus the difference ANB (Fig. 6.7); however, variations in the position of sella do not. If SNA is increased or reduced from the average value, this could be due to either a discrepancy in the position of the maxilla (as indicated by point A) or nasion. The

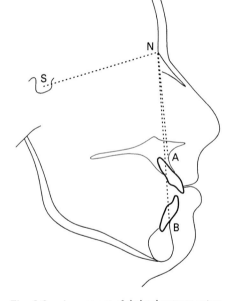

Fig. 6.6. Assessment of skeletal pattern using angles SNA and SNB: patient LH (male) aged 14 years.

	LH	**Mean**
SNA	78.5°	81° ± 3°
SNB	77°	78° ± 3°
ANB	1.5°	3° ± 2°

Corrected ANB = $1.5° + \dfrac{81° - 78.5°}{2}$ = 2.75°

This would normally be rounded to the nearest 0.5° giving a corrected value of 3° The ANB difference suggests a mild Class III skeletal pattern. However, if the ANB difference is corrected for the low value of SNA, this suggests a Class I skeletal pattern.

following (rather crude) modification is often used in order to make allowance for this:

Provided the angle between the maxillary plane and the sella–nasion line is within 5°–11°:

- if SNA is increased, for every degree that SNA is greater than 81°, subtract 0.5° from ANB;
- if SNA is reduced, for every degree that SNA is less than 81°, add 0.5° to ANB.

If the angle between the maxillary plane and the sella–nasion line is not within 5°–11°, this correction is not applicable.

Alternatively, an approach which avoids the cranial base (e.g. the Ballard conversion or the Wits analysis) can be used to supplement the above analysis, particularly where the cephalometric findings are at variance with the clinical assessment.

6.6.2. Ballard conversion (Fig. 6.8)

This analysis uses the incisors as indicators of the relative position of the maxilla and mandible. It is easy to confuse a Ballard conversion and a prognosis tracing (see Fig. 6.12), but in the former the aim is to tilt the teeth to their normal angles (thus eliminating any dento-alveolar compensation) with the result that the residual overjet will indicate the relationship of the maxilla to the mandible.

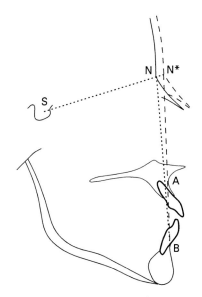

Fig. 6.7. Effect of variations in the position of nasion on angles SNA, SNB, and ANB:

SNA = 78.5°	SN*A = 81°
SNB = 77°	SN*B = 81°
ANB = 1.5°	AN*B = 0°

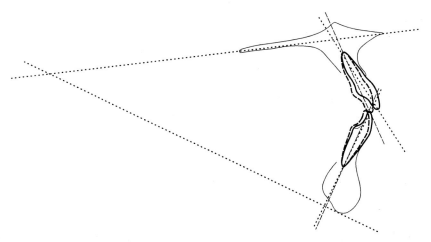

Fig. 6.8. Ballard conversion: average upper incisor angle to maxillary plane, 109°; lower incisor angle to mandibular plane, 120° – 31.5° = 88.5°.
The method is as follows.

1. Trace on a separate piece of tracing paper the outline of the maxilla, the mandibular symphysis, the incisors, and the maxillary and mandibular planes.
2. Mark the 'rotation points' of the incisors one-third of the root length away from the root apex.
3. By rotating around the point marked, reposition the upper incisor at an angle of 109° to the maxillary plane. Repeat for the lower incisor (allowing for the maxillary mandibular planes angle of 31.5° in this case).
4. The residual overjet reflects the underlying skeletal pattern. In this case the Ballard conversion indicates a mild Class III skeletal pattern as the repositioned incisors are nearly edge to edge.

6.6.3. Wits analysis (Fig. 6.9)

This analysis compares the relationships of the maxilla and mandible with the occlusal plane. There are several definitions of the occlusal plane, but for the purposes of the Wits analysis it is taken to be a line drawn between the cusp tips

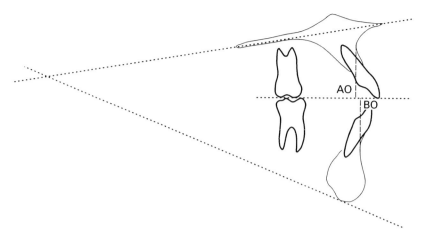

Fig. 6.9. Wits analysis: LH (male) aged 14 years. The method is as follows.

1. Draw in the functional occlusal plane (FOP).
2. Drop perpendiculars from point A and point B to the FOP to give points AO and BO.
3. Measure the distance between AO and BO.

The average value is +1 mm (± 1.9 mm) for males and 0 mm (± 1.77 mm) for females. The distance from AO to BO for LH (male) is +2 mm, suggesting a mild Class III skeletal pattern.

of the molars and premolars (or deciduous molars), which is known as the functional occlusal plane. Perpendicular lines from both point A and point B are dropped to the functional occlusal plane to give points AO and BO. The distance between AO and BO is then measured. The mean values are 1 mm (SD + 1.9 mm) for males and 0 mm (SD + 1.77 mm) for females.

The drawback to this approach is that the functional occlusal plane is not easy to locate, which obviously affects the accuracy and reproducibility of the Wits analysis. A slight difference in the angulation of the functional occlusal plane can have a marked effect on the relative positions of AO and BO.

6.7. VERTICAL SKELETAL PATTERN

Again there are many different ways of assessing vertical skeletal proportions. The more commonly used include the following.

● The Maxillary–Mandibular Planes Angle (Fig. 6.10). The average angle between the maxillary plane and the mandibular plane (MMPA) is 27° + 4°. Some analyses measure the angle between the Frankfort and the mandibular planes (average 28° + 4°). However, the maxillary plane is easier to locate accurately and therefore the MMPA is preferred.

● The Facial Proportion (Fig. 6.11). This is the ratio of the lower facial height to the total anterior facial height measured perpendicularly from the maxillary plane, calculated as a percentage:

$$\text{facial proportion (FP)} = \frac{\text{MxPl to Me}}{\text{MxPl to Me} + \text{MxPl to N}} \times 100.$$

If there appears to be a discrepancy between the results for these two measurements of vertical relationship, it should be remembered that the MMPA reflects both posterior lower facial height and anterior lower facial height. Therefore in

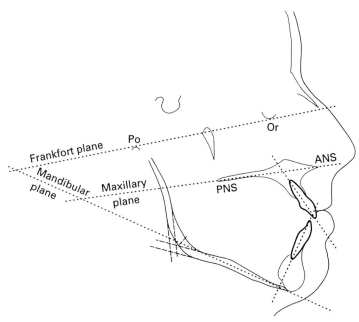

Fig. 6.10. Assessment of vertical skeletal pattern using the MMPA and FMPA: LH (male) aged 14 years.

	LH	**Mean**
MMPA	31.5°	27° ± 4°
FMPA	34.5°	28° ± 4°

Both the MMPA and the Frankfort mandibular planes angle are increased. This may be due to either an increased lower anterior face height or a reduced lower posterior face height.

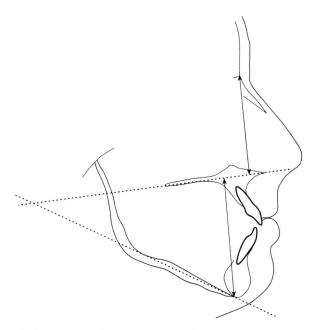

Fig. 6.11. Calculating the facial proportion: LH (male) aged 14 years.

$$\text{Facial proportion} = \frac{\text{MxPl to Me}}{(\text{MxPl to Me}) + (\text{MxPl to N})} \times 100$$

$$= \frac{70 \text{ mm}}{57.5 \text{ mm} + 70 \text{ mm}} = \frac{70 \text{ mm}}{127.5 \text{ mm}}$$

$$= 55\% \text{ (average value)}.$$

the case of patient LH who has an increased MMPA but an average facial proportion it would appear that the posterior lower facial height is reduced (as opposed to an increased anterior lower facial height).

6.8. INCISOR POSITION

The average value for the angle formed between the upper incisor and the maxillary plane is 109°. The 'normal' value for lower incisor angle given in Table 6.1 is for an individual with an average MMPA of 27°. However, there is a relationship between the MMPA and the lower incisor angle: as the MMPA increases, the lower incisors become more retroclined. As the sum of the average MMPA (27°) and the average lower incisor angle (93°) equals 120°, an alternative way of deriving the 'average' lower incisor angulation for an individual is to subtract the MMPA from 120°:

lower incisor angle = 120° − MMPA.

6.8.1. Prognosis tracing

Sometimes it is helpful to be able to determine the type and amount of incisor movement required to correct an increased or reverse overjet. Although the skeletal pattern will give an indication, on occasion compensatory proclination or retroclination (known as dento-alveolar compensation) of the incisors can confuse the issue. When planning treatment in such a case it may be helpful to carry out a prognosis tracing. This involves 'moving' the incisor(s) to mimic the movements achievable with different types of appliance therapy to help determine the best course of action for that patient. An example is shown in Fig. 6.12, where it can be seen that bodily retraction of the upper incisors would result in their being retracted out of the palatal bone — obviously not a practical treatment proposition.

A quick method of calculating the final upper incisor angle following tipping movements is to assume that for 2.5° of angular movement (about a point of rotation one-third of the way down the root from the apex) the upper incisor edge will translate approximately 1 mm. However, it should be stressed that both methods provide only a rough guide to the tooth movements required.

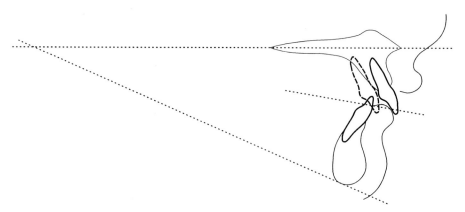

Fig. 6.12. Prognosis tracing: CP (female) aged 18 years.
From this diagram it can be seen that bodily movement of the upper incisors to reduce this patient's overjet would not be feasible. Therefore a surgical aproach was recommended.

6.8.2. A-Pogonion line (APog)

Raleigh Williams noted when he analysed the lateral cephalometric radiographs of individuals with pleasing facial appearances that one feature which they all had in common was that the tip of their lower incisor lay on or just in front of the line connecting point A with pogonion. He advocated using this position of the lower incisor as a treatment goal to help ensure a good facial profile. While this line may be useful when planning orthodontic treatment, it must be remembered that it is only a guideline to good facial aesthetics, and not an indicator of stability. If the lower incisors are moved from their pretreatment position of labiolingual balance, whatever the rationale, there is a likelihood of relapse following removal of appliances. This topic is discussed in more detail in Chapters 7 and 10.

6.9. SOFT TISSUE ANALYSIS

The major role of analysis of the soft tissues is in diagnosis and planning prior to orthognathic surgery (Chapter 20). As with other elements of cephalometric analysis, there are a large number of different analyses of varying complexity. The following are some of the more commonly used:

The Holdaway line

This is a line from soft tissue chin to the upper lip. In a well-proportioned face this line, if extended, should bisect the nose (Fig. 6.13).

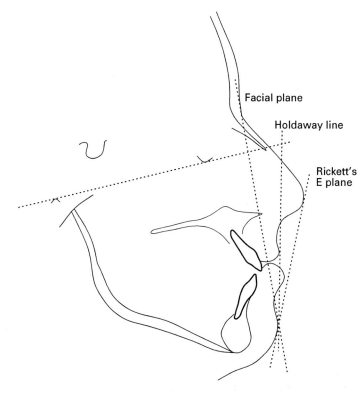

Fig. 6.13. Soft tissue analysis.

Rickett's E-plane

This line joins soft tissue chin and the tip of the nose. In a balanced face the lower lip should lie 2 mm (± 2 mm) anterior to this line with the upper lip positioned a little further posteriorly to the line (Fig. 6.13).

Facial plane

The facial plane is a line between the soft tissue nasion and the soft tissue chin. In a well-balanced face the Frankfort plane should bisect the facial plane at an angle of about 86° and point A should lie on it (Fig. 6.13).

As with other aspects of cephalometrics, but perhaps more pertinently, these analyses should be supplementary to a clinical examination, and it should also be remembered that beauty is in the eye of the beholder.

6.10. ASSESSING GROWTH AND TREATMENT CHANGES

The advantage of standardizing lateral cephalometric radiographs is that it is then possible to compare radiographs either of groups of patients for research purposes or of the same patient over time to evaluate growth and treatment changes. In some cases it may be helpful to monitor growth of a patient over time before deciding upon a treatment plan, particularly if unfavourable growth would result in a malocclusion that could not be treated by orthodontics alone. During treatment it can be helpful to determine the contributions that tooth movements and/or growth have made to the correction and to help ensure that, where possible, a stable result is achieved. For example, in a Class II division 1 malocclusion, correction of an increased overjet can occur by retroclination of the upper incisors and/or proclination of the lower incisors and/or forward growth of the mandible and/or restraint of forward growth of the maxilla. If the major part of the correction is due to proclination of the lower incisors there is an increased likelihood of relapse of the overjet following cessation of appliance therapy owing to soft tissue pressures. If this is determined before appliances are removed, it may be possible to take steps to rectify the situation.

However, in order to be able to compare radiographs accurately it is necessary to have a fixed point or reference line which does not change with time or growth. Unfortunately this poses a dilemma, as there are no natural fixed points or planes within the face and skull. This should be borne in mind when interpreting the differences seen using any of the superimpositions discussed below.

6.10.1 Cranial base

The SN line is taken in cephalometrics as approximating to the cranial base. However, growth does occur at nasion, and therefore superimpositions on this line for the purpose of evaluating changes over time should be based at sella. Unfortunately, growth at nasion does not always conveniently occur along the SN line — if nasion moves upwards or downwards with growth, this will of course introduce a rotational error in comparisons of tracings superimposed on SN. It is more accurate to use the outline of the cranial base (called de Coster's line) as little change occurs in the anterior cranial base after 7 years of age (see Chapter 4). However, a clear radiograph and a good knowledge of anatomy is required to do this reliably.

6.10.2. The maxilla

Growth of the maxilla occurs on all surfaces by periosteal remodelling. For the purpose of interpretation of growth and/or treatment changes the least affected surface is the anterior surface of the palatal vault, although the maxilla is commonly superimposed on the maxillary plane at PNS.

6.10.3. The mandible

It was noted above that there are no natural stable reference points within the face and skull. Bjork overcame this problem by inserting metal markers in the facial skeleton. Whilst this approach is obviously not applicable in the management of patients, it did provide considerable information on patterns of facial growth, indicating that in the mandible the landmarks which change least with growth are as follows (in order of usefulness):

- the innermost surface of the cortical bone of the symphysis;
- the tip of the chin;
- the outline of the inferior dental canal;
- the crypt of the developing third permanent molars from the time of commencement of mineralization until root formation begins.

PRINCIPAL SOURCES AND FURTHER READING

Brown, M. (1981). Eight methods of analysing a cephalogram to establish anteroposterior skeletal discrepancy. *British Journal of Orthodontics*, **8**, 139–46.
- This paper admirably illustrates the pitfalls and problems with cephalometric analysis, whilst also briefly presenting some alternative analyses.

Ferguson, J. W., Evans, R. I. W., and Cheng, L. H. H. (1992). Diagnostic accuracy and observer performance in the diagnosis of abnormalities in the anterior maxilla: a comparison of panoramic with intra-oral radiography. *British Dental Journal*, **173**, 265–71.

Gravely, J. F. and Murray Benzies, P. (1974). The clinical significance of tracing error in cephalometry. *British Journal of Orthodontics*, **1**, 95–101.
- A classical paper on tracing errors.

Guidelines for the use of radiographs in clinical orthodontics. British Orthodontic Society, London, 1994.

Houston, W. J. B. (1979). The current status of facial growth prediction. *British Journal of Orthodontics*, **6**, 11–17.

Houston, W. J. B. (1986). Sources of error in measurements from cephalometric radiographs. *European Journal of Orthodontics*, **8**, 149–51.

Jacobson, A. (1995). *Radiographic cephalometry: from basics to videoimaging.* Quintessence Publishing, USA.
- An authoratative book. Includes a very good section on how to trace a cephalometric radiograph with actual copy films and overlays to aid landmark identification.

Lewis, D. H. (1981). Basic tracing for lateral skull radiographs. *Dental Update*, **8**, 45–51.

Lewis, D. H. (1981). Lateral skull radiographs: growth and treatment changes. *Dental Update*, **8**, 193–99.
- These two papers by Lewis give an introduction to cephalometrics which is easy to follow.

Sandham, A. (1988). Repeatability of head posture recordings from lateral cephalometric radiographs. *British Journal of Orthodontics*, **15**, 157–62.

7 Treatment planning

7.1. INTRODUCTION

Without doubt, treatment planning is the most difficult, but also the most important, element of orthodontics. A knowledge of dental development, facial growth, psychology, and appliance mechanics are all prerequisites for success. Whilst much can be learnt from textbooks there is no substitute for clinical experience gained over time. Therefore, when in doubt, the less experienced should refer the patient to a specialist for advice.

Prior to planning treatment a thorough examination of the patient and their malocclusion should be carried out (Chapter 5). As soon as practicable after this assessment, the patient's records, including study models and radiographs, should be studied, preferably during a quiet period away from the clinical environment.

7.2. PATIENT MOTIVATION

In order for orthodontic treatment to be successful the patient's willing participation and cooperation are essential. Therefore time spent on assessing a patient's concerns regarding the alignment of their teeth and their motivation towards appliance treatment is never wasted. It may be wiser to achieve a compromise result successfully than to fail to complete an ideal treatment plan. In this respect it is important to counsel the patient regarding their role in the success of treatment. If motivation is at all in doubt, it is wiser not to proceed or at least to 'test the water' with a simple appliance before any irreversible steps, for example extractions, are undertaken. On occasion, a patient will seek perfection but will be unwilling to cooperate fully with the type of appliance necessary to achieve this. Faced with this situation, the wise clinician will not proceed.

7.3. LIMITATIONS OF ORTHODONTIC TREATMENT

When planning treatment the limitations of orthodontic appliances should be borne in mind. With an enthusiastic patient and favourable growth (which is more likely in children and in Class II rather than Class III malocclusions) compensation of moderately severe skeletal patterns can be achieved with functional and/or fixed appliances. However, where growth is likely to be unfavourable and/or the underlying skeletal pattern is severe, consideration should be given to using a combined surgical and orthodontic approach (see Chapter 20).

Conventional removable appliances (Chapter 16) are only suitable for malocclusions where tipping movements will suffice. Functional appliances (Chapter

18) are particularly useful in the management of Class II malocclusions in a growing patient.

7.4. TIMING OF TREATMENT

In the vast majority of cases definitive orthodontic treatment is best carried out in the early permanent dentition. The reasons for this include the following:

- Growth can be utilized to facilitate anteroposterior arch correction and overbite reduction.
- The tendency for spontaneous tooth movement is greatest during and shortly after tooth eruption, and while the patient is still growing.
- Active tooth movement cannot begin until after eruption.
- Patient cooperation reaches a peak in the early teens, but diminishes rapidly from around 14–15 years.
- Cellular reactions and bone remodelling in response to orthodontic forces are more rapid in children.

Orthodontic treatment is possible in adulthood but the range of malocclusions that can be tackled by orthodontics alone is diminished because of a lack of growth. In addition, tooth movement is initially slower than in children. Root resorption during treatment has been found to occur to a greater extent in adults. Nevertheless, once they have made the decision to go ahead with orthodontic treatment, adults usually make conscientious and cooperative patients.

7.5. AIMS OF TREATMENT

The first step in the planning process is to decide whether or not treatment is indicated. This issue has been discussed in detail in Chapter 1. In summary, appliances and/or extractions should only be embarked upon when a significant improvement in dental health or aesthetics can be achieved. It is better not to proceed than to run the risk of worsening a patient's occlusion or appearance.

Once it has been decided that treatment is indicated, consideration should be given to the aims of treatment. This involves visualizing the finished result and then evaluating what occlusal changes are required to achieve this. It is advisable to decide what the ideal aims should be and then, if necessary, to modify them in the light of other considerations such as patient cooperation. However, it is important to note in the patient's records any treatment plans discussed and why a particular set of treatment aims was finally selected.

When deciding upon the aims of treatment the less experienced operator may find it helpful to construct a brief summary of the patient's malocclusion (see Chapter 5, Section 5.9). This gives a 'problem list' from which those factors that are to be corrected can be selected. However, a logical approach is required. For example, of the two plans below, plan B is preferable as this is the sequence which practical treatment would take.

Plan A
1. Reduction of overjet.
2. Correction of crossbite $\underline{5}$.
3. Relief of crowding.
4. Reduction of overbite.

Fig. 7.1. Patient HW aged 12 years: (a)–(e) pretreatment; (f)–(j) post-treatment. HW had a Class II division 1 malocclusion on a Class II skeletal pattern with crowding. As proclination of the lower labial segment had helped to compensate for the Class II skeletal pattern, this malocclusion was treated by extraction of all four first premolars and upper removable appliances. Anchorage was reinforced with extra-oral anchorage.

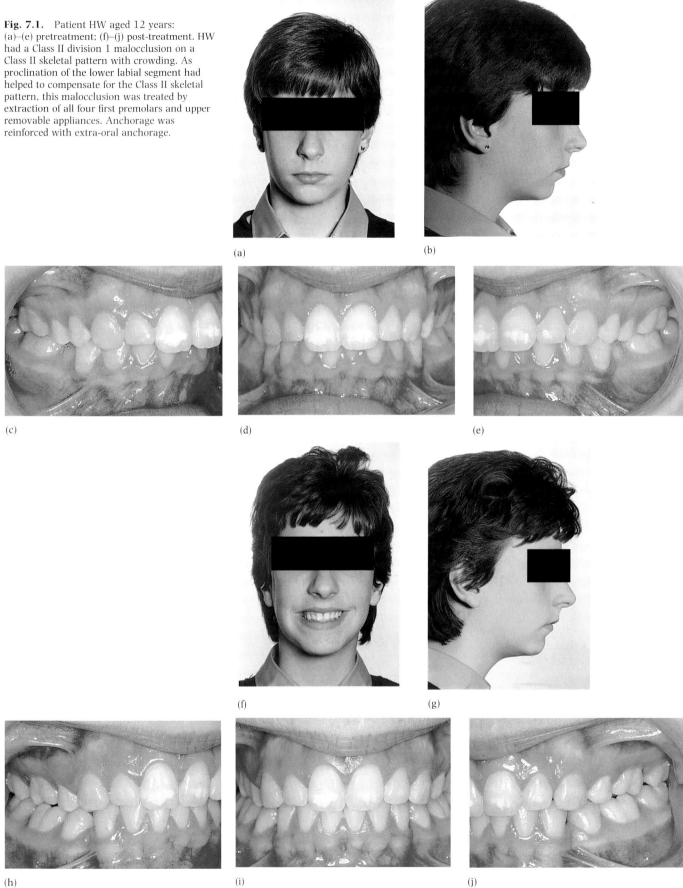

(a)

(b)

(c)

(d)

(e)

(f)

(g)

(h)

(i)

(j)

Plan B

1. Relief of crowding.
2. Reduction of overbite.
3. Correction of crossbite ⌋5.
4. Reduction of overjet.

It is important to remember that the planning process is flexible and that the initial aims selected may have to be re-evaluated and revised.

7.6. PRINCIPLES OF TREATMENT PLANNING

The approach to treatment planning outlined below will provide a logical basis for the management of most malocclusions (Fig. 7.1). However, this section should be read in conjunction with Chapters 8–15 for a fuller appreciation of management.

Mixed dentition problems are covered separately in Chapter 3.

7.6.1. The lower arch (Fig. 7.2)

It is accepted that in the majority of patients the lower labial segment lies in a zone of balance between the tongue and the cheeks. There are exceptions to this rule (see Chapter 10), but the management of such cases is the domain of the specialist and it is advisable for the inexperienced operator to consider the labiolingual position of the lower incisors as immutable. This precept has the advantage of providing a starting point around which treatment planning can be based.

The first step is to assess the alignment, including the presence of crowding or spacing, of the lower arch. If alignment is good or acceptable, then attention can be turned to the upper arch (Section 7.6.2). If the lower labial segment is either actually crowded, or crowding is expected following eruption of the canines (potential crowding), both the degree of crowding and the likelihood of its increasing significantly need to be considered. Once intercanine growth has slowed, at around 9 years of age, crowding of the lower labial segment is likely to increase, particularly if third permanent molars are developing and/or the patient is still actively growing. With practice the degree of crowding can often be assessed by eye. The less experienced may find it helpful to measure the arch circumference (from the mesial surface of the first permanent molars around the arch through the contact points) and compare this with the actual widths of the permanent teeth (Fig. 7.3).

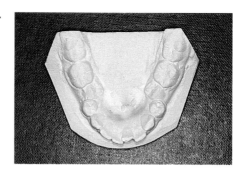

Fig. 7.2. Lower arch of HW showing proclination of lower labial segment with moderate crowding. Extraction of both lower first premolars was planned.

Fig. 7.3. (a) Arch circumference measured from the mesial aspect of the first permanent molars by means of the best fit through the contact points around the arch. A flexible piece of wire (for example copper or fuse wire) should be used. (b) The widths of each individual tooth (anterior to the first molars) are measured using dividers. Each dimension is indented onto a ruled line on a piece of paper to give the space required to accommodate all the teeth anterior to the first permanent molars in alignment. (c) Comparison of the sum total of the combined widths with the actual space available (the arch circumference) gives an exact measurement of the crowding present.

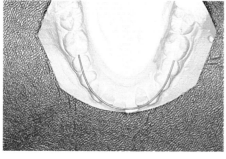

(a)

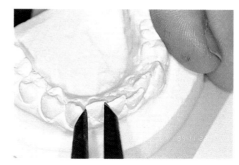

(b)

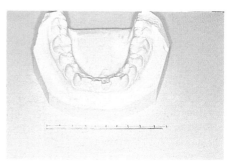

(c)

If the crowding is very mild it may be wiser to accept this. If mid-arch extractions are carried out, residual spacing may remain or if if fixed appliances are used to try and close any residual space, some lingual retraction of the incisors may occur which is generally undesirable.

If the overbite is increased, account must also be taken of the space required to level the curve of Spee. An averagely increased curve of Spee will require approximately a quarter unit of space for leveling.

Planning space requirements is discussed in greater detail in Section 7.7. In summary, space can be provided by the following manoeuvres:

- distal movement of the molars, which is commonly considered for the upper arch but very rarely in the lower arch;

- expansion;

- extractions (see Section 7.7.1), which is the most commonly used approach.

Once relief of crowding, if indicated, has been decided upon, the next step in the treatment planning process is to consider what tooth movements are required to align the lower arch. Spontaneous tooth movements are greatest as the teeth are erupting in growing patients but cannot be relied upon to produce complete alignment. Changes are greatest for the first 6 months following relief of crowding.

Mesially inclined canines and lingually inclined lower premolars will usually become upright if space is made available provided that there are no occlusal interferences, although this occurs less readily in an older patient who is not growing. If the canines are distally inclined or any teeth are rotated, fixed appliances are usually required to achieve satisfactory alignment. Also, if extraction of the second premolars or first molars is indicated, fixed appliances are usually necessary to achieve alignment and to close space by bodily movement (Section 7.7.1).

If there is a centreline discrepancy in a crowded lower arch, some spontaneous correction may be achieved by staggering the extractions. However, if the discrepancy is greater than half a tooth width, complete correction is unlikely and fixed appliances will be required if the centrelines are to be coordinated.

7.6.2. The upper arch (Fig. 7.4)

Once alignment of the lower arch has been planned, it is often helpful to envisage the anticipated position of the lower canine before focusing on building the upper arch around the lower arch. The first step in this process is mentally to reposition the maxillary canine into a Class I relationship with the lower canine. This will not only give an indication of whether space has to be created, but will also indicate the amount and type of movement required. Allowance should be made for spacing of the lower labial segment, if present, and for tooth-size discrepancies, for example peg-shaped lateral incisors.

If the aim of the treatment is to produce a Class I incisor and molar relationship, then in most cases with crowding it is usual to plan to extract the same tooth in the upper arch as is planned in the mandibular arch. This makes coordination of space closure and appliance mechanics between the arches considerably easier. The major exceptions to this rule occur when extractions are planned to aid dento-alveolar compensation in malocclusions with a skeletal component. For example, in Class II malocclusions extractions in the upper arch alone leading to a Class II buccal segment relationship may be indicated if the lower arch is well aligned, or extraction of the first premolars in the upper arch may be

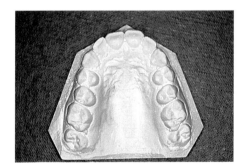

Fig. 7.4. Upper arch of HW showing mild crowding. It was decided to extract both upper first premolars to provide space for retraction of upper canines into Class I relationship with the corrected position of lower canines.

matched by the extraction of the second premolars in the lower arch to alter the anchorage balance (see Chapters 9 and 10).

The tooth movements needed to align the upper labial segment, and therefore the type of appliance required, should be considered in conjunction with correction of the incisor relationship.

7.6.3. Correction of the incisor relationship (Fig. 7.5)

Correction of Class II divisions 1 and 2, and Class III incisor relationships are discussed in greater detail in Chapters 9, 10, and 11. Functional appliances are most useful in the correction of Class II malocclusions in the growing patient. If bodily, de-rotation, intrusion, or extrusion movements are required, fixed appliances are indicated.

It is also important to consider the incisor relationship in the vertical dimension, i.e. overbite. This is particularly pertinent in Class II malocclusions, where the overbite is increased, and in Class III malocclusions where proclination of the upper incisors alone will reduce the overbite and the chances of stability of the corrected incisor relationship.

7.6.4. The buccal segments (Fig. 7.6)

Once the labial segments have been planned, attention should be focused on the buccal segments and the molar relationship. If no extractions are planned, no teeth are congenitally absent, or matched extractions in both arches are indicated, the molar relationship at the end of treatment should be Class I. If extractions are carried out in the upper arch only, the buccal segments should be Class II; conversely, if only lower arch extractions are planned, a Class III molar relationship should result.

It is important to consider how the desired molar relationship will be achieved. Following loss of the lower second deciduous molar, the first permanent molar will drift mesially into the leeway space, but apart from this little spontaneous change can be anticipated. Therefore if correction of the buccal segment relationship is desirable, active change using appliances is necessary. Methods of changing the molar relationship include the following:

● intramaxillary forces (for example space closure with a fixed appliance);
● intermaxillary forces (for example Class II elastic traction or a functional appliance);
● extra-oral traction;
● anchorage loss, although by definition this is molar movement in an undesirable direction.

7.6.5. Anchorage

This topic is considered in more detail in Chapter 15. However, during treatment planning it may be helpful to view it in terms of the balance between the available space and the desired tooth movements. Consideration of the amount of space and the type of movement required to achieve alignment and/or correction of the incisor relationship in the steps above will give an indication of the anchorage requirements of a particular malocclusion. Obviously, if most or all of the space created by extractions is needed to retract the canines and align the incisors, no forward movement of the buccal segment teeth can be permitted and

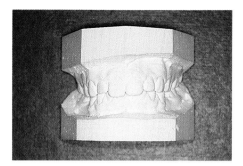

Fig. 7.5. Correction of HW's incisor relationship required reduction of the overbite and then the overjet. As proclination of the lower incisors had helped to compensate for the mild Class II skeletal pattern, reduction of the overjet by tipping the upper incisors palatally was feasible. An upper removable appliance with a flat anterior bite plane and canine retraction springs was prescribed. A second appliance was used for overjet reduction once the overbite had been reduced and the upper canines retracted into a Class I relationship with the lower arch.

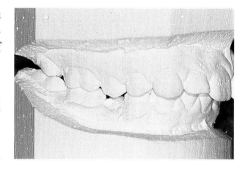

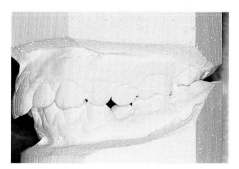

Fig. 7.6. HW's molar relationship was Class I therefore no correction of the buccal segments was required.

anchorage will have to be reinforced (see Chapter 15). In addition, the effect of the type of tooth movement required on anchorage must be taken into consideration. For example, bodily retraction of the upper incisors to reduce an increased overjet will place a greater strain on anchorage than tipping movements (i.e. the former will tend to drag the molars mesially).

It has been observed that space closure occurs more rapidly in patients with increased vertical skeletal proportions than in those with reduced vertical proportions. In practice this means that anchorage loss following extractions is more likely to be a problem in the patient with a tendency to a vertical growth pattern.

The effect of any planned tooth movement upon the patient's facial profile also needs to be estimated. Closure of spacing (either present before treatment or created by extractions) will have the effect of retracting the anterior teeth and moving the buccal segment teeth forwards. The extent to which one of these predominates within each arch should be determined during treatment planning, as should the actual mechanics of appliance therapy necessary. Where retraction of the anterior teeth would be detrimental to the profile, specialist advice should be sought before extractions are carried out.

7.6.6. Retention

It is imperative that retention is considered at the treatment planning stage and presented to the patient as a vital part of the overall treatment package. Treatment should always aim to leave the teeth in a stable position on completion, but a period of retention is necessary to allow consolidation of newly formed bone, remodelling of the periodontal fibres, and soft tissue adaptation. Permanent retention is occasionally required, but such cases should be the province of the specialist.

Retention is discussed in more detail in Chapter 15 and also in Chapters 8–13 in relation to the correction of each type of malocclusion. In general, a regime of at least 3 months full-time wear and then 3 months nights-only wear is advisable following treatment with removable appliances. Most operators double the time period following treatment with fixed appliances.

7.6.7. Potential pitfalls

Consideration should be given to referring a patient for specialist advice where any doubt exists or if any of the following features are noted:

- marked skeletal discrepancies in the anteroposterior, vertical, or transverse dimension;
- deep overbite associated with reduced vertical skeletal proportions;
- the molar relationship is a full unit Class II and the lower arch is crowded;
- Class II division 1 malocclusions where the overjet is greater than 10 mm and/or the overjet is increased and the upper incisors are upright;
- first permanent molars of poor prognosis and a Class II or Class III incisor relationship;
- asymmetrical crowding;
- generalized spacing which concerns the patient.

7.7. CREATING SPACE

Space to relieve crowding and/or to compensate for a skeletal discrepancy can be gained by the following procedures:

- extractions
- expansion
- distal movement of the buccal segment teeth
- reduction of tooth width
- a combination of any or all of the above.

7.7.1. Extractions

Before planning the extraction of any permanent teeth it is important to ensure that all remaining teeth are present and developing in a satisfactory position. The factors governing the choice of teeth for extraction include the following:

- Prognosis.
- Position.
- Amount of space required and where. Provided that relief of crowding only is indicated, the following is a general guide: 1–2 mm per quadrant, first pre-molar extractions should be avoided and a specialist opinion sought; 3–5 mm per quadrant, often indicates premolar extractions; more than 5 mm per quadrant, extractions and space maintenance, or even the extraction of more than one tooth per quadrant, may be necessary.
- The incisor relationship (see Chapters 8–11).
- Anchorage requirements and desired buccal segment relationship at the end of treatment.
- Appliances to be used.
- Patient's profile.

If extractions are required in both arches, forward movement of the buccal segments to close space spontaneously will be facilitated if the same tooth is removed in both the maxilla and the mandible. This is less important if fixed appliances are to be used, and indeed extracting further forward in the upper arch in Class II and in the lower arch of Class III malocclusions may aid in the correction of skeletal discrepancies.

The position of the tooth being extracted within the arch will affect the anchorage balance between the teeth anterior and posterior to the extraction site. This means that extraction of first premolars will give greater space for alignment and/or retraction of the incisors than extraction of second pre-molars, which in turn provides more space than extraction of first molars, and so on.

Incisors

Extraction of a lower incisor tends to result in lingual tilting of the remaining lower labial segment teeth and a reduction in intercanine width, which will produce an increase in overbite and often an increase in crowding, particularly in a growing child. Occasionally, if the lower canines are distally inclined and the lower labial segment crowded in a child who refuses fixed appliance treatment, an acceptable compromise can be reached by extraction of one or two lower incisors. If a lower incisor is excluded from the arch, its extraction may result in satisfactory alignment, but often a sectional lower fixed appliance is indicated to achieve good root paralleling.

In the adult, removal of a lower incisor may be helpful if the incisor and buccal segment relationship is Class I and the lower labial segment is crowded. However, a sectional fixed appliance is usually necessary to achieve satisfactory alignment and to close space by bodily movement (Fig. 7.7), although it is wise to defer this approach until after the third permanent molars have erupted or been removed.

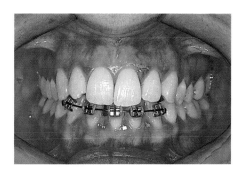

Fig. 7.7. Sectional fixed appliance to align lower labial segment.

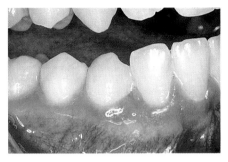

(a)

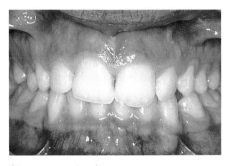

(b)

Fig. 7.8. (a) Result following removal of displaced lower canine; (b) patient who had both upper palatally displaced canines extracted.

Fig. 7.9. (a)–(c) Class I malocclusion with moderate upper and lower crowding, treated by extraction of all four first premolars; (d)–(f) occlusion a year after extractions.

Upper incisors are rarely the teeth of choice for extraction, but where trauma or morphology have reduced their prognosis, or an incisor is grossly displaced, there may be no alternative. Management of missing/enforced extraction of upper incisors is discussed in greater detail in Chapter 8, Section 8.3.2.

Canines

Because of their position as the cornerstone of the arch, canines are usually only considered for extraction if they are severely displaced and/or crowded out of the arch. Occasionally, in cases with severe crowding, the first premolar erupts into contact with the lateral incisor. This can be aesthetically acceptable (Fig. 7.8), which is a great bonus, particularly in the upper arch, as the canine is broader than the first premolar and extraction of the latter alone would not provide sufficient space for alignment of the former. However, the occlusion should be checked to ensure that no displacing contacts are present on lateral excursions. Otherwise, fixed appliance therapy is usually required following removal of a canine to achieve a satisfactory contact between the lateral incisor and the first premolar. Canines are discussed further in Chapter 14.

First premolars

First premolars are the teeth of choice for relief of moderate to severe crowding in either arch. By virtue of their position within the arch, extraction of the first premolars provides space for alignment and retraction of the labial segments, as well as relief of buccal segment crowding. Extraction of a first premolar in either arch usually gives the best chance of spontaneous occurrence of acceptable alignment (Fig. 7.9). Also, if space closure is complete, a good contact between the canine and first premolar can often be achieved. This is of particular value in the lower arch where, provided that the canine is mesially inclined, spontaneous alignment of the lower labial segment may occur. This is most rapid within the

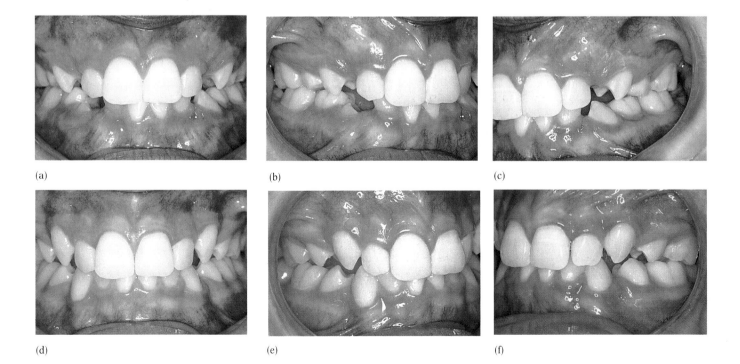

(a)

(b)

(c)

(d)

(e)

(f)

initial 6 months following extraction. If the canines are distally inclined, they will not upright spontaneously into the extraction space and fixed appliances will be required for their retraction.

In the upper arch the first premolars usually erupt prior to the maxillary canine and maximum spontaneous improvement in the position of this tooth can be achieved if the first premolar is extracted just before its emergence. However, if space is at a premium, a space maintainer should be fitted first.

If the crowding is mild, extraction of first premolars may result in residual spacing. If fixed appliances are then used to close the remaining space, there is a danger of over-retracting the labial segments, which may have deleterious effects upon the profile. In cases with mild crowding, consideration should be given to extracting teeth further distal in the arch (Fig. 7.10).

Second premolars

The indications for extraction of second premolars include the following:

- congenital absence of the second premolars and crowding of the arch;
- hypoplasia of the second premolars and crowding of the arch;
- severe displacement of the second premolar;
- mild to moderate crowding (2–4 mm per quadrant);
- where space closure by forward movement of the molars rather than retraction of the labial segments is indicated.

Extraction of the second premolars is preferable to extraction of the first premolars in cases with mild to moderate crowding as their extraction alters the anchorage balance, favouring space closure by forward movement of the molars. In order to facilitate this and to ensure a satisfactory contact between the first premolar and the first molar, fixed appliances are required, particularly in the lower arch.

Early loss of the second deciduous molars can result in crowding of the second premolars palatally in the upper arch and lingually in the lower arch (Fig. 7.11). In the upper arch extraction of the displaced second premolars on eruption is often indicated. Conversely, in the lower arch extraction of the first premolars is usually easier and in most cases uprighting of the second premolars occurs spontaneously following relief of crowding.

First permanent molars

First permanent molars are never an orthodontist's first choice. However, their extraction may be indicated if their prognosis is compromised to such an extent that they are unlikely to last for a reasonable time. Extraction of the first permanent molars is discussed in greater detail in Chapter 3.

Second permanent molars

Extraction of second permanent molars has become more popular in recent years. Concern raised by some practitioners about the 'deleterious' effect upon the profile of premolar extractions (see Section 7.8) has led to a fashionable revival of 'non-extraction' treatment. This term is confusing because in many such cases second permanent molars are extracted as part of the treatment.

Indications for extraction of second permanent molars include the following:

- facilitation of distal movement of the upper buccal segments;
- relief of mild lower premolar crowding;

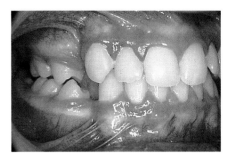

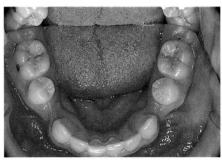

Fig. 7.10. Residual spacing in a patient with mild crowding who had all four first premolars removed.

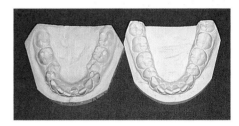

Fig. 7.11. The model on the left (patient HW) shows lingual crowding of the lower second premolars. The model on the right illustrates the improvement that occurred in the position of the lower second premolars following extraction of the first premolars (see also Fig. 7.2).

Fig. 7.12. Patient with mild lower arch crowding who had both lower second molars removed in an attempt to prevent a further increase in crowding: (a) DPT radiograph prior to extraction of both lower second molars (the upper second molars were not extracted because of concerns over the prognosis for the upper first molars); (b) DPT radiograph two years after the extractions showing eruption of both lower third molars.

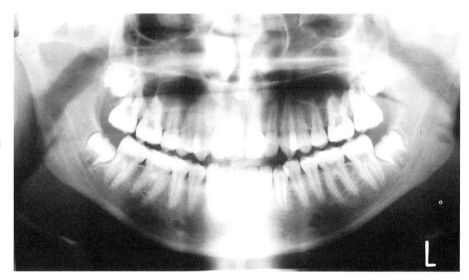

(a)

(b)

- provision of additional space for the third permanent molars and thus reduction of the likelihood of their impaction;
- prevention of lower labial segment crowding.

Because of the greater tendency for mesial drift in the upper arch, extraction of second permanent molars will not provide space for the relief of premolar or labial segment crowding without using appliances. Timing of the extraction of second molars in the upper arch is less critical than in the lower arch, and generally the upper third molar will erupt into a good position. In the lower arch removal of a second permanent molar will yield, on average, around 1–2 mm of space in the premolar region and will provide additional space for eruption of third permanent molar. However, space alone will not ensure that the (unpredictable) lower third permanent molar will erupt into a satisfactory position. The likelihood that the lower third permanent molar will erupt into occlusion is increased if the following factors (as seen on an orthopantomographic (DPT), or lateral oblique radiograph) are satisfied (Fig. 7.12):

- the angle between the third permanent molar tooth germ and the long axis of the second molar is between 10° and 30°;

- the crypt of the developing third molar overlaps the root of the second molar;
- the third permanent molar is developed to the bifurcation.

Even if these criteria are satisfied, eruption of the lower third molar into occlusion cannot be guaranteed, and it should be made clear to the patient that a course of fixed appliance treatment to upright or align the third molar may be necessary.

Third permanent molars

Early extraction of these teeth has been advocated in the past to prevent lower labial segment crowding. However, most oral surgeons are now unwilling to remove symptomless wisdom teeth. Research into the role of the third permanent molar in lower labial segment crowding has not demonstrated a clear-cut case of cause and effect. Studies have shown that patients with absent third molars are less likely to exhibit crowding, but are also likely to have smaller teeth than average. This topic is discussed in more detail in Chapter 8.

7.7.2. Expansion

Space can be created by expanding an arch laterally, but this is only an option in malocclusions where a unilateral crossbite exists; otherwise the expansion is likely to be unstable. Expansion of a narrow upper arch to correct a unilateral crossbite with displacement is straightforward. If the upper arch is crowded, it is prudent to complete the expansion first before assessing whether extractions are also indicated. Expansion of the lower arch may be indicated if a lingual crossbite of the lower premolars and/or molars exists, but management of this type of malocclusion is the province of the specialist. Crossbites are discussed in more detail in Chapter 13.

7.7.3. Distal movement of molars

Distal movement of the first permanent molar in the lower arch is attempted very rarely, but can be considered if extraction of the lower second permanent molar is planned owing to displacement or space considerations. This can be achieved with a removable screw appliance, or a lip bumper; however, fixed appliances are more commonly used.

Distal movement of the molars in the upper arch may be indicated in the following situations:

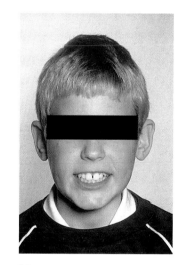

(a)

Fig. 7.13. Because of the presence of an upper midline diastema it was decided to gain space to align the upper arch by distal movement of the upper buccal segments: (a), (b) pretreatment; (c) upper fixed appliance *in situ*. In these cases it is wise to take the molar further distally than required; (d) post-treatment.

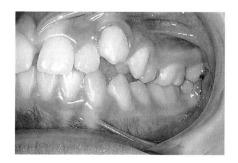

(b)

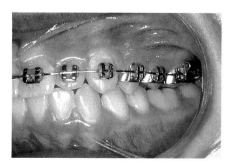

(c)

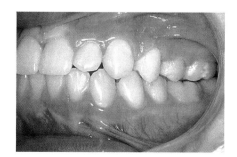

(d)

- Class I with mild upper arch crowding, or mild Class II division 1 with a well-aligned lower arch and molar relationship less than half a unit Class II (Fig. 7.13).
- Where extraction of both upper first premolars does not give sufficient space to complete alignment and/or overjet reduction in the upper arch (Fig. 7.14).
- Where early unilateral loss of a deciduous molar has resulted in mesial drift of the first permanent molar.
- Where the upper arch is crowded but a median diastema is present (Fig. 7.13). Extraction of premolars in this situation may result in a worsening of the diastema.
- Where the prognosis for stability of overjet reduction is doubtful, it may be wiser to create space for retraction of the upper labial segment by DMUBS rather than extractions.

Distal movement of the upper buccal segment teeth usually involves headgear as the motive force. A screw appliance can be used for unilateral movement, but, except in Class III cases, care is required to ensure that anchorage is not lost and it is wise to include extra-oral anchorage in the appliance design.

7.7.4. Enamel stripping

Removal of a small amount of enamel from the mesial and distal surfaces of the lower incisor teeth is known as enamel stripping or reproximation. It is really a 'last ditch' method and should only be considered in adults where the lower labial segment is mildly crowded. No more than 1–2 mm of space in total should be gained in this way, and the teeth should be treated topically with fluoride following reduction of the enamel.

7.8. STABILITY VERSUS PROFILE

Wide smiles, with a tendency towards bimaxillary proclination, are fashionable in the USA, where there is a trend for alignment to be achieved by expansion and/or proclination. The drawback to this approach is that movement of the teeth outside their zone of labiolingual balance increases the likelihood of relapse.

It has been suggested by some orthodontists that extractions have a deleterious effect upon the profile. This view is more prevalent in the USA, and as a result, an enormous amount of research to investigate these claims has been carried out. This work suggests that the effect of extractions upon the profile is minimal. For example, in one study (see section on further reading) it was found that the lips of patients who had undergone premolar extractions followed by fixed appliance treatment were retracted only 1–2 mm further on average than those of patients managed by removal of second molars and fixed appliances. Individual variation in soft tissue thickness and growth pattern was noted to be of greater significance.

7.9. PRESENTATION OF THE TREATMENT PLAN TO THE PATIENT

The last step of treatment planning is to present the proposed treatment to the patient and, if appropriate, their parent or guardian. Often there is more than one possible option and each should be presented to the patient with an explanation of the relative merits. It is helpful if this explanation can be accompanied by colour pictures of the appliances to be used.

The nature of the patient's role in orthodontic treatment should be explained carefully at this stage, particularly the increased likelihood of decalcification and

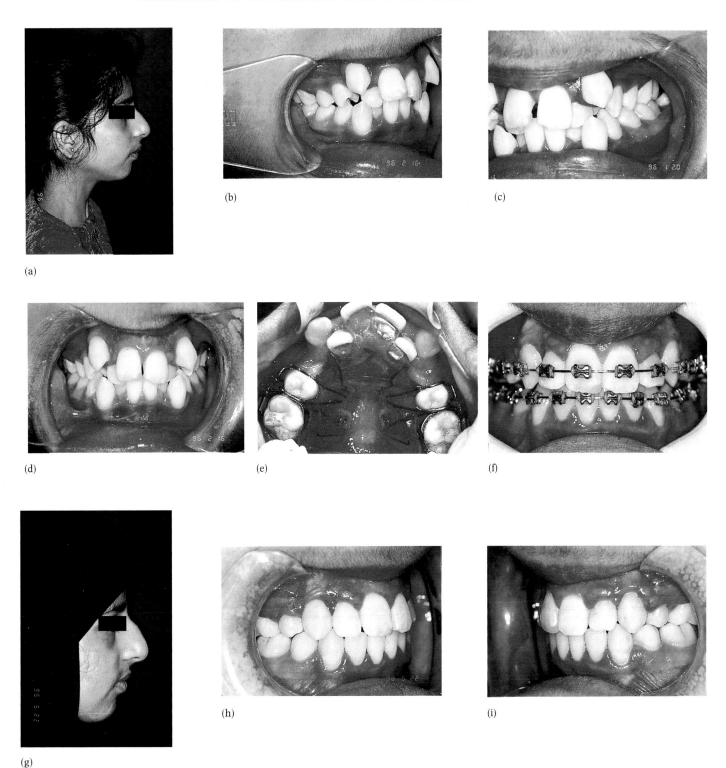

Fig. 7.14. Patient NM aged 13 years. Class II skeletal pattern (ANB=7°). Upper and lower arch crowding. Buccal segment relationship a full unit Class II left and right. Therefore, this was a maximum anchorage case: (a)–(d) pretreatment. Because the extraction of one premolar in each quadrant would not give enough space to relieve the crowding and reduce the overjet, distal movement of the buccal segments with headgear was indicated. A nudger appliance (see section 16.4.6) was used to aid distal movement (e). Once the upper molars had been moved into a Class I relationship with the lower arch fixed appliances were used to complete alignment and reduction of the overbite and overjet (f); (g)–(i) post-treatment. (NB: The patient still had a Class II skeletal pattern at the end of treatment — dental camouflage was used to compensate for this.)

periodontal damage if toothbrushing and dietary advice is not followed. If the treatment involves headgear or elastic traction, this should also be discussed. It is wise to overestimate treatment times, even taking into account appliance breakages, holidays, etc. If treatment is completed more quickly the patient will be impressed with your skill. However, in the unlikely event that unforeseen circumstances prolong treatment there will be time to recover.

As in all branches of medicine and dentistry, orthodontic treatment has potential risks. These should be explained to the patient so that their informed consent to the treatment is obtained. However, it is important not to be alarmist and any risks should be put in context. This topic is discussed in greater detail in Chapter 1.

It may be helpful if some written material is provided to back up the information that is given at the consultation, and the patient is allowed some time to reflect upon the proposed treatment at home before reaching a decision on whether or not to go ahead.

PRINCIPAL SOURCES AND FURTHER READING

Bishara, S. E. and Burkey, P. S. (1986). Second molar extractions: a review. *American Journal of Orthodontics*, **89**, 415–24.
- An informative review.
British Orthodontic Society (1996). *Young practitioner's guide to Orthodontics*. BOS Office, 291 Grays Inn Road, London.
- This is a well-illustrated simple introduction to orthodontics.
Dacre, J. T. (1985). The long-term effects of one lower incisor extraction. *European Journal of Orthodontics*, **7**, 136–44.
Dacre J. T. (1987). The criteria for lower second molar extraction. *British Journal of Orthodontics*, **14**, 1–9.
Drysdale, C. *et al.* (1996). Orthodontic management of root-filled teeth. *British Journal of Orthodontics*, **23**, 255–60.
Lee, R. T. (1999). Arch width and form: A review. *American Journal of Orthodontics and Dentofacial Orthopedics*, **115**, 305–13.
Morse, P. H. and Webb, W. G. (1973). The indication for distal movement of upper buccal segments. *British Journal of Orthodontics*, **1**, 18–26.
NHS Centre for Reviews and Dissemination, York (1998). Prophylactic removal of impacted third molars: is it justified? *British Journal of Orthodontics*, **26**, 149–51.
- Recommended reading for all dentists and orthodontists.
Richardson, M. E. and Richardson, A. (1993). Lower third molar development subsequent to second molar extraction. *American Journal of Orthodontics and Dentofacial Orthopedics*, **104**, 566–74.
- This article suggests that the criteria for second molar extraction do not need to be as strict as previously thought. However, the author advises the inexperienced orthodontist to limit extraction of lower second molars to those cases satisfying the criteria outlined in Section 7.7.1.
Staggers J. A. (1990) A comparison of second molar and first premolar extraction treatment. *American Journal of Orthodontics and Dentofacial Orthopedics*, **98**, 430–6.
- The author reports that the facial profile resulting after extraction of second molars was not statistically different from that resulting after extraction of first premolars, despite further retraction of the incisors in the latter group. Well worth reading.
Swessi, D. M. and Stephens, C. D. (1993). The spontaneous effect of lower first premolar extraction on the mesio-distal angulation of adjacent teeth and the relationship of this to extraction space closure in the long-term. *European Journal of Orthodontics*, **15**, 503–11.
- The title is fairly self-explanatory regarding the aims of this study. The authors found that excessive tipping of the canine and second premolar was the exception rather than the rule when lower first premolars were extracted and no appliances used.
Tulloch, J. F. C. (1978). Treatment following loss of second premolars. *British Journal of Orthodontics*, **5**, 29–34.

Young, T. M. and Smith, R. J. (1993) Effects of orthodontics on the facial profile: a comparison of changes during non-extraction and premolar extraction treatment. *American Journal of Orthodontics and Dentofacial Orthopedics*, **103**, 452–8.
- '... the results provide additional evidence that it is simplistic and incorrect to blame undesirable facial aesthetics after orthodontic treatment on the extraction of premolars'.

8 Class I

A Class I incisor relationship is defined by the British Standards incisor classification as follows: 'the lower incisor edges occlude with or lie immediately below the cingulum plateau of the upper central incisors'. Therefore Class I malocclusions include those where the anteroposterior occlusal relationship is normal and there is a discrepancy either within the arches and/or in the transverse or vertical relationship between the arches.

8.1. AETIOLOGY

8.1.1. Skeletal

In Class I malocclusions the skeletal pattern is usually Class I, but it can also be Class II or Class III with the inclination of the incisors compensating for the underlying skeletal discrepancy (Fig. 8.1), i.e. dento-alveolar compensation. Marked transverse skeletal discrepancies between the arches are more commonly associated with Class II or Class III occlusions, but milder transverse discrepancies are often seen in Class I cases. Increased vertical skeletal proportions and anterior open bite can also occur where the anteroposterior incisor relationship is Class I.

8.1.2. Soft tissues

In most Class I cases the soft tissue environment is favourable (for example resulting in dento-alveolar compensation) and is not an aetiological factor. The major exception to this is bimaxillary proclination, where the upper and lower incisors are proclined. This may be racial in origin and can also occur because lack of lip tonicity results in the incisors being moulded forwards under tongue pressure.

Fig. 8.1. (a) Class I incisor relationship on Class I skeletal pattern; (b) Class I incisor relationship on a Class II skeletal pattern; (c) Class I incisor relationship on a Class III skeletal pattern.

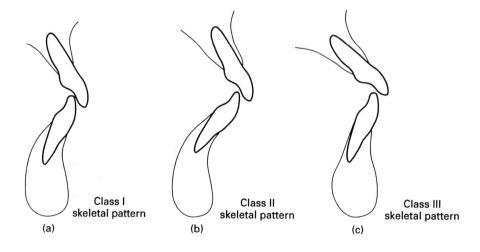

8.1.3. Dental factors

Dental factors are the main aetiological agent in Class I malocclusions. The most common are tooth/arch size discrepancies, leading to crowding or, less frequently, spacing.

The size of the teeth is genetically determined and so, to a great extent, is the size of the jaws. Environmental factors can also contribute to crowding or spacing. For example, premature loss of a deciduous tooth can lead to a localization of any pre-existing crowding.

Local factors also include displaced or impacted teeth, and anomalies in the size, number, and form of the teeth, all of which can lead to a localized malocclusion. However, it is important to remember that these factors can also be found in association with Class II or Class III malocclusions.

8.2. CROWDING

Crowding occurs where there is a discrepancy between the size of the teeth and the size of the arches. Approximately 60 per cent of Caucasian children exhibit crowding to some degree. In a crowded arch loss of a permanent or deciduous tooth will result in the remaining teeth tilting or drifting into the space created. This tendency is greatest when the adjacent teeth are erupting.

Crowding can either be accepted or relieved. Before deciding between these alternatives the following should be considered:

- the position, presence, and prognosis of remaining permanent teeth;
- the degree of crowding which is usually calculated in millimetres per arch or quadrant;
- the patient's malocclusion and any orthodontic treatment planned, including anchorage requirements;
- the patient's age and the likelihood of the crowding increasing or reducing with growth;
- the patient's profile.

These aspects of treatment planning are considered in more detail in Chapter 7, Sections 7.6 and 7.7.

In a Class I case with mild crowding (1–2 mm per quadrant) acceptance, or perhaps extraction of second molars, should be considered unless a significant increase in crowding is anticipated. In cases with moderate crowding (3–5 mm per quadrant) extraction of premolars is usually indicated. Where the crowding is severe (more than 5 mm per quadrant) space maintenance is definitely indicated prior to the extraction of, probably, the first premolars. Occasionally the extraction of two teeth per quadrant is indicated, but this severity of crowding is the province of the specialist.

After relief of crowding a degree of natural spontaneous movement will take place. In general, this is greater under the following conditions:

- in a growing child;
- if the extractions are carried out just prior to eruption of the adjacent teeth;
- where the adjacent teeth are favourably positioned to upright if space is made available (for example considerable improvement will often occur in a crowded lower labial segment provided that the mandibular canines are mesially inclined);
- there are no occlusal interferences with the anticipated tooth movement.

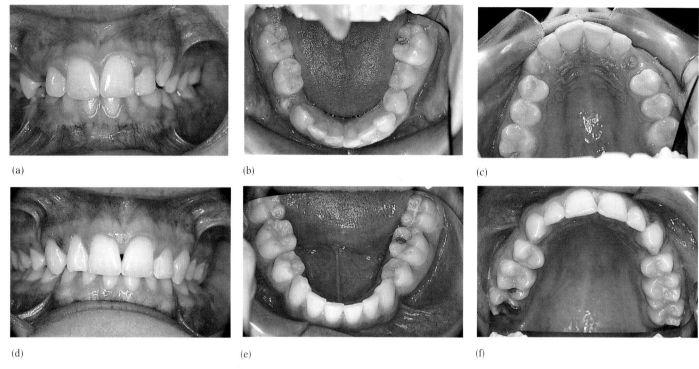

(a)   (b)   (c)

(d)   (e)   (f)

Fig. 8.2. Class I malocclusion treated by extraction of all four first premolars and no appliances: (a)–(c) prior to extractions; (d)–(f) 3 years after extractions.

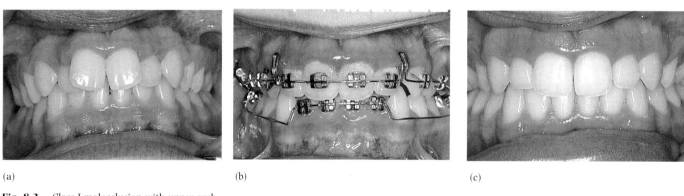

(a)   (b)   (c)

Fig. 8.3. Class I malocclusion with upper arch crowding, treated by extraction of upper first premolars and use of fixed appliances: (a) pretreatment; (b) during treatment; (c) 1 year after the end of retention.

Most spontaneous improvement occurs in the first 6 months after the extractions. If alignment is not complete after 1 year, then further improvement will require active tooth movement with appliances. Figure 8.2 shows a case which was treated by extraction of all four first premolars without appliances, and Fig. 8.3 shows a patient whose management required the extraction of upper first premolars and the use of fixed appliances.

8.2.1. Late lower incisor crowding

In most individuals intercanine width increases up to around 12 to 13 years of age, and this is followed by a very gradual diminution throughout adult life. The rate of decrease is most noticeable during the mid to late teens. This reduction in intercanine width results in an increase of any pre-existing lower labial crowding, or the emergence of crowding in arches which were well aligned or even spaced in the early teens. Therefore, to some extent, lower incisor crowding can be considered as an age change. Certainly, patients who have undergone orthodontic treatment (including extractions) are not immune from lower labial segment crowding unless steps are taken to retain alignment subsequently; for example with a bonded lingual retainer.

The aetiology of late lower incisor crowding is not fully understood, and considerable controversy still exists as to the role of the third permanent molar. Most authors acknowledge that the aetiology is multifactorial. Nevertheless the following have all been proposed as major influences in the development of this phenomenon:

● Forward growth of the mandible (either horizontally or manifesting as a growth rotation) when maxillary growth has ceased, together with soft tissue pressures, which result in a reduction in lower arch perimeter and labial segment crowding.

● Mesial migration of the posterior teeth owing to forces from the interseptal fibres and/or from the anterior component of the forces of occlusion.

● The presence of an erupting third molar pushes the dentition anteriorly, i.e. the third molar plays an active role.

● The presence of a third molar prevents pressure developed anteriorly (due to either mandibular growth or soft tissue pressures) from being dissipated distally around the arch, i.e. the third molar plays a passive role.

Reviews of the many studies that have been carried out indicate that the third permanent molar has a statistically weak association with late lower incisor crowding.

Removal of symtomless lower third molars has been advocated in the past in order to prevent lower labial segment crowding. A recent prospective study found that there was a (non-significant) reduction in the presence of crowding in patients who had had the lower wisdom teeth extracted, but concluded that removing the lower third molar to reduce the degree of lower labial segment crowding could not be justified. Management of lower labial segment crowding should be considered together with other aspects of the malocclusion (see Chapter 7), bearing in mind the propensity of this problem to worsen with age. However, lower labial segment crowding is occasionally seen in arches, which are otherwise well aligned with a good Class I buccal segment interdigitation and a slightly increased overbite (Fig. 8.4). These cases are best kept under observation until the late teens when the fate of the third permanent molars, if present, has been determined. At that stage mild lower labial segment crowding can be accepted. If the crowding is more marked and upper extractions are contraindicated, it may be better to consider extraction of the most displaced lower incisor and use of a sectional fixed appliance to align and upright the remaining lower labial segment teeth (Fig. 8.5). However, patients should be warned that this may result in the labial segments dropping lingually, to the detriment of alignment in the upper arch.

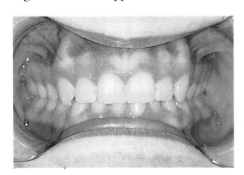
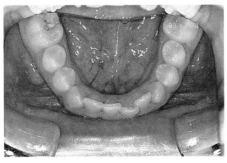

Fig. 8.4. Class I occlusion with acceptable mild lower labial segment crowding.

Fig. 8.5. Adult with severe lower labial segment crowding despite the previous loss of a lower incisor. Management involved the extraction of the most displaced incisor and a lower sectional fixed appliance: (a), (b) pretreatment; (c), (d) post-treatment.

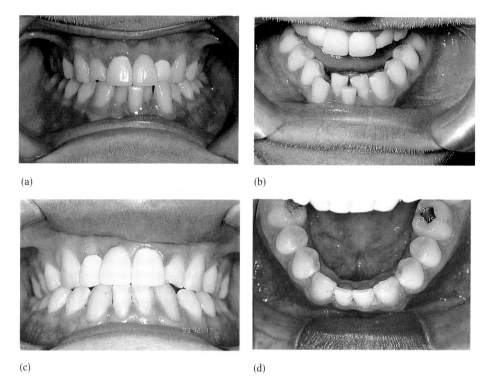

(a)

(b)

(c)

(d)

8.3. SPACING

Generalized spacing is rare and is due to either hypodontia or small teeth in well-developed arches. Interestingly, an association between small teeth and hypodontia has been demonstrated. Orthodontic management of generalized spacing is frequently difficult as there is usually a tendency for the spaces to reopen unless permanently retained. In milder cases it may be wiser to encourage the patient to accept the spacing, or if the teeth are narrower than average, acid-etch composite additions or porcelain veneers can be used to widen them and thus improve aesthetics. In severe cases of hypodontia a combined orthodontic–restorative approach to localize space for the provision of prostheses, or perhaps implants, may be required (Fig. 8.6).

Localized spacing may be due to hypodontia or loss of a tooth as a result of trauma, or because extraction was indicated because of displacement, morphology, or pathology. This problem is most noticeable if an upper incisor is missing as the symmetry of the smile is affected, a feature which is usually noticed more by the lay public than other aspects of a malocclusion.

Fig. 8.6. Patient with hypodontia (the upper right second premolar and all four lateral incisors were absent) treated with fixed appliances to localize space for prosthetic replacement of the lateral incisors: (a) pretreatment; (b) fixed appliance; (c) post-treatment, before replacement of the lateral incisors by dentures cum retainers.

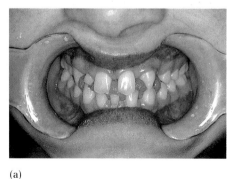

(a)

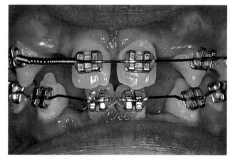

(b)

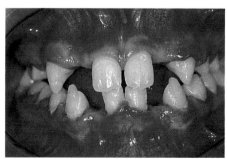

(c)

8.3.1. Median diastema

A median diastema is a space between the central incisors, which is more common in the upper arch (Fig. 8.7). A diastema is a normal physiological stage in the early mixed dentition when the fraenal attachment passes between the upper central incisors to attach to the incisive papilla. In normal development, as the lateral incisors and canines erupt this gap closes and the fraenal attachment migrates labially to the labial attached mucosa. If the upper arch is spaced or the lateral incisors are dimunitive or absent, there is less pressure forcing the upper central incisors together and the diastema will tend to persist. Rarely, the fraenal attachment appears to prevent the central incisors from moving together. In these cases, blanching of the incisive papilla can be observed if tension is applied to the fraenum, and on radiographic examination a V-shaped notch of the inter-dental bone can be seen between the incisors indicating the attachment of the fraenum (see Chapter 3, Fig. 3.26).

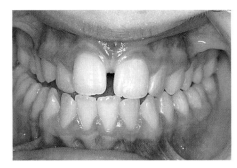

Fig. 8.7. Upper midline diastema.

Management (see also Chapter 3, Section 3.3.9)

It is important to take a periapical radiograph to exclude the presence of a super-numerary tooth which, if present, should be removed before closure of the diastema is undertaken. As median diastemas tend to reduce or close with the eruption of the canines, management can be subdivided as follows.

- Before eruption of the permanent canines intervention is only necessary if the diastema is greater than 3 mm and there is a lack of space for the lateral incisors to erupt. Care is required not to cause resorption of the incisor roots against the unerupted canines.
- After eruption of the permanent canines space closure is usually straightfor-ward. Either fixed or removable appliances are used as indicated by the angula-tion of the incisors. Prolonged retention is usually necessary as diastemas exhibit a great tendency to reopen, particularly if there is a familial tendency; the upper arch is spaced or the initial diastema was greater than 2 mm. In view of this it may be better to accept a minimal diastema, particularly if no other orthodontic treatment is required. Alternatively, if the central incisors are narrow a restora-tive solution, for example veneers, can be considered (Fig. 8.8).

If it is thought that the fraenum is an contributory factor, then fraenectomy is best carried out during space closure as scar tissue contraction will aid space closure.

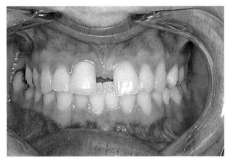

(a)

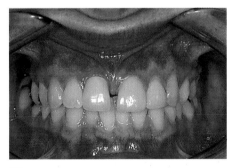

(b)

Fig. 8.8. Adult with narrow proclined upper central incisors with a midline diastema. An upper removable appliance was used to reduce the overbite, and then to retract and move 1/1 a little closer together: (a) pretreatment; (b) at the completion of active appliance therapy, following veneering of 21/1.

8.3.2. Management of missing upper incisors

Upper central incisors are rarely congenitally absent. They can be lost as a result of trauma, or occasionally their extraction may be indicated because of dilacera-tion. Upper lateral incisors are congenitally absent in approximately 2 per cent of a Caucasian population, but can also be lost following trauma. Both can occur unilaterally, bilaterally, or together. Whatever the reason for their absence, there are two treatment options:

- closure of the space
- opening of the space and placement of a denture or a bridge.

The choice for a particular patient will depend upon a number of factors, which are listed below. However, this is a difficult area of treatment planning and specialist advice should be sought.

- Skeletal relationship: if the skeletal pattern is Class III, space closure in the upper labial segment may compromise the incisor relationship; conversely,

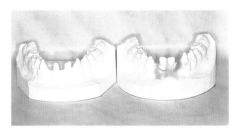

Fig. 8.9. Trial (Kesling's) set-up.

for a Class II division 1 pattern space closure may be preferable as it will aid overjet reduction.

- Presence of crowding or spacing.
- Colour and form of adjacent teeth: if the permanent canines are much darker than the incisors and/or particularly caniniform in shape, modification to make them resemble lateral incisors will be difficult; also, if a lateral incisor is to be brought forward to replace a missing single upper central incisor, an aesthetically pleasing result will only be possible if the lateral is fairly large and has a good gingival circumference.
- The inclination of adjacent teeth, as this will influence whether it is easier to open or close the space.
- The desired buccal segment occlusion at the end of treatment; for example if the lower arch is well aligned and the buccal segment relationship is Class I, space opening is preferable.
- The patient's wishes and ability to cooperate with complex treatment: some patients have definite ideas about whether they are willing to proceed with appliance treatment, and whether they wish to have the space closed or opened for a prosthetic replacement.

Trial (Kesling's) set-up

To investigate the feasibility of different options a trial set-up can be carried out using duplicate models. The teeth to be moved are cut off the model and repositioned in the desired place using wax (Fig. 8.9). This allows any number of options to be tested and also gives an opportunity to evaluate in more detail the amount and nature of any orthodontic and restorative treatment required by a particular option. This exercise is often helpful in describing the outcome of different options to the patient.

After assessment of the above factors a provisional plan can be discussed with the patient. It is often possible to draw up more than one plan and these should all be thoroughly discussed, including the advantages and disadvantages, and the long-term maintenance of any prosthetic replacements.

Space closure

This can be facilitated by early extraction of any deciduous teeth to allow forward movement of the first permanent molars in that quadrant(s). In crowded mouths, if this step is carried out early it may be possible to achieve a satisfactory result without appliances, but usually fixed appliances are necessary to correct the axial inclinations. If any masking procedures (for example contouring a canine incisally, palatally, and interproximally to resemble a lateral incisor) or acid-etch composite additions are required, these should be carried out prior to the placement of appliances to facilitate final tooth alignment. Placement of a bonded retainer post-treatment is advisable in the majority of cases (Fig. 8.10).

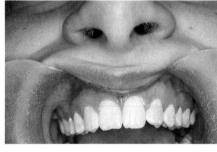

(a)

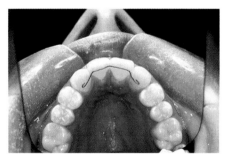

(b)

Fig. 8.10. (a) Patient with missing lateral incisors treated by space closure and modification of the upper canines. (b) Occlusal view of same patient to show bonded retainer.

Space maintenance or opening

If an incisor is extracted electively or a patient seen soon after loss has occurred, ideally a space maintenance should be fitted forthwith. In cases where space closure has occurred as a result either of early tooth loss or congenital absence, appliances will be required to open the space. The angulation of the adjacent teeth will determine whether fixed or removable appliances are required

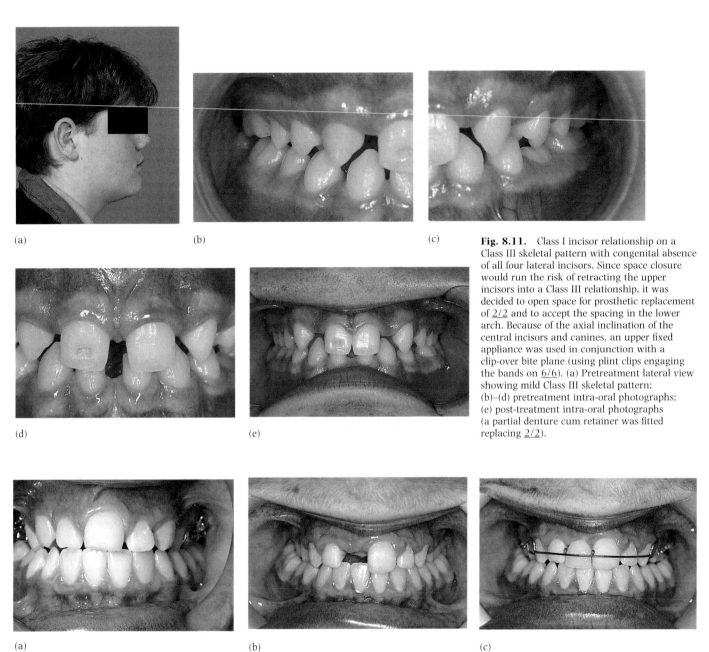

(a)   (b)   (c)

Fig. 8.11. Class I incisor relationship on a Class III skeletal pattern with congenital absence of all four lateral incisors. Since space closure would run the risk of retracting the upper incisors into a Class III relationship, it was decided to open space for prosthetic replacement of 2/2 and to accept the spacing in the lower arch. Because of the axial inclination of the central incisors and canines, an upper fixed appliance was used in conjunction with a clip-over bite plane (using plint clips engaging the bands on 6/6). (a) Pretreatment lateral view showing mild Class III skeletal pattern; (b)–(d) pretreatment intra-oral photographs; (e) post-treatment intra-oral photographs (a partial denture cum retainer was fitted replacing 2/2).

(d)   (e)

(a)   (b)   (c)

Fig. 8.12. (a) Patient with early traumatic loss of 1/ and partial space closure. Space for prosthetic replacement of 1/ was gained using a fixed appliance. (b) Result on completion of active treatment. (c) Partial denture cum retainer (NB: Stops were placed mesial to both 2/ and /1 to help prevent relapse).

(Fig. 8.11). Whenever space is opened prior to bridgework, it is important to retain with a partial denture for at least 3 to 6 months (Fig. 8.12), particularly if an adhesive acid-etch retained bridge is to be used. Research has shown that acid-etch bridges placed immediately after the completion of tooth movement have a greater incidence of failure than those placed following a period of retention with a removable retainer.

Implant technology is improving rapidly and it is hoped that it will become cheaper in the future, allowing this option to be more readily available.

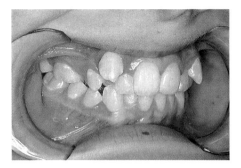

Fig. 8.13. Class I malocclusion with mild lower and marked upper arch crowding. In crowded arches the last teeth in a segment to erupt, in this case the upper canines, are the most likely to be short of space. The maxillary second premolars are also crowded, probably owing to early loss of the upper second deciduous molars.

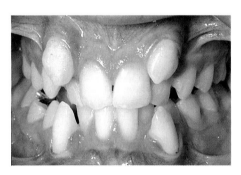

(a)

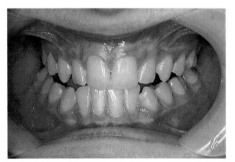

(b)

Fig. 8.14. Occasionally it may be prudent to extract the most displaced tooth. In this case all four canines were extracted: (a) prior to extractions; (b) after extractions. (NB: Patient is posturing forwards to show lower arch alignment.)

8.4. DISPLACED TEETH

Teeth can be displaced for a variety of reasons including the following:

- Abnormal position of the tooth germ: canines (Chapter 14) and second premolars are the most commonly affected teeth. Management depends upon the degree of displacement. If this is mild, extraction of the associated primary tooth plus space maintenance, if indicated, may result in an improvement in position in some cases. Alternatively, exposure and the application of orthodontic traction may be used to bring the mildly displaced tooth into the arch. If the displacement is severe, extraction is usually necessary.

- Crowding: lack of space for a permanent tooth to erupt within the arch can lead to or contribute to displacement. Those teeth that erupt last in a segment, for example upper lateral incisors, upper canines (Fig. 8.13), second premolars, and third molars, are most commonly affected. Management involves relief of crowding, followed by active tooth movement where necessary. However, if the displacement is severe it may be prudent to extract the displaced tooth (Fig. 8.14).

- Retention of a deciduous predecessor: extraction of the retained primary tooth should be carried out as soon as possible provided that the permanent successor is not displaced.

- Secondary to the presence of a supernumerary tooth or teeth (see Chapter 3): management involves extraction of the supernumerary followed by tooth alignment, usually with fixed appliances. Displacements due to supernumeraries have a tendency to relapse and prolonged retention is required.

- Caused by a habit (see Chapter 9).

- Secondary to pathology, for example a dentigerous cyst. This is the rarest cause.

8.5. VERTICAL DISCREPANCIES

Variations in the vertical dimension can occur in association with any anteroposterior skeletal relationship. Increased vertical skeletal proportions are discussed in Chapter 9 in relation to Class II division 1; in Chapter 11 in relation to Class III, and in Chapter 12 on anterior open bite.

8.6. TRANSVERSE DISCREPANCIES

A transverse discrepancy between the arches results in a crossbite and can occur in association with Class I, Class II, and Class III malocclusions. Classification and management of crossbite is discussed in Chapter 13.

8.7. BIMAXILLARY PROCLINATION

As the name suggests, bimaxillary proclination is the term used to describe occlusions where both the upper and lower incisors are proclined. Bimaxillary proclination is seen more commonly in some racial groups (for example Afro-Caribbean)), and so when an assessment is carried out the patient should be assessed bearing in mind what is normal for their ethnic background. This is particularly pertinent in cephalometric analysis.

When bimaxillary proclination occurs in a Class I malocclusion the overjet is increased because of the angulation of the incisors (Fig. 8.15). Management is difficult because both upper and lower incisors need to be retroclined to reduce the overjet. Retroclination of the lower labial segment will encroach on tongue space and therefore has a high likelihood of relapse following removal of appliances. For these reasons, treatment of bimaxillary proclination should be approached with caution and consideration should be given to accepting the incisor relationship. If the lips are incompetent, but have a good muscle tone and are likely to achieve a lip-to-lip seal if the incisors are retracted, the chances of a stable result are increased. However, the patient should still be warned that the prognosis for stability is guarded. Where bimaxillary proclination is associated with competent lips, or with grossly incompetent lips which are unlikely to retain the corrected incisor position, it may be wiser not to proceed. However, if, treatment is decided upon, permanent retention is advisable.

Bimaxillary proclination can also occur in association with Class II division 1 and Class III malocclusions.

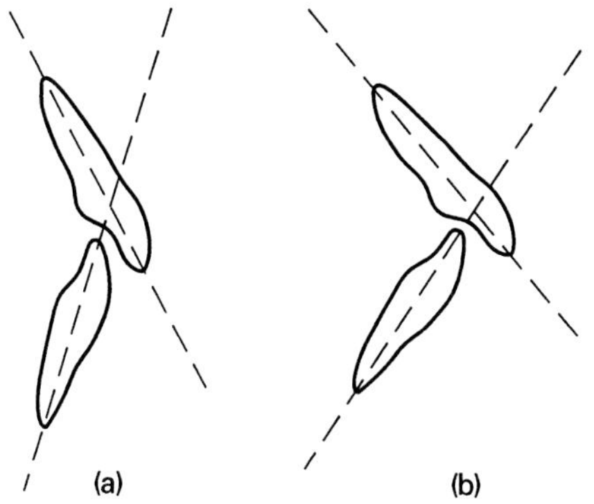

Fig. 8.15. (a) Class I incisor relationship with normal axial inclination (inter-incisal angle is 137°); (b) Class I incisor relationship with bimaxillary inclination showing increased overjet (inter-incisal angle is 107°).

PRINCIPAL SOURCES AND FURTHER READING

Bishara, S. E. (1999). Third molars: a dilemma: Or is it? *American Journal of Orthodontics and Dentofacial Orthopedics*, **115**, 628–33.

Harradine, N. W. T., Pearson, M. H., and Toth, B. (1998). The effect of extraction of third molars on late lower incisor crowding: A randomised controlled trial. *British Journal of Orthodontics*, **25**, 117–22.

● This excellent study is essential reading.

Little, R. M., Reidel, R. A., and Artun, J. (1981). An evaluation of changes in mandibular anterior alignment from 10–20 years postretention. *American Journal of Orthodontics and Dentofacial Orthopedics*, **93**, 423–8.

● Classic paper. The authors found that lower labial segment crowding tends to increase even following extractions and appliance therapy.

Richardson, M. E. (1989). The role of the third molar in the cause of late lower arch crowding: a review. *American Journal of Orthodontics and Dentofacial Orthopedics*, **95**, 79–83.

● The evidence in support of the theory that the presence of a third molar is one of the aetiological factors in late lower incisor crowding is reviewed in this paper.

Shashua, D. and Artun, J. (1999). Relapse after orthodontic correction of maxillary median diastema: a follow-up evaluation of consecutive cases. *The Angle Orthodontist*, **69**, 257–63.

Stephens, C. D. (1989). The use of natural spontaneous tooth movement in the treatment of malocclusion. *Dental Update*, **16**, 337–42.

● An interesting paper in which the role of interceptive extractions in Class I malocclusions is discussed.

Vasir, N. S., and Robinson, R. J. (1991). The mandibular third molar and late crowding of the mandibular incisors — a review. *British Journal of Orthodontics*, **18**, 59–66.

● An unbiased review of the literature regarding the role of third molars in late lower incisor crowding. The authors conclude that the wisdom tooth has a small, but variable, effect.

9   Class II division 1

The British Standards classification defines a Class II division 1 incisor relationship as follows: 'the lower incisor edges lie posterior to the cingulum plateau of the upper incisors, there is an increase in overjet and the upper central incisors are usually proclined'. In a Caucasian population the incidence of Class II division 1 incisor relationship is approximately 15–20 per cent.

Prominent upper incisors, particularly when the lips are incompetent, are at increased risk of being traumatized. It has been shown that children with an overjet greater than 9 mm are twice as likely to have suffered trauma involving their upper incisor teeth as are those with normal or reduced overjets.

9.1. AETIOLOGY

9.1.1. Skeletal pattern

A Class II division 1 incisor relationship is usually associated with a Class II skeletal pattern, commonly due to a retrognathic mandible (Fig. 9.1). However, proclination of the upper incisors and/or retroclination of the lower incisors by a habit or the soft tissues can result in an increased overjet on a Class I (Fig. 9.2), or even a Class III skeletal pattern.

Fig. 9.1. A Class II division 1 incisor relationship on a Class II skeletal pattern with a retrognathic mandible.

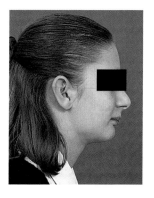
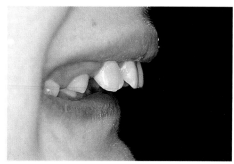

Fig. 9.2. A Class II division 1 incisor relationship on a Class I skeletal pattern.

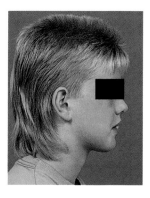
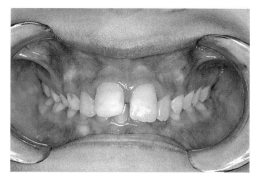

A Class II division 1 incisor relationship is found in association with a range of vertical skeletal patterns. Management of those patients with significantly increased or significantly reduced vertical proportions is usually difficult and is the province of the specialist.

9.1.2. Soft tissues

The influence of the soft tissues on a Class II division 1 malocclusion is mainly mediated by the skeletal pattern, both anteroposteriorly and vertically, and also by the patient's efforts to achieve an anterior oral seal.

In a Class II division 1 malocclusion the lips are typically incompetent owing to the prominence of the upper incisors and/or the underlying skeletal pattern. If the lips are incompetent, the patient will try to achieve an anterior oral seal in one of the following ways:

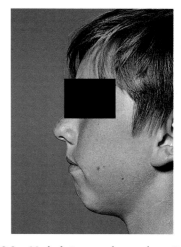

Fig. 9.3. Marked circumoral muscular activity is visible as this patient attempts to achieve an anterior oral seal by a lip-to-lip seal.

- circumoral muscular activity to achieve a lip-to-lip seal (Fig. 9.3);
- the mandible is postured forwards to allow the lips to meet at rest;
- the lower lip is drawn up behind the upper incisors (Fig. 9.4);
- the tongue is placed forwards between the incisors to contact the lower lip, often contributing to the development of an incomplete overbite;
- a combination of these.

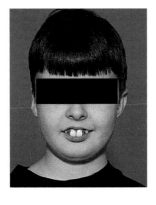
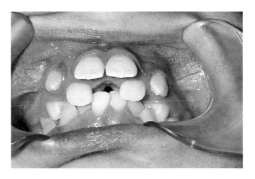

Fig. 9.4. In this patient with a Class II division 1 malocclusion the lower lip functions behind the upper central incisors, which have been proclined, and in front of the lateral incisors, which have been retroclined as a result.

Where the patient can achieve lip-to-lip contact by circumoral muscle activity or the mandible is postured forwards, the influence of the soft tissues is often to moderate the effect of the underlying skeletal pattern by dento-alveolar compensation. More commonly a seal is achieved by the lower lip being drawn up behind the upper incisors, which leads to retroclination of the lower labial segment and/or proclination of the upper incisors with the result that the incisor relationship is more severe than the underlying skeletal pattern.

However, if the tongue comes forward to contact the lower lip during swallowing, proclination of the lower incisors may occur, helping to compensate for the underlying skeletal pattern. This type of soft tissue behaviour is often associated with increased vertical skeletal proportions and/or grossly incompetent lips, or a habit which has resulted in an increase in overjet and an anterior open bite. In practice, it is often difficult to determine the degree to which this is adaptive tongue behaviour, or whether a rarer endogenous tongue thrust exists (see Chapter 12).

Infrequently, a Class II division 1 incisor relationship occurs owing to retroclination of the lower incisors by a very active lower lip (Fig. 9.5).

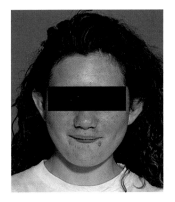

(a)

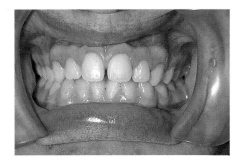

(b)

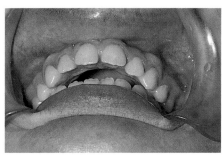

(c)

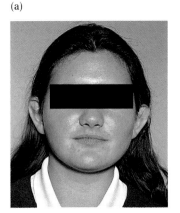

(d)

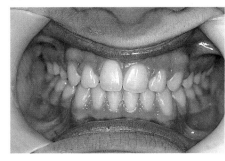

(e)

Fig. 9.5. A Class II division 1 malocclusion due mainly to retroclination of the lower labial segment by an active lower lip. This patient achieved an anterior oral seal by contact between the tongue and the lower lip. (a)–(c) pretreatment; (d), (e) post-treatment.

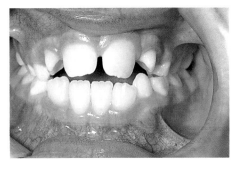

(a)

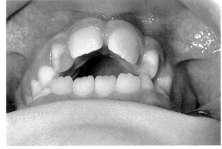

(b)

Fig. 9.6. The effects of a persistent digit sucking habit upon the occlusion: the upper incisors have been proclined and the lower incisors retroclined.

9.1.3. Dental factors

A Class II division 1 incisor relationship may occur in the presence of crowding or spacing. Where the arches are crowded, lack of space may result in the upper incisors being crowded out of the arch labially and thus to exacerbation of the overjet. Conversely, crowding of the lower labial segment may help to compensate for an increased overjet in the same manner. In such cases, extractions anterior to the second premolars in the lower arch may result in the lower labial segment dropping lingually with a concomitant worsening of the incisor relationship.

9.1.4. Habits

A persistent digit-sucking habit will act like an orthodontic force upon the teeth if indulged in for more than a few hours per day. The severity of the effects produced will depend upon the duration and the intensity, but the following are commonly associated with a determined habit (Fig. 9.6):

- proclination of the upper incisors;
- retroclination of the lower labial segment;
- an incomplete overbite or a localized anterior open bite;
- narrowing of the upper arch thought to be mediated by the tongue taking up a lower position in the mouth and the negative pressure generated during sucking of the digit.

The first two effects will contribute to an increase in overjet.

The effects of a habit will be superimposed upon the child's existing skeletal pattern and incisor relationship, and thus can lead to an increased overjet in a child with a Class I or Class III skeletal pattern, or can exacerbate a pre-existing Class II malocclusion. The effects may be asymmetric if a single finger or thumb is sucked (Fig. 9.7).

9.2. OCCLUSAL FEATURES

The overjet is increased, and the upper incisors may be proclined, perhaps as the result of a habit or an adaptive swallow; or upright, with the increased overjet reflecting the skeletal pattern. The overbite is often increased, but may be incomplete as a result of an adaptive tongue-forward swallow, a habit, or increased vertical skeletal proportions. If the latter two factors are marked, an anterior open bite may result. If the lips are grossly incompetent and are habitually apart at rest, drying of the gingivae may lead to an exacerbation of any pre-existing gingivitis.

The molar relationship usually reflects the skeletal pattern unless early deciduous tooth loss has resulted in mesial drift of the first permanent molars.

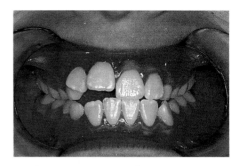

Fig. 9.7. An asymmetrical increase in overjet in a patient with a habit of sucking one finger.

9.3. ASSESSMENT OF, AND TREATMENT PLANNING IN, CLASS II DIVISION 1 MALOCCLUSIONS

Before deciding upon a definitive treatment plan the following factors should be considered:

The patient's age

This is of importance in relation to facial growth: first whether further facial growth is to be expected, and second, if further growth is anticipated, whether this is likely to be favourable or unfavourable. In the 'average' growing child, forward growth of the mandible occurs during the pubertal growth spurt and the early teens. This is advantageous in the management of Class II malocclusions. However, correction of the incisor relationship in a child with increased vertical skeletal proportions and a backward-opening rotational pattern of growth has a poorer prognosis for stability. This is because the anteroposterior discrepancy will worsen with growth, and in addition an increase in the lower face height may reduce the likelihood of lip competence at the end of treatment.

In the adult patient, a lack of growth will reduce the range of skeletal Class II malocclusions that can be treated by orthodontic means alone and will also make overbite reduction more difficult.

The difficulty of treatment

The skeletal pattern is the major determinant of the difficulty of treatment. Those cases with a marked anteroposterior discrepancy and/or significantly increased or reduced vertical skeletal proportions will require careful evaluation, an experienced orthodontist, and possibly surgery for a successful result.

The results of a recent retrospective study of over 1200 consecutively treated Class II division 1 malocclusions found that patients with large overjets and more upright incisors were less likely to achieve an excellent outcome.

The likely stability of overjet reduction

The soft tissues are the major determinant of stability following overjet reduction. Before planning treatment it is often helpful to try to determine those factors that have contributed to the development of that particular Class II division 1 maloccusion and the degree to which they can be modified or corrected by treatment. For example, the patient shown in Fig. 9.8 has an increased overjet on a Class I skeletal pattern with a lower lip trap. In the absence of a habit, it is probable that the upper incisors were deflected labially as they erupted, and it is likely that

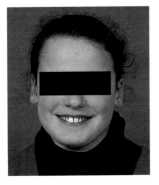

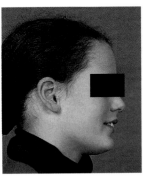

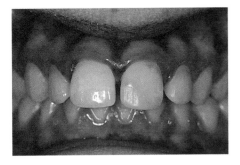

Fig. 9.8. Following overjet reduction, this patient's lips will probably be competent. Therefore the prognosis for stability is good.

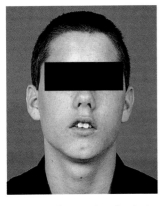

Fig. 9.9. Class II division 1 malocclusion with a poor prognosis for overjet reduction owing to the markedly incompetent lips and increased vertical proportions.

retraction of the upper incisors within the control of the lower lip would be stable as the lips would then be competent. In contrast, the patient shown in Fig. 9.9 has a Class II skeletal pattern with increased vertical skeletal proportions and markedly incompetent lips. An anterior oral seal was achieved by contact between the tongue and lower lip. In this case overjet reduction is unlikely to be stable as, following retraction, the upper labial segment would not be controlled by the lower lip and the forward tongue swallow would probably continue.

Ideally, at the end of overjet reduction the lower lip should act on the incisal one-third of the upper incisors and be able to achieve a competent lip seal. If this is not possible, it should be considered whether treatment is necessary and, if indicated, whether prolonged retention or even surgery is required.

The patient's facial appearance

In some cases a consideration of the profile may help to make the decision between two alternative modes of treatment. For example, in a case with a Class II skeletal pattern due to a retrusive mandible, a functional appliance may be preferable to distal movement of the upper buccal segments with headgear. The profile may also influence the decision whether or not to relieve mild crowding by extractions.

Occasionally, although management by orthodontics alone is feasible, this will be to the detriment of the facial appearance and acceptance of the increased overjet or a surgical approach may be preferred. Features which may lead to this scenario include an obtuse nasolabial angle or excessive upper incisor show (Fig. 9.10).

9.3.1. Practical treatment planning

Treatment planning in general is discussed in Chapter 7. Class II division 1 malocclusions are commonly associated with increased overbite, which must be reduced before the overjet can be reduced. Overbite reduction requires space (about 1–2 mm for an averagely increased overbite) and allowance for this must be made when planning space requirements in the lower arch. Significantly increased overbites will require more space and fixed appliances, or even surgery. Overbite reduction is also considered in more detail in Chapter 10, Section 10.3.1.

If extractions are required in the lower arch, both spontaneous and active tooth movement are facilitated by removal of the corresponding tooth in the upper arch. The actual choice of extraction site will depend upon the presence of crowding, the tooth movements planned, and their anchorage requirements. However, in the treatment of moderately severe Class II division 1 malocclusions with fixed appliances, lower second premolars and upper first premolars may be chosen. This extraction pattern favours forward movement of the lower molar to aid correction of the molar relationship and retraction of the upper labial segment.

Where the lower arch is well aligned and the molar relationship is Class II, space for overjet reduction can be gained by distal movement of the upper buccal segments or by extractions. Where possible, a Class I buccal segment relationship is preferable. If extractions are carried out in the upper arch only, the molar relationship at the end of treatment will be Class II. This is functionally satisfactory, but as half a molar width is narrower than a premolar, some residual space often remains in the upper arch. If fixed appliances are used, the upper first molar can be rotated mesiopalatally to take up this space by virtue of its rhomboid shape.

Distal movement is discussed in more detail in Chapter 7, Section 7.7.3, and is usually considered if the molar relationship is half a unit Class II or less, although a full unit of space can be gained in a cooperative, growing patient. If the prognosis for overjet reduction is guarded, it may be advisable to gain space

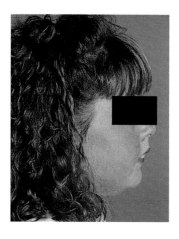 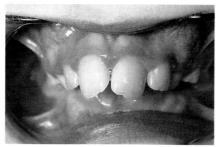

Fig. 9.10. Patient with an obtuse nasolabial angle and incompetent lips. This patient also showed an excessive amount of upper incisor show at rest and when smiling.

in the upper arch by distal movement of the upper buccal segments rather than by extractions. Then should relapse occur this will not result in a reopening of the extraction space.

Treatment in the following situations is difficult and is best managed by a specialist:

● The molar relationship is Class II and the lower arch is crowded as the extraction of one unit in each quadrant in the upper arch will not give sufficient space for relief of crowding and overjet reduction (see Fig. 7.14).

● The molar relationship is greater than one unit Class II.

Management of these cases may involve the extraction of four teeth from the upper arch; distal movement of the upper buccal segments; or a functional appliance used initially to gain a degree of anteroposterior correction. Upper and lower fixed appliances are then usually required to complete alignment.

9.4. EARLY TREATMENT

Given the susceptibility of prominent incisors to trauma, early treatment is a tempting proposition. In addition, the child's parents are often concerned and are keen for early treatment. However, there are a number of factors that need to be considered:

● In younger children the lips are often incompetent, thus reducing the chances of stability following overjet reduction. Therefore, if treatment is carried out in the early mixed dentition, very prolonged retention may be required until the permanent dentition is established, with obvious implications for dental health.

● Because of space considerations it may not be possible to reduce the overjet fully, thus increasing the chances of relapse.

● If the upper incisors are retracted before the maxillary permanent canines have erupted, there is a risk of root resorption or deflection of the canines.

● In practice, if overjet reduction is carried out in the early mixed dentition, further treatment is often required once the permanent dentition is established, by which time the patient's co-operation is flagging.

In America a large, randomized, controlled clincial trial has been set up to look at the timing of treatment for Class II malocclusions. Pre-adolescent children were randomized to either observation or to early treatment with either a functional appliance or headgear. Following this phase patients in all three groups

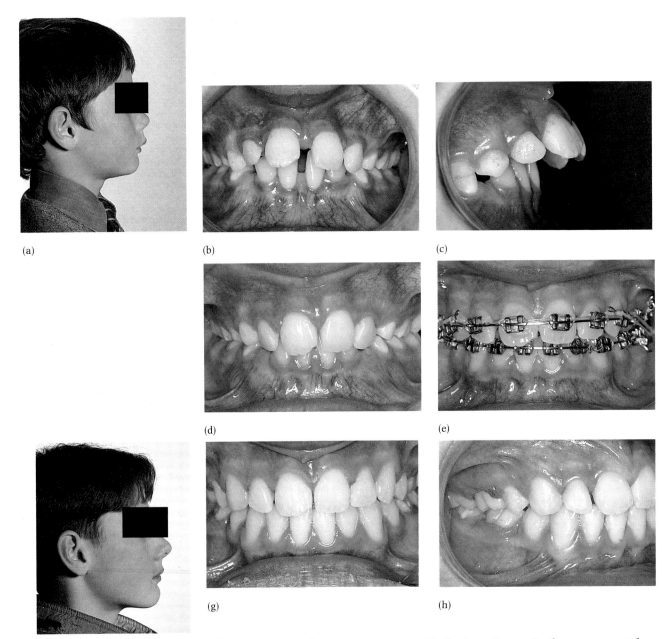

(a)   (b)   (c)

(d)   (e)

(f)   (g)   (h)

Fig. 9.11. Boy aged 9 years with a Class II division 1 malocclusion on a Class II skeletal pattern. As the upper incisors were at risk of trauma, treatment was started early with a functional appliance. Following eruption of the permanent dentition, definitive treatment involving the extraction of all four second premolars and the use of fixed appliances was carried out to correct the inter-incisal angle and alleviate the crowding: (a)–(c) pretreatment (age 9); (d) at end of treatment with functional appliance (note the retroclination of the upper incisors as most of the reduction of the overjet has been achieved by dento-alveolar change); (e) following extraction of second premolars fixed appliances were placed; (f)–(h) following removal of fixed appliances (age 15).

underwent comprehensive treatment with fixed appliances in the permanent dentition. The preliminary data from this study indicates that the early skeletal effects from functional or headgear appliance treatment are not maintained long-term and that following completion of fixed appliance therapy in the permanent dentition, little difference, if any, remained between the early treatment and control (observation) groups. Although, on average, the time in fixed appliances was reduced for children who underwent early treatment the overall treatment time was considerably longer if the early treatment time was included.

At present many clinicians feel that treatment is best deferred until the eruption of the secondary dentition where space can be gained for relief of crowding and reduction of the overjet by the extraction of permanent teeth (if indicated), and soft tissue maturity increases the likelihood of lip competence. In the interim a custom-made mouthguard can be worn for sports. However, if the upper incisors are thought to be at particular risk of trauma during the mixed dentition, treatment with a functional appliance can be considered (Fig. 9.11).

9.5. MANAGEMENT OF AN INCREASED OVERJET ASSOCIATED WITH A CLASS I OR MILD CLASS II SKELETAL PATTERN

Fixed appliances, with extractions if indicated, will give good results in skilled hands in this group (Fig. 9.12).

Provided the skeletal pattern is Class I, that fixed appliances are not indicated for other features of the malocclusion, and that the increased overjet can be reduced by tilting of the upper labial segment, a removable appliance can be considered (Fig. 9.13). The feasibility of using tilting movements to reduce an overjet can be evaluated with a prognosis tracing from a lateral cephalometric radiograph (see Chapter 6, Section 6.8).

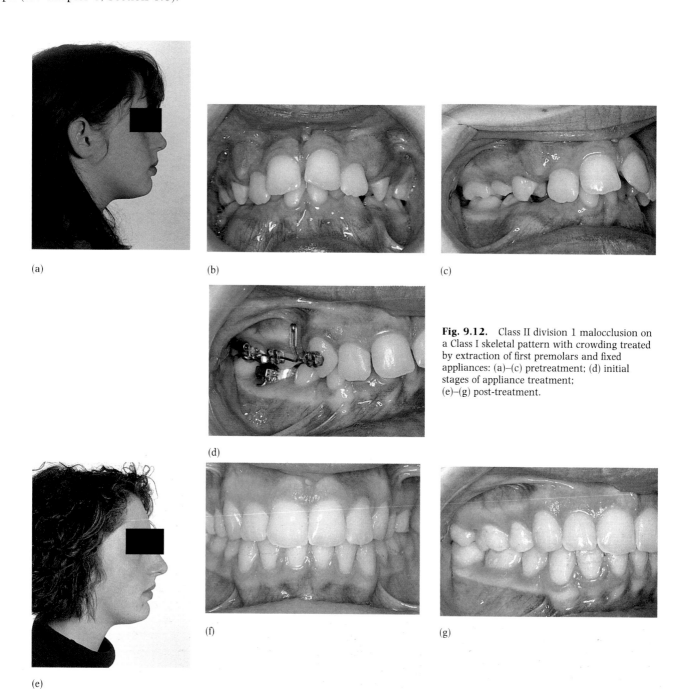

(a)

(b)

(c)

(d)

(e)

(f)

(g)

Fig. 9.12. Class II division 1 malocclusion on a Class I skeletal pattern with crowding treated by extraction of first premolars and fixed appliances: (a)–(c) pretreatment; (d) initial stages of appliance treatment; (e)–(g) post-treatment.

Fig. 9.13. Class II division 1 malocclusion managed with removable appliances. The patient suffered from recurrent ulceration due to cyclic neutropenia and therefore the patient's medical practitioner requested an appliance which could be removed if the ulceration became severe: (a), (b) pretreatment; (c) showing removable appliance with palatal finger springs to retract the canines and a flat anterior bite plane for overbite reduction; (d) post-treatment.

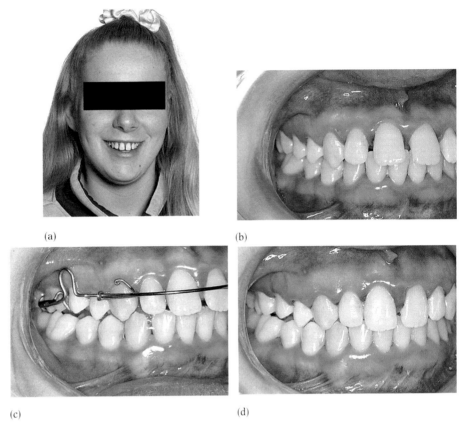

(a)

(b)

(c)

(d)

If lower arch extractions are required, the likelihood that good spontaneous alignment of the lower arch will occur during treatment with an upper removable appliance is increased if moderate crowding is managed by extraction of the first premolars in a growing child. If the crowding is mild, consideration should be given to either accepting the crowding, perhaps with the extraction of second molars, or extracting the second premolars and using fixed appliances (see Chapter 7, Section 7.7).

A functional appliance can be used to reduce an overjet in a cooperative child with well-aligned arches and a mild to moderate skeletal Class II pattern, provided that treatment is timed for the pubertal growth spurt (Chapter 18). If the arches are crowded, anteroposterior correction can be achieved with a functional appliance followed by extractions, and then fixed appliances can be used to achieve alignment and to detail the occlusion.

9.6. MANAGEMENT OF AN INCREASED OVERJET ASSOCIATED WITH A MODERATE TO SEVERE CLASS II SKELETAL PATTERN

Management of the more severe case is the province of the experienced operator. There are three possible approaches to treatment:

1. **Growth modification** by attempting restraint of maxillary growth, by encouraging mandibular growth, or by a combination of the two (Fig. 9.14). In practice, the amount of change that can be produced is small and success is dependent upon favourable growth and an enthusiastic patient. Prolonged retention until growth is complete is desirable. Headgear can be used to try and restrain growth of the maxilla horizontally and/or vertically, depending upon the direction of force relative to the maxilla. Functional appliances

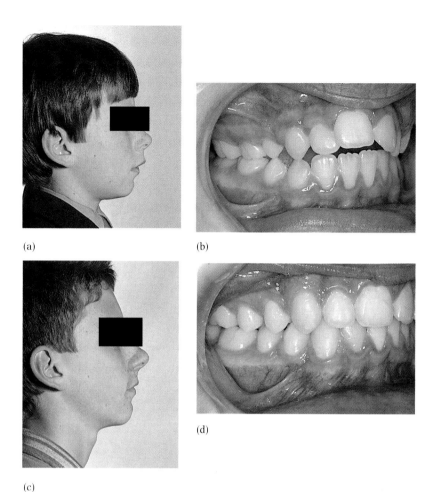

(a)

(b)

(c)

(d)

Fig. 9.14. Patient treated by growth modification. Because correction required a combination of restraint of vertical and forward growth of the maxilla and encouragement of forward growth of the mandible, a functional appliance with high-pull headgear was used: (a), (b) pretreatment aged 12 years; (c), (d) at the end of retention aged 15 years.

appear to produce restraint of maxillary growth whilst encouraging mandibular growth.

2. **Orthodontic camouflage** using fixed appliances to achieve bodily retraction of the upper incisors (Fig. 9.15). The severity of the case that can be approached in this way is limited by the availability of cortical bone palatal to the upper incisors and by the patient's facial profile. If headgear is used in conjunction with this approach, a degree of growth modification may also be produced in favourably growing children.

3. **Surgical correction** (see Chapter 20).

As mandibular growth predominates over maxillary growth during the pubertal growth spurt, more Class II malocclusions than Class III malocclusions can be managed with orthodontics alone. Research indicates that the amount of growth modification that can be achieved is limited, but even a small amount of skeletal change can be helpful. In practice, the child with a moderately severe Class II skeletal pattern can often be managed by a combination of approaches 1 and 2, provided that growth is not unfavourable. This usually involves an initial phase of functional appliance therapy carried out during the pubertal growth spurt, followed by a second phase of fixed appliance treatment plus extractions if indicated.

Orthodontic camouflage can also be achieved by proclination of the lower labial segment. In the main this movement is inherently instable, but it can be stable in a small number of cases where the lower incisors have been trapped lingually by an increased overbite or pushed lingually by a habit or by a lower lip

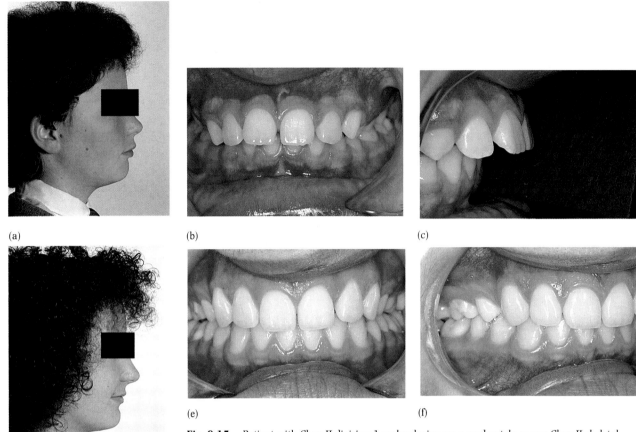

Fig. 9.15. Patient with Class II division 1 malocclusion on a moderately severe Class II skeletal pattern treated by orthodontic camouflage in which both upper first premolars were extracted to gain space for overjet reduction and fixed appliances were used for bodily retraction of the upper incisors: (a)–(c) pretreatment (note the upright upper incisors); (d)–(f) post-retention.

trap. Diagnosis of these cases is difficult and the inexperienced operator should avoid proclination of the lower labial segment at all costs. Occasionally, some proclination of the lower labial segment and permanent retention is felt by the adult patient and operator to be preferable to a surgical option.

Unfortunately, gummy smiles associated with increased vertical skeletal proportions and/or a short upper lip will often worsen as the incisors are retracted. Therefore active steps should be taken to manage this problem. Milder cases are best managed by either the use of high-pull headgear to a functional type of appliance or a fixed appliance to try and restrain maxillary vertical development while the rest of the face grows. In severe cases of vertical maxillary excess or where there is an excessive amount of upper incisor show in an adult patient, surgery to impact the maxilla is advisable.

In cases with a severe Class II skeletal pattern, particularly where the lower facial height is significantly increased or reduced, a combination of orthodontics and surgery may be required to produce an aesthetic and stable correction of the malocclusion (see Chapter 20). The threshold for surgery is lower in adults because of a lack of growth.

9.7. RETENTION

A common mistake is to stop treatment before overjet reduction is fully completed. In many cases the patient continues to retract the lower lip behind the upper incisors to achieve an anterior oral seal, with a subsequent relapse in incisor position. Therefore full reduction of the overjet and the achievement of lip competence is advisable.

Unfortunately no amount of retention will make an inherently unstable tooth position become stable, and so retention must be considered during treatment planning. Provided that the upper incisors have been retracted to a position of soft tissue balance and are controlled by the lower lip, only a short period of retention is required to allow for adaptation of the periodontal fibres and soft tissues. One exception to this is functional appliance therapy where retention until growth is complete is advisable (Chapter 18).

PRINCIPAL SOURCES AND FURTHER READING

Aelbers, C. M. F and Dermaut, L. R. (1996). Orthopedics in orthodontics: fiction or reality. A review of the literature. *American Journal of Orthodontics and Dentofacial Orthopedics*, **110**, 513–19 and 667–71.

Banks, P. A. (1986). An analysis of complete and incomplete overbite in Class II division 1 malocclusions (an analysis of overbite incompleteness). *British Journal of Orthodontics*, **13**, 23–32.

Battagel, J. M. (1989). Profile changes in Class II division 1 malocclusions: a comparison of the effects of Edgewise and Frankel appliance therapy. *European Journal of Orthodontics*, **11**, 243–53.

Burden D. J. *et al.* (1999). Predictors of outcome among patients with Class II division 1 malocclusion treated with fixed appliances in the permanent dentition. *American Journal of Orthodontics and Dentofacial Orthopedics*, **116**, 452–59.

King, G. J., Keeling, S. D., Hocevar, R. A., and Wheeler, T. T. (1990). The timing of treatment for Class II malocclusions in children: a literature review. *Angle Orthodontist*, **60**, 87–97.

• The arguments for and against early treatment of Class II division 1 malocclusions.

Tulloch, C. J. F., Phillips, C., and Proffit, W. R. (1998). Benefit of early Class II treatment: progress report of a two-phase randomised clinical trial. *American Journal of Orthodontics and Dentofacial Orthopedics*, **113**, 62–72.

• The results of this important trial are essential reading for any clinician involved in treating patients with Class II malocclusions.

10 Class II division 2

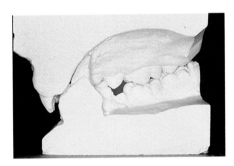

Fig. 10.1. A cross-sectional view through the study models of a patient with a very severe Class II division 2 incisor relationship. Lack of an occlusal stop allowed the incisors to continue erupting, leading to a significantly increased overbite.

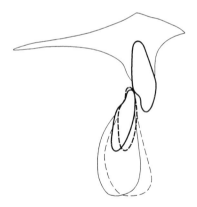

Fig. 10.2. Diagram showing how, despite a forward pattern of facial growth, the overbite can become worse in an untreated Class II division 2 incisor relationship.

A Class II incisor relationship is defined by the British Standards classification as being present when the lower incisor edges occlude posterior to the cingulum plateau of the upper incisors. Class II division 2 includes those malocclusions where the upper central incisors are retroclined. The overjet is usually minimal, but may be increased. The prevalence of this malocclusion in a Caucasian population is approximately 10 per cent.

10.1. AETIOLOGY

The majority of Class II division 2 malocclusions arise as a result of a number of interrelated skeletal and soft tissue factors.

10.1.1. Skeletal pattern

Class II division 2 malocclusion is commonly associated with a mild Class II skeletal pattern, but may also occur in association with a Class I or even a Class III dental base relationship. Where the skeletal pattern is more markedly Class II the upper incisors usually lie outside the control of the lower lip, resulting in a Class II division 1 relationship, but where the lower lip line is high relative to the upper incisors a Class II division 2 malocclusion can result.

The vertical dimension is also important in the aetiology of Class II division 2 malocclusions, and typically is reduced. A reduced lower face height occurring in conjunction with a Class II jaw relationship often results in the absence of an occlusal stop to the lower incisors, which then continue to erupt leading to an increased overbite (Fig. 10.1).

A reduced lower facial height is associated with a forward rotational pattern of growth. This usually means that the mandible becomes more prognathic with growth (Fig. 10.2). While this pattern of growth is helpful in reducing the severity of a Class II skeletal pattern, it also has the effect of increasing overbite unless an occlusal stop is created by treatment to limit further eruption of the lower incisors and to shift the axis of growth rotation to the lower incisal edges.

10.1.2. Soft tissues

The influence of the soft tissues in Class II division 2 malocclusions is usually mediated by the skeletal pattern. If the lower facial height is reduced, the lower lip line will effectively be higher relative to the crown of the upper incisors (more than the normal one-third coverage). A high lower lip line will tend to retrocline the upper incisors (Fig. 10.3; see also Fig. 5.9). In some cases the upper lateral incisors, which have a shorter crown length, will escape the action of the lower lip and therefore lie at an average inclination, whereas the central incisors are retroclined (Fig. 10.4).

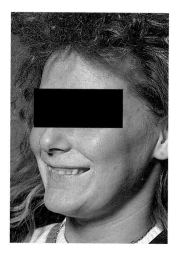

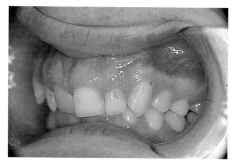

Fig. 10.3. Class II division 2 malocclusion with retroclination of all the upper incisors owing to a high lower lip line which is evident in the view of the patient smiling.

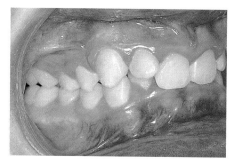

Fig. 10.4. Typical Class II division 2 malocclusion with retroclination of the upper central incisors. The lateral incisors, which are shorter, escape the effect of the lower lip and lie at an average inclination, albeit slightly mesiolabially rotated and crowded.

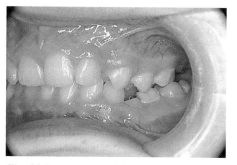

Fig. 10.5. Patient with bimaxillary retroclination due to the action of the lips.

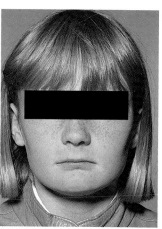

Class II division 2 incisor relationships may also result from bimaxillary retroclination caused by active muscular lips (Fig. 10.5), irrespective of the skeletal pattern.

10.1.3. Dental factors

As with other malocclusions, crowding is commonly seen in conjunction with a Class II division 2 incisor relationship. In addition, any pre-existing crowding is exacerbated because retroclination of the upper central incisors results in their being positioned in an arc of smaller circumference. In the upper labial segment this usually manifests in a lack of space for the upper lateral incisors which are crowded and are typically rotated mesiolabially out of the arch. In the same manner lower arch crowding is often exacerabated by retroclination of the lower labial segment. This can occur because the lower labial segment becomes 'trapped' lingually to the upper labial segment by an increased overbite (Fig. 10.6).

Lack of an effective occlusal stop to eruption of the lower incisors may result in their continued development, giving rise to an increased overbite. This may be due to a Class II skeletal pattern or retroclination of the incisors as a result of the action of the lips, leading to an increased inter-incisal angle. In addition, it has been found that in some Class II division 2 cases the upper central incisors

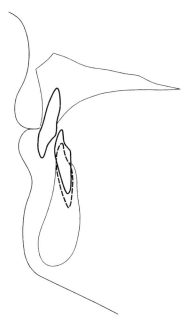

Fig. 10.6. 'Trapping' of the lower incisor teeth behind the cingulum of the upper incisors in a Class II division 2 malocclusion. Note the space created labial to the lower incisor crown by reduction of the overbite (the dotted line) within the soft tissue environment.

exhibit a more acute crown and root angulation. However, rather than being the cause, this crown root angulation could itself be due to the action of a high lower lip line causing deflection of the crown of the tooth relative to the root after eruption.

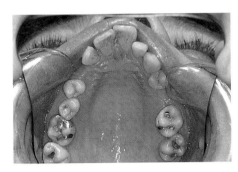

Fig. 10.7. Ulceration of the palatal mucosa of 1/1 caused by the occlusion of the lower incisor edges — an example of a traumatic overbite.

10.2. OCCLUSAL FEATURES

Classically, the upper central incisors are retroclined and the lateral incisors are at an average angulation or are proclined, depending upon their position relative to the lower lip (see Fig. 10.4). Where the lower lip line is very high the lateral incisors may be retroclined (see Fig. 10.3). The more severe malocclusions occur either where the underlying skeletal pattern is more Class II or where the lip musculature is active, causing bimaxillary retroclination.

In mild cases the lower incisors occlude with the upper incisors, but in patients with a more severe Class II skeletal pattern the overbite may be complete onto the palatal mucosa. In a small proportion of cases the lower incisors may cause ulceration of the palatal tissues (Fig. 10.7), and in some patients retroclination of the upper incisors leads to stripping of the labial gingivae of the lower incisors (Fig. 10.8). In these cases the overbite is described as traumatic, but fortunately both are comparatively rare.

Another feature associated with a more severe underlying Class II skeletal pattern is lingual crossbite of the first and occasionally the second premolars (Fig. 10.9) owing to the relative positions and widths of the arches, and possibly to trapping of the lower labial segment within a retroclined upper labial segment.

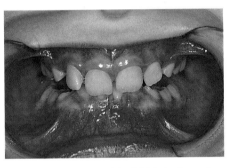

Fig. 10.8. Stripping of the labial gingivae of the lower incisors caused by the severely retroclined upper incisors — an example of a traumatic overbite.

10.3. MANAGEMENT

In the mild Class II division 2 malocclusion, where the lower incisors occlude with the upper incisors, treatment can be limited to achievement of alignment and the incisor relationship accepted.

Stable correction of a Class II division 2 incisor relationship is difficult as it requires not only reduction of the increased overbite (discussed in Section 10.3.1), but also reduction of the inter-incisal angle which classically is increased (Fig. 10.10). If re-eruption of the incisors and therefore an increase in overbite is to be resisted, the inter-incisal angle needs to be reduced, preferably to between 125° and 135°, so that an effective occlusal stop is created (Fig. 10.11).

The inter-incisal angle in a Class II division 2 malocclusion can be reduced in a number of ways:

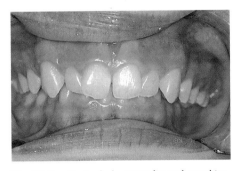

Fig. 10.9. Particularly severe lingual crossbite of the entire left buccal segment owing to a Class II skeletal pattern resulting in wider portion of upper arch occluding with narrower section of lower arch.

- Torquing the incisor roots palatally/lingually with a fixed appliance (Fig. 10.12).
- Proclination of the lower labial segment (Fig. 10.13). This approach should only be employed by the experienced as, although it provides additional space for alignment of the lower incisor teeth, proclination of the lower labial segment will only be stable if it has been trapped lingually by the upper labial segment.
- Proclination of the upper labial segment followed by use of a functional appliance to reduce the resultant overjet and achieve intermaxillary correction (Fig. 10.14).
- A combination of the above approaches.

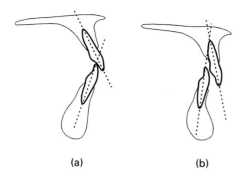

Fig. 10.10. (a) A Class I incisor relationship with an average inter-incisal angle of around 135°; (b) a Class II division 2 relationship where the inter-incisal angle is increased.

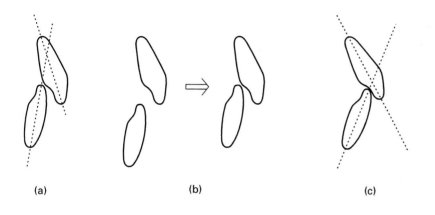

Fig. 10.11. If a Class II division 2 incisor relationship is to be corrected not only the overbite but also the inter-incisal angle must be reduced to prevent re-eruption of the incisors post-treatment: (a) Class II division 2 incisor relationship; (b) reduction of the overbite alone will not be stable as the incisors will re-erupt following removal of appliances ; (c) reduction of the inter-incisal angle in conjunction with reduction of the overbite has a greater chance of stability.

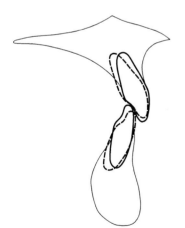

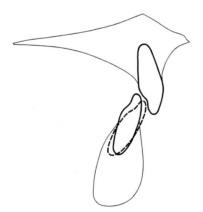

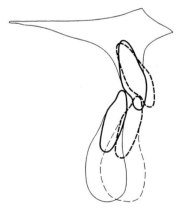

Fig. 10.12. Correction of a Class II division 2 incisor relationship by reducing the overbite and torquing the incisors lingually/palatally. Fixed appliances are necessary.

Fig. 10.13. Correction of a Class II division 2 incisor relationship by proclination of the lower labial segment.

Fig. 10.14. Correction of a Class II division 2 incisor relationship by an initial phase involving proclination of the upper incisors, followed by reduction of the resultant overjet with a functional appliance.

The treatment approach chosen for a particular patient will depend upon the aetiology of the malocclusion, the presence and degree of crowding, the patient's profile, and their probable compliance.

Once the decision has been made to accept or correct the incisor relationship, consideration should be given as to whether extractions are required to relieve crowding and to provide space for incisor alignment. Some practitioners have argued that closure of excess extraction space in a Class II division 2 malocclusion will result in further retroclination of the labial segments and a 'dished-in profile'. This claim is usually made in association with the presentation of isolated case reports. However, research using groups of carefully matched patients has shown that there is little difference in the amount of retraction of the lips between extraction and non-extraction treatment approaches (see Chapter 7, Section 7.8). Nevertheless, it would seem advisable in the management of Class II division 2 malocclusions to minimize lingual movement of the lower incisors in order to avoid any possibility of worsening the patient's overbite; indeed, it may be preferable to accept a degree of lower arch crowding rather than run this risk. Certainly, extraction of permanent teeth in the lower arch in Class II division 2 maloccclusions should be approached with caution, and if any doubt exists specialist advice should be sought. In addition, clinical experience suggests that space closure occurs less readily in patients with reduced vertical skeletal proportions, which are commonly associated with Class II division 2 malocclusions, than in those with increased lower face heights.

In general, proclination of the lower labial segment should be considered unstable, but it has been argued that in some Class II division 2 malocclusions the lower labial segment is trapped behind the upper labial segment, resulting in retroclination of the lower incisors and constriction of the lower intercanine width. This means that a limited increase in intercanine width and a degree of proclination of the lower labial segment can be stable, although it is important to assess the lower labial supporting tissues to avoid iatrogenic gingival recession. However, proclination of the lower incisors is helpful in reducing both overbite and the inter-incisal angle.

In view of the above comments, it is not surprising that Class II division 2 malocclusions are managed more frequently on a non-extraction basis, particularly in the lower arch, than are other types of malocclusion.

This discussion has highlighted some of the difficulties inherent in planning treatment of Class II division 2 incisor relationships. Except for the mild case, where management is to be limited to alignment of the upper arch, correction of Class II division 2 incisor relationships is best left to the specialist.

10.3.1. Approaches to the reduction of overbite

Intrusion of the incisors

Actual intrusion of the incisors is difficult to achieve. Fixed appliances are necessary and the mechanics employed pit intrusion of the incisors against extrusion of the buccal segment teeth; as it is easier to move the molars occlusally than to intrude the incisors into bone, the former tends to predominate. In practice, the effects achieved are relative intrusion, where the incisors are held still while vertical growth of the face occurs around them, plus extrusion of the molars. High-pull headgear can be hooked onto the anterior segment of the archwire of an upper fixed appliance to try and achieve intrusion of the upper labial segment; however, this approach has become less popular due to concerns over headgear safety and root resorption.

Increasing the anchorage unit posteriorly by including second permanent molars (or even third molars in adults) will aid intrusion of the incisors and help to limit extrusion of the molars. Arches which bypass the canines and premolars to pit the incisors against the molars, for example the utility arch (Fig. 10.15), are employed with some success to reduce overbite by intrusion of the incisors, although some molar extrusion does occur.

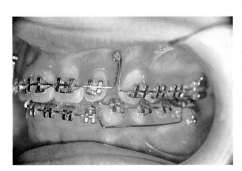

Fig. 10.15. Lower utility arch for overbite reduction. Note the difference in level between the lower incisor brackets and the buccal segment teeth.

Eruption of the molars

Use of a flat anterior bite-plane on an upper removable appliance to free the occlusion of the buccal segment teeth will, if worn conscientiously, limit further occlusal movement of the incisors and allow the lower molars to erupt, thus reducing the overbite. This method requires a growing patient to accommodate the increase in vertical dimension that results, otherwise the molars will reintrude under the forces of occlusion once the appliance is withdrawn. However, this tendency can be resisted to a degree if the treatment creates a stable incisor relationship.

Extrusion of the molars

As mentioned above, the major effect of attempting intrusion of the incisors is often extrusion of the molars. This may be advantageous in Class II division 2 cases as this type of malocclusion is usually associated with reduced vertical proportions. Again, vertical growth is required if the overbite reduction achieved in this way is to be stable.

Proclination of the lower incisors

Advancement of the lower labial segment anteriorly will result in a reduction of overbite as the incisors tip labially. This approach should only be carried out by the experienced orthodontist (see Section 10.3.2). However, in a few cases where the lower incisors have been trapped behind the upper labial segment by an increased overbite, fitting of an upper bite-plane appliance may allow the lower labial segment to procline spontaneously (Fig. 10.16).

Surgery

In adults with a markedly increased overbite and those patients where the underlying skeletal pattern is more markedly Class II, a combination of orthodontics and surgery is required.

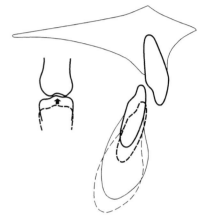

Fig. 10.16. Diagram to show spontaneous proclination of the lower labial segment following placement of a flat anterior bite-plane which has reduced the overbite by eruption of the lower molars.

10.3.2. Practical management

The incisor relationship is to be accepted

In milder cases where the lower incisors occlude onto tooth tissue it may be possible to accept the increased overbite, limiting treatment to alignment, particularly of the upper lateral incisors.

As discussed above, it may be preferable to accept mild to moderate lower arch crowding rather than run the risk of extractions leading to lingual movement of the lower labial segment and a worsening of the overbite. If the crowding is marked, extraction of lower first premolars may be required. However, if lower arch extractions run the risk that the lower incisors may tilt lingually and come to occlude with the palatal gingivae behind the upper incisors, it may be preferable to use fixed appliances and correct the incisor relationship instead (see below).

Space for alignment of the upper arch can be created by extractions (Chapter 7, Section 7.7.1) or by distal movement of the upper buccal segment teeth (Chapter 7, Section 7.7.3). Extraction of the upper first premolars is usually indicated if the first premolars have been lost in the lower arch or the buccal segment relationship is greater than half a unit Class II. Extraction of second premolars will give less space anteriorly and can be considered if upper arch crowding is mild and/or

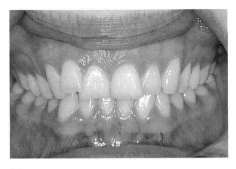

(a)

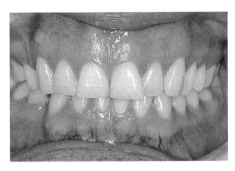

(b)

Fig. 10.17. A mild Class II division 2 incisor relationship with mild upper and lower arch crowding. The patient requested treatment to align 2/. Treatment involved the extraction of 4/7, 4/7 to relieve the crowding, followed by an upper removable appliance to retract 3/ and align 2/: (a) pretreatment; (b) post-treatment.

distal movement of the molars is not indicated or the patient is unwilling to wear headgear.

Distal movement of the upper buccal segments can be considered where the lower arch alignment is to be accepted and the molar relationship is not greater than half a unit Class II. Extraction of the upper second molars may be required to facilitate distal movement, provided that upper third molars of a good size are present and in a favourable position. In some cases removable appliances can be used to achieve upper arch alignment. Although a removable appliance cannot be used to de-rotate rotated upper lateral incisors, relief of crowding and retraction of these teeth into the line of the arch may provide sufficient improvement (Fig. 10.17). The appliance should incorporate a flat anterior bite-plane to free the occlusion of the lower labial segment and achieve some overbite reduction.

When planning treatment in these cases it is important to bear in mind that, if the upper incisors are retroclined, the upper canines should only be retracted sufficiently to provide space for alignment of the incisors. This is because retroclined upper incisors occupy less arch length than upright incisors; therefore if the maxillary canines are retracted to Class I, excess space will be created in the upper labial segment. This may leave the upper canines buccally positioned relative to the arch in a half-unit Class II relationship with the lower canines, in which case consideration should be given to correcting the incisor relationship with fixed appliances.

If use of a removable appliance will not produce an acceptable result then fixed appliances are indicated.

The incisor relationship is to be corrected

Correction of the incisor relationship is indicated where the overbite is complete to the palatal soft tissues, or is liable to become so following extractions in the lower arch to relieve crowding. In some patients, reduction of overbite is necessary in order to be able to treat other features of a malocclusion. Certainly, correction of the incisor relationship should be given priority if the overbite is traumatic.

It will be apparent from the discussion at the beginning of Section 10.3 that there are three possible treatment modalities as described below.

Fixed appliances

When fixed appliances are used the inter-incisal angle can be reduced by palatal/lingual root torque or by proclination of the lower incisors. The relative role of these two approaches in the management of a particular malocclusion is a matter of fine judgement.

Torquing of incisor apices is dependent upon the presence of sufficient cortical bone palatally/lingually and places a considerable strain on anchorage. This type of movement is also more likely to result in resorption of the root apices than other types of tooth movement.

Mild crowding in the lower arch may be eliminated by forward movement of the lower labial segment. If crowding is marked, extractions will be required and a lower fixed appliance used to ensure that space closure occurs without movement of the lower incisor edges lingually (Fig. 10.18). Space for correction of the incisor relationship can be gained by upper arch extractions or by distal movement of the upper buccal segments. If headgear is used for anchorage or distal movement, a direction of pull below the occlusal plane (cervical pull) is usually indicated in Class II division 2 malocclusions as the vertical facial proportions are reduced. A lingual crossbite, if present, usually affects the first premolars only. If extraction of the upper first premolars is not indicated, or if the second premolars

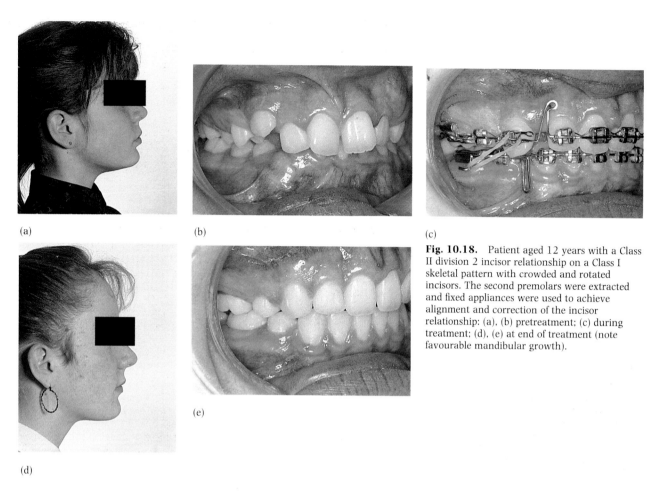

(a)

(b)

(c)

(d)

(e)

Fig. 10.18. Patient aged 12 years with a Class II division 2 incisor relationship on a Class I skeletal pattern with crowded and rotated incisors. The second premolars were extracted and fixed appliances were used to achieve alignment and correction of the incisor relationship: (a), (b) pretreatment; (c) during treatment; (d), (e) at end of treatment (note favourable mandibular growth).

are involved, elimination of the crossbite will involve a combination of contraction across the affected upper teeth and expansion of the lower premolar width. Following treatment, the prognosis for the corrected position is good as cuspal interlock will help to prevent relapse.

On completion of treatment it is prudent to retain with a upper removable appliance incorporating a bite-plane. Ideally, retention should be continued until growth is complete to try and prevent a return of the overbite. Whilst this is not always practicable, one approach is to retain for about 6 months full time, followed by 6 months nights only. If proclination of the lower labial segment is decided upon, an assessment of the stability of this movement needs to be made at the planning stage and permanent retention instituted where indicated.

Functional appliances

Functional appliances can be utilized in the correction of Class II division 2 malocclusions in growing patients with a mild to moderate Class II skeletal pattern and a relatively well-aligned lower arch (Fig. 10.19). Reduction of the interincisal angle is achieved mainly by proclination of the upper incisors, although some proclination of the lower labial segment may occur as a result of the functional appliance. If an activator type of functional appliance is used, then a prefunctional phase is required to procline any retroclined incisors and to expand the upper arch (to ensure the correct buccolingual arch relationship at the end of treatment). This can be achieved using a removable appliance (Fig. 10.20); this design is known as an ELSAA (Expansion and Labial Segment Alignment Appliance). If a twin-block functional is used, then a spring to procline the

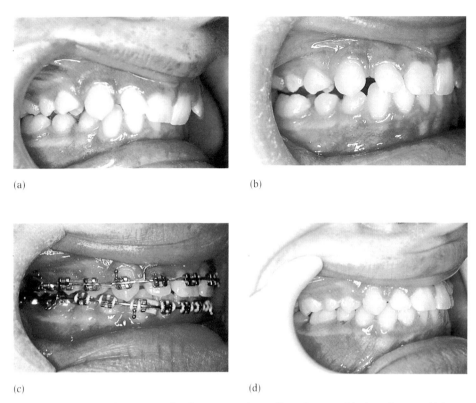

(a)

(b)

(c)

(d)

Fig. 10.19. Class II division 2 malocclusion treated initially with a twin-block appliance, which incorporated a double cantilever spring to procline the retroclined upper central incisors. Then fixed appliances were used to detail the occlusion: (a) pretreatment; (b) at end of the functional phase; (c) fixed appliance phase; (d) end of active treatment.

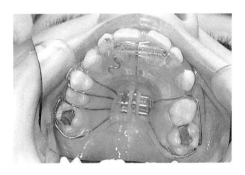

Fig. 10.20. An upper removable appliance used to expand the upper arch and procline retroclined upper incisors prior to functional appliance therapy.

Fig. 10.21. Adult patient with severe Class II division 2 malocclusion on a marked Class II skeletal pattern with reduced vertical proportions. It was decided that a combined orthodontic and orthognathic surgery appproach was required to correct this malocclusion.

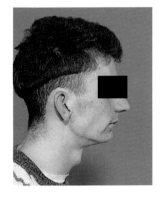

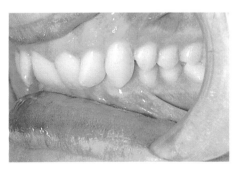

incisors can be incorporated into the upper appliance. Finally, fixed appliances are often required to detail the occlusion. If the lower incisors have been proclined, the stability of their position should be assessed and, if doubtful, permanent retention (or at least retention until growth is complete) should be instituted.

Surgery (see Chapter 20)

A stable aesthetic orthodontic correction may not be possible in patients with an unfavourable skeletal pattern anteroposteriorly and/or vertically, particularly if growth is complete (Fig. 10.21). In these cases surgery may be necessary. A phase of presurgical orthodontics is required to align the teeth. However, arch levelling is usually not completed as extrusion of the molars is much more easily accomplished after surgery. Where the overbite is particularly marked, the lower labial segment may have to be set down surgically, in which case space will have to be created distal to the lower canines for the surgical cuts to be made.

PRINCIPAL SOURCES AND FURTHER READING

Burstone, C. R. (1977) Deep overbite correction by intrusion. *American Journal of Orthodontics*, **72**, 1–22.
● A useful paper for the more experienced orthodontist using fixed appliances.
Lee, R. T. (1999). Arch width and form: a review. *American Journal of Orthodontics and Dentofacial Orthopedics*, **115**, 305–13.
Leighton, B. C. and Adams, C. P. (1986). Incisor inclination in Class II division 2 malocclusions. *European Journal of Orthodontics*, **8**, 98–105.
Kim, T. W. and Little, R. M. (1999). Post retention assessment of deep overbite correction in Class II division 2 malocclusion. *Angle Orthodontist*. **69**, 175–86.
Rutter, R. R. and Witt, E. (1990). Correction of Class II division 2 malocclusions through the use of the Bionator appliance. Report of two cases. *American Journal of Orthodontics and Dentofacial Orthopedics*, **97**, 106–12.
Selwyn-Barnett, B. J. (1991). Rationale of treatment for Class II division 2 malocclusion. *British Journal of Orthodontics*, **18**, 173–81.
● This paper contains a carefully constructed argument for management of Class II division 2 malocclusion by proclination of the lower labial segment rather than extractions, in order to avoid detrimental effects upon the profile.
Selwyn-Barnett, B. J. (1996). Class II division 2 malocclusion: a method of planning and treatment. *British Journal of Orthodontics*, **23**, 29–36.

11 Class III

The British Standards definition of Class III incisor relationship includes those malocclusions where the lower incisor edge occludes anterior to the cingulum plateau of the upper incisors. Class III malocclusions affect around 3 per cent of Caucasians.

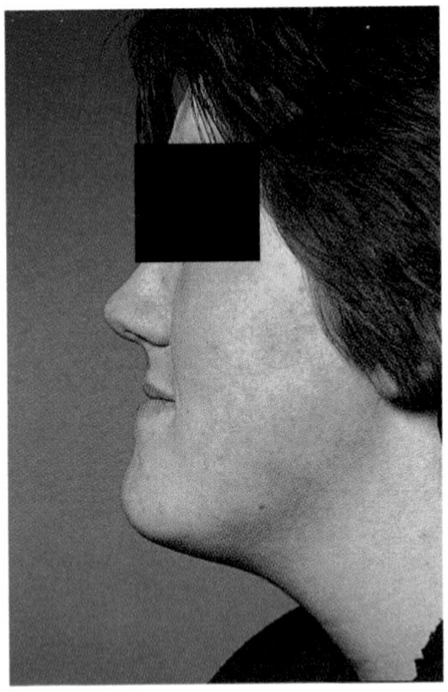

11.1. AETIOLOGY

11.1.1. Skeletal pattern

The skeletal relationship is the most important factor in the aetiology of most Class III malocclusions, and the majority of Class III incisor relationships are associated with an underlying Class III skeletal relationship. Cephalometric studies have shown that, compared with Class I occlusions, Class III malocclusions exhibit the following:

* increased mandibular length;
* a more anteriorly placed glenoid fossa so that the condylar head is positioned more anteriorly leading to mandibular prognathism;
* reduced maxillary length;
* a more retruded position of the maxilla leading to maxillary retrusion.

The first two of these factors are the most influential. Figure 11.1 shows a patient with a Class III malocclusion with mandibular prognathism and Fig. 11.2 illustrates maxillary retrognathia (maxillary retrusion).

Class III malocclusions occur in association with a range of vertical skeletal proportions, ranging from increased to reduced. A backward opening rotation pattern of facial growth will tend to result in a reduction of overbite; however, a forward rotating pattern of facial growth will lead to an increase in the prominence of the chin.

11.1.2. Soft tissues

In the majority of Class III malocclusions the soft tissues do not play a major aetiological role. In fact the reverse is often the case, with the soft tissues tending to tilt the upper and lower incisors towards each other so that the incisor relationship is often less severe than the underlying skeletal pattern. This dento-alveolar compensation occurs in Class III malocclusions because an anterior oral seal can frequently be achieved by upper to lower lip contact. This has the effect of moulding the upper and lower labial segments towards each other. The main exception occurs in patients with increased vertical skeletal proportions where the lips are more likely to be incompetent and an anterior oral seal is often accomplished by tongue to lower lip contact.

Fig. 11.1. Patient with mandibular prognathism

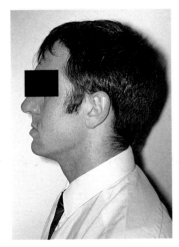

Fig. 11.2. Patient with maxillary retrognathia.

11.1.3. Dental factors

Class III malocclusions are often associated with a narrow upper arch and a broad lower arch, with the result that crowding is seen more commonly, and to a greater degree, in the upper arch than in the lower. Frequently, the lower arch is well aligned or evenly spaced.

11.2. OCCLUSAL FEATURES

By definition Class III malocclusions occur when the lower incisors are positioned more labially relative to the upper incisors. Therefore an anterior crossbite of one or more of the incisors is a common feature of Class III malocclusions. As with any crossbite, it is essential to check for a displacement of the mandible on closure from a premature contact into maximal interdigitation. In Class III malocclusions this can be ascertained by asking the patient to try to achieve an edge-to-edge incisor position. If such a displacement is present, the prognosis for correction of the incisor relationship is more favourable. In the past it was thought that such a displacement led to overclosure and greater prominence of the mandible, with the condylar head displaced forward. In fact cephalometric studies suggest that in most cases, although there is a forward displacement of the mandible to disengage the premature contact of the incisors as closure into occlusion occurs, the mandible moves backwards until the condyles regain their normal position within the glenoid fossa (Fig. 11.3).

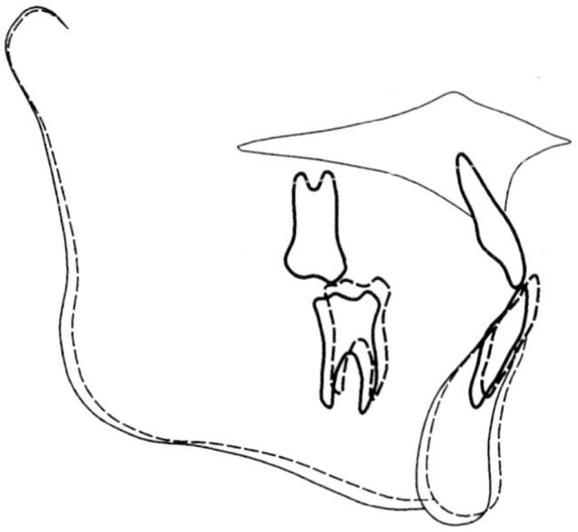

Another common feature of Class III malocclusions is buccal crossbite, which is usually due to a discrepancy in the relative width of the arches. This occurs because the lower arch is positioned relatively more anteriorly in Class III malocclusions and is often well developed, while the upper arch is narrow. This is also reflected in the relative crowding within the arches, with the upper arch commonly more crowded (Fig. 11.4).

As mentioned above, Class III malocclusions often exhibit dento-alveolar compensation with the upper incisors proclined and the lower incisors retroclined, which reduces the severity of the incisor relationship (Fig. 11.5).

11.3. TREATMENT PLANNING IN CLASS III MALOCCLUSIONS

A number of factors should be considered before planning treatment.

The **patient's opinion** regarding their occlusion and facial appearance must be taken into account. This subject needs to be approached with some tact.

The **severity of the skeletal pattern** both anteroposteriorly and vertically should be assessed. This is the major determinant of the difficulty and prognosis of orthodontic treatment.

The **expected pattern of future growth** both anteroposteriorly and vertically should be considered. It is important to remember that average growth will tend to result in a worsening of the relationship between the arches, and a significant deterioration can be anticipated if growth is unfavourable. When evaluating the likely direction and extent of facial growth, the patient's age, sex, and facial pattern should be taken into consideration (see Chapter 4). Children with increased vertical skeletal proportions often continue to exhibit a vertical pattern of growth, which will have the effect of reducing incisor overbite. Obviously for patients on the borderline between different management regimes it is wise to err on the side of pessimism (as growth will often prove this to be correct).

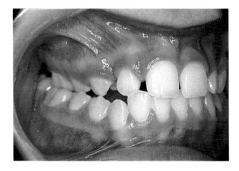

Fig. 11.3. Diagram illustrating the path of closure in a Class III malocclusion from an edge-to-edge incisor relationship into maximal occlusion. Although the mandible is displaced forwards from the initial contact of the incisors to achieve maximal interdigitation, the condylar head is not displaced out of the glenoid fossa.

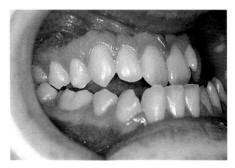

Fig. 11.4. A Class III malocclusion with a narrow crowded upper arch and a broader less crowded lower arch with associated buccal crossbite.

Fig. 11.5. Dento-alveolar compensation.

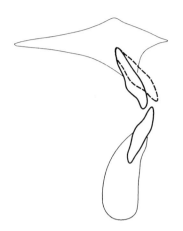

Fig. 11.6. Diagram to show how proclination of the upper incisors results in a reduction of overbite.

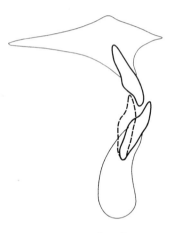

Fig. 11.7. Diagram to show how retroclination of the lower incisors results in an increase of overbite.

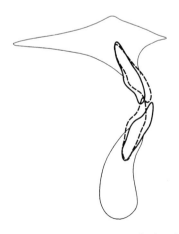

Fig. 11.8. A prognosis tracing which indicates that a combination of retroclination of the lower incisors and proclination of the upper labial segment is required to correct the incisor relationship.

In Class III malocclusions a normal or increased **overbite** is an advantage, as a vertical overlap of the upper incisors with the lower incisors post-treatment is vital for stability.

If the patient can achieve an edge-to-edge incisor position, this increases the prognosis for correction of the incisor relationship.

In general, orthodontic management of Class III malocclusion will aim to increase **dento-alveolar compensation**. Therefore, if considerable dento-alveolar compensation is already present, trying to increase it further may not be an aesthetic or stable treatment option.

The **degree of crowding** in each arch should be considered. In Class III malocclusions crowding occurs more frequently, and to a greater degree, in the upper arch than in the lower. Extractions in the upper arch only should be resisted as this will often lead to a worsening of the incisor relationship. Where upper arch extractions are necessary, it is advisable to extract at least as far forwards in the lower arch.

Orthodontic correction of a Class III incisor relationship can be achieved by either proclination of the upper incisors alone or retroclination of the lower incisors with or without proclination of the upper incisors. The approach applicable to a particular malocclusion is largely determined by the skeletal pattern and the amount of overbite present before treatment, as proclination of the upper incisors reduces the overbite (Fig. 11.6) whereas retroclination of the lower incisors helps to increase overbite (Fig. 11.7). A prognosis tracing (see Chapter 6, Section 6.8) may be helpful in deciding between the two approaches (Fig. 11.8).

If the lower arch is moderately crowded, consideration should be given to extracting the lower first premolars to allow the lower labial segment to drop lingually, thereby aiding dento-alveolar compensation. This can result in residual space in the lower arch if fixed appliances are not used.

Additional space for relief of crowding in the upper arch can often be gained by expansion of the arch anteriorly to correct the incisor relationship and/or buccolingually to correct buccal segment crossbites. Therefore, where possible, it may be prudent to delay permanent extractions until after the crossbite is corrected and the degree of crowding is reassessed. Expansion of the upper arch to correct a crossbite will have the effect of reducing overbite, which is a disadvantage in Class III cases. This reduction in overbite occurs because expansion of the upper arch is achieved primarily by tilting the upper premolars and molars buccally, which results in the palatal cusps of these teeth swinging down and 'propping open' the occlusion. Therefore, if upper arch expansion is indicated and the overbite is reduced, fixed appliances should be used to try and limit tilting of the upper molars buccally during the expansion.

Distal movement of the upper buccal segments with headgear to gain space for alignment is inadvisable as this will have the effect of restraining growth of the maxilla. However, in Class III cases with mild to moderate mid-arch crowding, space can be made by a combination of forward movement of the incisors as well as some distal movement of the remaining buccal segment teeth. This can be accomplished by using a removable appliance with a screw positioned at the site of crowding or with fixed appliances.

Another approach is to use a functional appliance, but it is difficult for patients to posture posteriorly to achieve an active working bite. Therefore functional appliances are less widely used in Class III malocclusions, although they can be useful in mild cases in the mixed dentition where a combination of proclination of the upper incisors together with retroclination of the lower incisors is required.

In patients with a severe Class III skeletal pattern and/or reduced overbite, the possibility that a surgical approach may ultimately be required must be considered, particularly before any permanent extractions are undertaken (see Section 11.4.4).

11.4. TREATMENT OPTIONS

11.4.1. Accepting the incisor relationship

In mild Class III malocclusions, particularly those cases where the overbite is minimal, it may be preferable to accept the incisor relationship and direct treatment towards achieving arch alignment (Fig. 11.9).

Occasionally patients with more severe Class III incisor relationships are unconcerned about their malocclusion, particularly if the remainder of the family have a similar facial appearance. In this situation, and also where a patient is unwilling to undergo the fixed appliance treatment necessary to correct the incisor relationship, treatment can be limited to achieving alignment only.

Sometimes upper arch crowding results in the lateral incisors erupting palatally and the canines buccally. If the upper lateral incisors are markedly displaced then their extraction may make treatment more straightforward (Fig. 11.10). Some patients are happy to accept a smile with the canines adjacent to the central incisors. However, veneers can be used to make the canines resemble lateral incisors more closely.

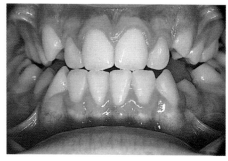

Fig. 11.9. Mild Class III case where it was decided to accept the incisor relationship and direct treatment towards alignment of the arches only.

11.4.2. Proclination of the upper labial segment

Correction of the incisor relationship by proclination of the upper incisors only can be considered in cases with the following features:

- a Class I or mild Class III skeletal pattern
- the upper incisors are not already significantly proclined
- an adequate overbite will be present at the end of treatment to retain the corrected position of the upper incisors, given that a reduction of overbite will occur as the incisors are tipped labially (see Section 11.3 and Fig. 11.6).

If indicated, this approach is often best carried out in the mixed dentition when the unerupted permanent canines are high above the roots of the upper lateral incisors (Fig. 11.11). Extraction of the lower deciduous canines at the same time may allow the lower labial segment to move lingually slightly, thereby aiding correction of the incisor relationship. Early correction of a Class III incisor relationship has the additional advantage that further forward mandibular growth may be counterbalanced by dento-alveolar compensation (Fig. 11.12).

Later in the mixed dentition, when the developing permanent canines drop down into a buccal position relative to the lateral incisor root, there may be a risk of resorption if the incisors are moved labially. In this situation correction is best deferred until the permanent canines have erupted.

Where the upper labial segment is mildly crowded, permanent extractions should be delayed until after the incisor relationship is corrected as proclination of the upper incisors will provide additional space. If the lower arch is at all crowded, consideration should be given to relieving the crowding by extractions as this will allow some lingual movement of the lower labial segment teeth.

Proclination of the upper labial segment can often be accomplished successfully with a removable appliance, particularly as buccal capping can be incorporated to free the occlusion with the lower arch. A screw type design is particularly useful in the mixed dentition as then the upper incisors can be utilized for retention of the appliance (see Chapter 16). Fixed appliances can also be

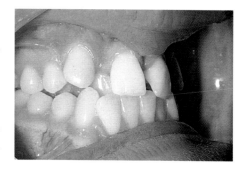

(a)

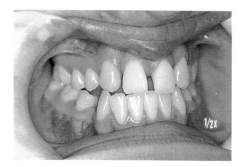

(b)

Fig. 11.10. Patient whose Class III malocclusion with marked upper arch crowding was managed by extraction of the palatally displaced upper lateral incisors and the lower first premolars: (a) prior to extractions; (b) 6 months after extractions and prior to fixed appliance therapy.

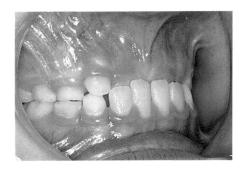 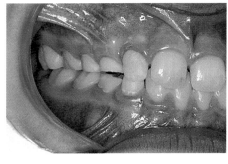

(a)   (b)

Fig. 11.11. Mild Class III malocclusion that was treated in the mixed dentition by proclination of the upper labial segment with a removable appliance: (a) pretreatment; (b) post-treatment.

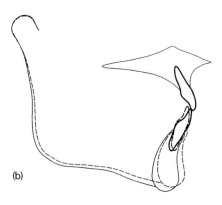

Fig. 11.12. (a) Forward growth rotation is the most common pattern of mandibular growth. In a Class III malocclusion this will lead to a worsening of the skeletal pattern and the incisor relationship. (b) If a Class III incisor relationship is corrected in the mixed dentition, dento-alveolar compensation may help to mask the effects of further growth provided that this is not marked.

used to advance the upper labial segment and are useful when other features of the malocclusion dictate their use.

11.4.3. Retroclination of the lower labial segment with or without proclination of the upper labial segment

In those cases with a mild to moderate Class III skeletal pattern, or where there is a reduced overbite, a combination of retroclination of the lower incisors and proclination of the upper incisors will achieve correction of the incisor relationship (see Fig. 11.8). Although the pitfalls of significant movement of the lower labial segment have been emphasized in earlier chapters, in the correction of Class III malocclusions the positions of the upper and lower incisors are changed around within the zone of soft tissue balance and, provided that there is an adequate overbite and further growth is not unfavourable, the corrected incisor relationship has a good chance of stability. Although removable and functional appliances can be used to advance the upper incisors and retrocline the lower incisors, in practice these tooth movements are accomplished more efficiently with fixed appliances.

Space is required in the lower arch for retroclination of the lower labial segment, and extractions are required unless the arch is spaced naturally. Use of a round archwire in the lower arch and a rectangular arch in the upper arch along with judicious space closure can be used to help correct the incisor relationship (Fig. 11.13).

Intermaxillary Class III elastic traction (see Chapter 15, Section 15.6.1) from the lower labial segment to the upper molars (Fig. 11.14) can also be used to help move the upper arch forwards and the lower arch backwards, but care is required to avoid extrusion of the molars which will reduce overbite.

Reverse-pull headgear, also known as a face-mask (Fig. 11.15), is used to apply an anteriorly directed force, via elastics, on the maxillary teeth and maxilla. Although some have claimed that this appliance can change the position of the maxilla, a very cooperative patient is necessary in view of the prolonged daily wear required, often over several years. Nevertheless, this technique is occasionally useful in the management of Class III malocclusions, particularly those associated with a cleft lip and palate anomaly, and also in cases of hypodontia where forward movement of the buccal segment teeth to close space is desirable.

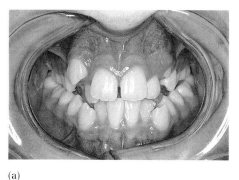

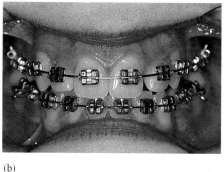

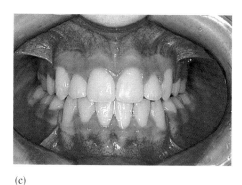

(a)   (b)   (c)

Fig. 11.13. Correction of a Class III malocclusion by retroclination of the lower incisors and proclination of the upper incisors using fixed appliances with relief of crowding by the extraction of all four first premolars: (a) pretreatment; (b) fixed appliances *in situ.* (note the use of rectangular archwire in the upper arch and a round wire in the lower arch during space closure to help achieve the desired movements); (c) post-treatment result.

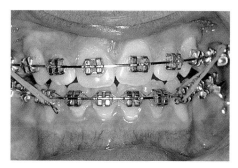

Fig. 11.14. Class III intermaxillary traction.

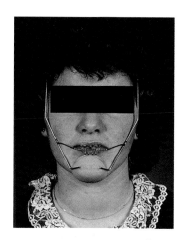

Fig. 11.15. Face-mask.

11.4.4. Surgery

In some cases the severity of the skeletal pattern and/or the presence of a reduced overbite or an anterior open bite precludes orthodontics alone, and surgery is necessary to correct the underlying skeletal discrepancy. It is impossible to produce hard and fast guidelines as to when to choose surgery rather than orthodontics, but it has been suggested that surgery is almost always required if the value for the ANB angle is below – 4° and the inclination of the lower incisors to the mandibular plane is less than 83°. However, the cepahalometric findings should be considered in conjunction with other features of the malocclusion and the patient's facial appearance.

For those patients where orthodontic treatment will be challenging owing to the severity of the skeletal pattern and/or a lack of overbite, a surgical approach should be explored before any permanent extractions are carried out, and preferably before any appliance treatment. The reason for this is that management of Class III malocclusions by orthodontics alone involves dento-alveolar compensation for the underlying skeletal pattern. However, in order to achieve a satisfactory occlusal and facial result with a surgical approach, any dento-alveolar compensation must first be removed or reduced (Fig. 11.16). For example, if

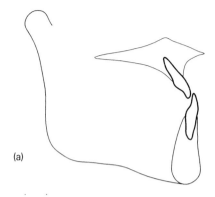
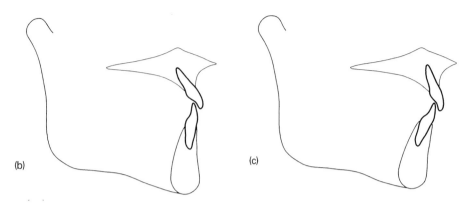

Fig. 11.16. (a) Severe Class III malocclusion with dento-alveolar compensation. (b) Without reduction of the dento-alveolar compensation, surgery to produce a Class I incisor relationship will only achieve a limited correction of the underlying skeletal pattern, thus constraining the overall aesthetic result. (c) Decompensation of the incisors to bring them nearer to their correct axial inclination allows a complete correction of the underlying skeletal pattern.

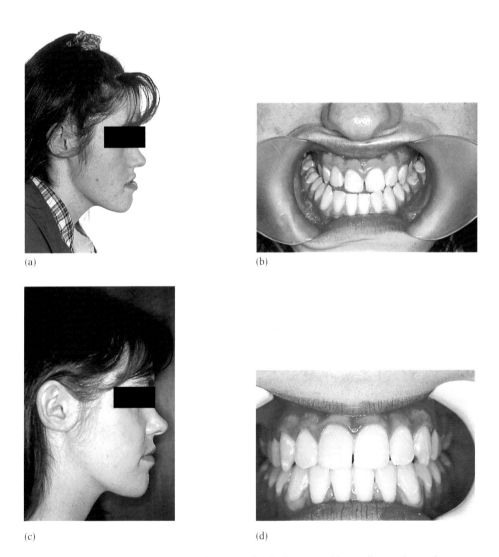

Fig. 11.17. Patient treated with a combination of orthodontics and bimaxillary orthognathic surgery: (a), (b) pretreatment; (c), (d) post-treatment.

lower premolars are extracted in an attempt to retract the lower labial segment but this fails and a surgical approach is subsequently necessary, the presurgical orthodontic phase will probably involve proclination of the incisors to a more average inclination with reopening of the extraction spaces. This is a frustrating experience for both patient and operator.

Some patients with marked skeletal III malocclusions are unwilling to wear appliances. Management by surgery alone is unsatisfactory as the resulting occlusion is poor, and in addition a full correction of the underlying skeletal problem is not possible without dento-alveolar decompensation. Therefore patients should be encouraged to undergo the appliance therapy necessary for the best result.

An example of a patient treated by a combination of orthodontics and surgery is shown in Fig. 11.17. Surgical approaches to the correction of Class III malocclusions are considered in Chapter 20.

PRINCIPAL SOURCES AND FURTHER READING

Battagel, J. M. (1993). Discriminant analysis: a model for the prediction of relapse in Class III children treated orthodontically by a non-extraction technique. *European Journal of Orthodontics*, **15**, 199–209.

Battagel, J. M. (1993). The aetiological factors in Class III malocclusion. *European Journal of Orthodontics*, **15**, 347–70.

Battagel, J. M. and Orton, H. S. (1993). Class III malocclusion: the post-retention findings following a non-extraction treatment approach. *European Journal of Orthodontics*, **15**, 45–55.

Bryant, P. M. F. (1981). Mandibular rotation and Class III malocclusion. *British Journal of Orthodontics*, **8**, 61–75.

● This paper is worth reading for the introduction alone, which contains a very good discussion of growth rotations. The study itself looks at the effect of growth rotations and treatment upon Class III malocclusions.

Dibbets, J. M. (1996). Morphological differences between the Angle classes. *European Journal of Orthodontics*, **18**, 111–18.

Gravely, J. F. (1984). A study of the mandibular closure path in Angle Class III relationship. *British Journal of Orthodontics*, **11**, 85–91.

● A very readable and clever article which examines the displacement element of Class III malocclusions.

Kerr, W. J. S. and Tenhave, T. R. (1988) A comparison of three appliance systems in the treatment of Class III malocclusion. *European Journal of Orthodontics*, **10**, 203–14.

Kerr, W. J. S., Miller, S., and Dawber, J. E. (1992). Class III malocclusion: surgery or orthodontics? *British Journal of Orthodontics*, **19**, 21–4.

● An interesting study which compares the pretreatment lateral cephalometric radiographs of two groups of Class III cases treated by either surgery or orthodontics alone. The authors report the thresholds for three cephalometric values which would indicate when surgery is required.

Kim, J. H. *et al.* (1999). The effectiveness of protraction face mask therapy: a meta-analysis. *American Journal of Orthodontics and Dentofacial Orthopedics*, **115**, 675–85.

12 Anterior open bite and posterior open bite

12.1. DEFINITIONS

- **Anterior open bite** (AOB): there is no vertical overlap of the incisors when the buccal segment teeth are in occlusion (Fig. 12.1).
- **Posterior open bite** (POB): when the teeth are in occlusion there is a space between the posterior teeth (Fig. 12.2).
- **Incomplete overbite**: the lower incisors do not occlude with the upper incisors or the palatal mucosa (Fig. 12.3). The overbite may be decreased or increased.

12.2. AETIOLOGY OF ANTERIOR OPEN BITE

In common with other types of malocclusion, both inherited and environmental factors are implicated in the aetiology of anterior open bite. These factors include skeletal pattern, soft tissues, habits, and localized failure of development. In many cases the aetiology is multifactorial, and in practice it can be difficult to determine the relative roles of these influences as the presenting malocclusion is similar. However, a thorough history and examination, perhaps with a period of observation, may be helpful.

12.2.1. Skeletal pattern

Individuals with a tendency to vertical rather than horizontal facial growth exhibit increased vertical skeletal proportions (see Chapter 4). Where the lower face height is increased there will be an increased inter-occlusal distance between the maxilla and mandible. Although the labial segment teeth appear to be able to compensate for this to a limited extent by further eruption, where the inter-occlusal distance exceeds this compensatory ability an anterior open bite will result. If the vertical, downwards, and backwards, pattern of growth continues, the anterior open bite will become more marked.

In this group of patients the anterior open bite is usually symmetrical and in the more severe cases may extend distally around the arch so that only the posterior molars are in contact when the patient is in maximal interdigitation (Fig. 12.4). The vertical devlopment of the labial segments results in typically extended alveolar processes when viewed on a lateral cephalometric radiograph (Fig. 12.5).

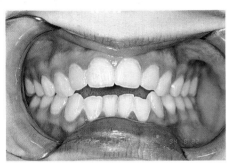

Fig. 12.1. Anterior open bite.

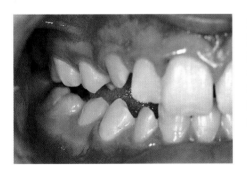

Fig. 12.2. Posterior open bite.

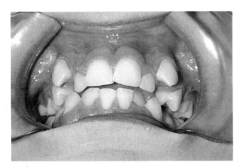

Fig. 12.3. Incomplete overbite.

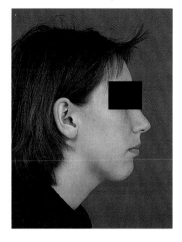

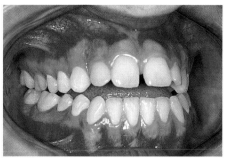

Fig. 12.4. Patient with increased vertical skeletal proportions and an anterior open bite.

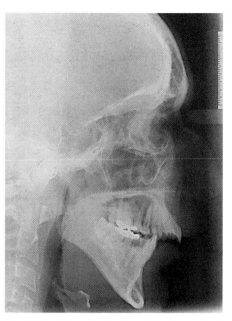

Fig. 12.5. Lateral cephalometric radiograph of a patient with a marked Class II division 1 malocclusion on a Class II skeletal pattern with increased vertical skeletal proportions. Note the thin dento-alveolar processes.

12.2.2. Soft tissue pattern

In order to be able to swallow it is necessary to create an anterior oral seal. In younger children the lips are often incompetent and a proportion will achieve an anterior seal by positioning their tongue forward between the anterior teeth during swallowing. Individuals with increased vertical skeletal proportions have an increased likelihood of incompetent lips and may continue to achieve an anterior oral seal in this manner even when the soft tissues have matured. This type of swallowing pattern is also seen in patients with an anterior open bite due to a digit-sucking habit (see Section 12.2.3). In these situations the behaviour of the tongue is adaptive. An endogenous or primary tongue thrust is rare, but it is difficult to distinguish it from an adaptive tongue thrust as the occlusal features are similar (Fig. 12.6). However, it has been suggested that an endogenous tongue thrust is associated with sigmatism (lisping), and in some cases the both the upper and lower incisors are proclined by the action of the tongue.

12.2.3. Habits

The effects of a habit depend upon its duration and intensity. If a persistent digit-sucking habit continues into the mixed and permanent dentitions, this can result in an anterior open bite due to restriction of development of the incisors by the finger or thumb (Fig. 12.7). Characteristically, the anterior open bite produced is asymmetrical (unless the patient sucks two fingers) and it is often associated with a posterior crossbite. Constriction of the upper arch is believed to be caused by cheek pressure and a low tongue position.

After a sucking habit stops the open bite tends to resolve, although this may take several years. During this period the tongue may come forward during swallowing to achieve an anterior seal. In a small proportion of cases where the habit has continued until growth is complete the open bite may persist.

12.2.4. Localized failure of development

This is seen in patients with a cleft of the lip and alveolus (Fig. 12.8), although rarely it may occur for no apparent reason.

12.2.5. Mouth breathing

It has been suggested that the open-mouth posture adopted by individuals who habitually mouthbreathe, either due to nasal obstruction or habit, results in

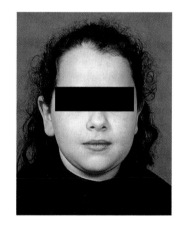

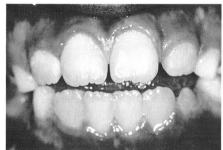

Fig. 12.6. Patient with an anterior open bite which was believed to be due to an endogenous tongue thrust. Despite the lips being competent, the tongue was thrust forward between the incisors during swallowing. Both upper and lower incisors were proclined. The patient did not have a digit-sucking habit.

Fig. 12.7. The occlusal effects of a persistent digit-sucking habit. Note the anterior open bite and the unilateral posterior crossbite.

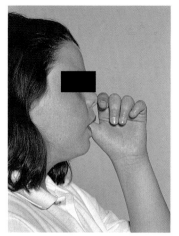
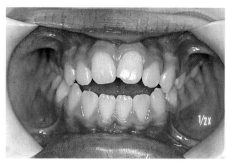

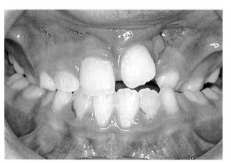

Fig. 12.8. A patient with a repaired cleft involving the lip and palate showing typical localized limitation of vertical development in the region of the cleft alveolus.

overdevelopment of the buccal segment teeth. This leads to an increase in the height of the lower third of the face and consequently a greater incidence of anterior open bite. In support of this it has been shown that patients referred for tonsillectomy and adenoidectomy had significantly increased lower facial heights compared with controls, and that post-operatively the disparity between the two groups diminished. However, the differences demonstrated were small. Other workers have shown that children referred to ear, nose, and throat clinics exhibit the same range of malocclusions as the normal population, and no relationship has been demonstrated between nasal airway resistance and skeletal pattern in normal individuals.

On balance, it would appear that mouthbreathing *per se* does not play a significant role in the development of anterior open bite in most patients.

12.3. MANAGEMENT OF ANTERIOR OPEN BITE

Notwithstanding the difficulties faced in determining aetiology, treatment of anterior open bite is one of the more challenging aspects of orthodontics. Management of an anterior open bite due purely to a digit-sucking habit can be straightforward, but where the skeletal pattern, growth, and/or soft tissue environment are unfavourable, correction without resort to orthognathic surgery may not be possible.

In the mixed dentition, a digit-sucking habit that has resulted in an anterior open bite should be gently discouraged. If a child is keen to stop, a removable appliance can be fitted to act as a reminder. However, if the child derives support from his habit, forcing him to wear an appliance to discourage it is unlikely to be successful. Although a number of barbaric designs have been described (involving wire projections for example), a simple plate with a long labial bow for anterior retention will usually suffice if a habit-breaker is indicated. After fitting, the acrylic behind the upper incisors should be trimmed to allow any spontaneous alignment. Once the permanent dentition is established, more active steps can be taken, although this can often be combined with treatment for other aspects of the malocclusion.

A period of observation may be helpful in the management of patients with an anterior open bite which is not associated with a digit-sucking habit. In some cases an anterior open bite may reduce spontaneously, possibly because of maturation of the soft tissues and improved lip competence, or favourable growth.

Skeletal open bites with increased vertical proportions are often associated with a downward and backward rotation of the mandible with growth. Obviously, if growth is unfavourable, it is better to know this before planning treatment rather than experiencing difficulties once treatment is under way.

Previously, it was thought that extracting molars in cases with increased vertical skeletal proportions would help to 'close down the bite'. However, this was not based on scientific evidence.

12.3.1. Approaches to the management of anterior open bite

There are three possible approaches to management.

Acceptance of the anterior open bite

In this case treatment is aimed at relief of any crowding and alignment of the arches. This approach can be considered in the following situations (particularly if the AOB does not present a problem to the patient):

- mild cases;
- where the soft tissue environment is not favourable, for example where the lips are markedly incompetent and/or an endogenous tongue thrust is suspected;
- in more marked malocclusions where the patient is not motivated towards surgery.

Orthodontic correction of the anterior open bite

If growth and the soft tissue environment are favourable, an orthodontic solution to the anterior open bite can be considered. A careful assessment should be carried out, including the anteroposterior and vertical skeletal pattern, the feasibility of the tooth movements required, and post-treatment stability.

Extrusion of the incisors to close an anterior open bite is inadvisable, as the condition will relapse once the appliances are removed. Rather, treatment should aim to try and intrude the molars, or at least control their vertical development. Intrusion of the molars can be attempted with high-pull headgear and/or by using buccal capping on a removable appliance.

In the milder malocclusions the use of high-pull headgear during conventional treatment may suffice. In cases with a more marked anterior open bite associated with a Class II skeletal pattern, a removable appliance or a functional appliance incorporating buccal blocks and high-pull headgear can be used to try to restrain vertical maxillary growth. In order to achieve true growth modification it is necessary to apply an intrusive force to the maxilla for at least 14–16 hours per day during the pubertal growth spurt, continuing until growth is complete. This is only achievable with excellent patient cooperation and favourable growth. The maxillary intrusion splint and the buccal intrusion splint are removable appliances which were developed by Orton and are now widely adopted. The maxillary intrusion splint incorporates acrylic coverage of all the teeth in the upper arch and high-pull headgear (Fig. 12.9). The buccal intrusion splint is similar, except that only the buccal segment teeth are capped. Functional appliances used for Class II malocclusions with increased vertical proportions include the twin-block appliance (Fig. 12.10) and the van Beek appliance (Fig. 12.11). Both incorporate high-pull headgear and buccal capping. In many cases fixed appliances are then used to complete arch alignment, together with extractions if indicated.

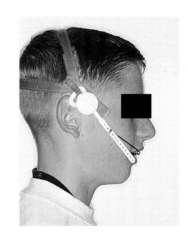

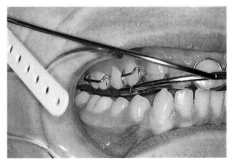

Fig. 12.9. A patient wearing a maxillary intrusion splint and high-pull headgear. The face-bow of the headgear slots into tubes embedded in the acrylic of the occlusal capping, which extends to cover all the maxillary teeth.

Fig. 12.10. Upper and lower twin-blocks.

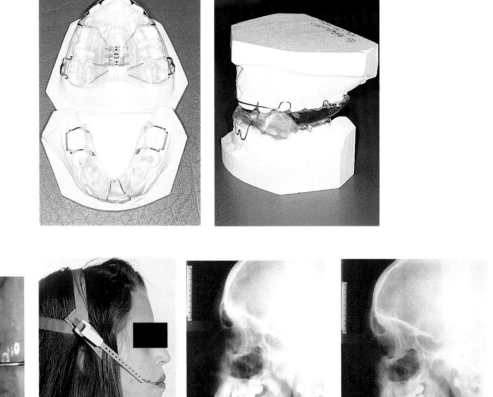

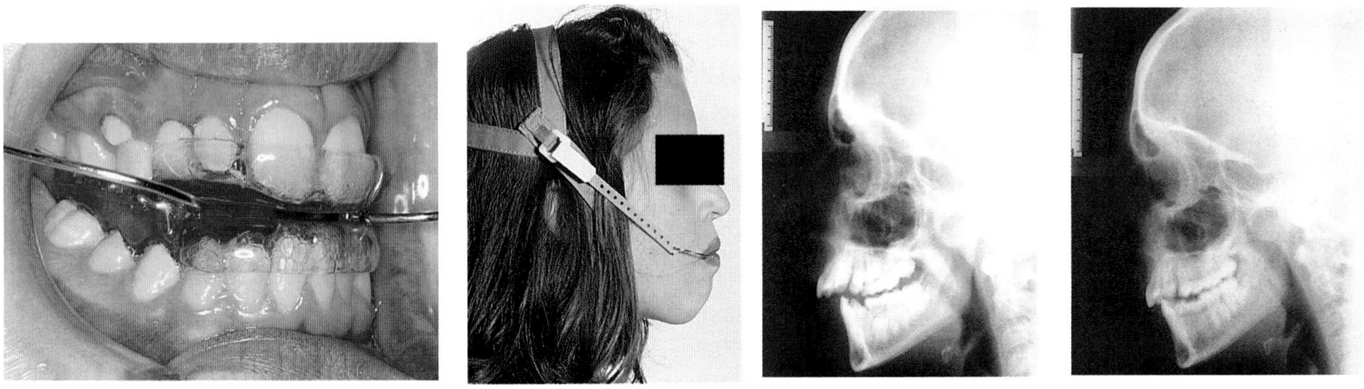

(a)   (b)   (c)   (d)

Fig. 12.11. (a) Intra-oral view of a van Beek appliance; (b) extra-oral view showing the high-pull headgear; (c) lateral cephalometric radiograph of the patient prior to treatment; (d) lateral cephalometric radiograph of the same patient 1 year later.

In cases with bimaxillary crowding and proclination, relief of crowding and alignment of the incisors can result in reduction of an open bite (Fig. 12.12). Stability of this correction is more likely if the lips were incompetent prior to treatment but become competent following retroclination of the incisors.

If it is difficult to ascertain the exact aetiology of an anterior open bite but a primary tongue thrust is suspected, even though these are uncommon, it is wise to err on the side of caution regarding treatment objectives and to warn patients of the possibility of relapse.

Surgery

This option can be considered once growth is complete for severe problems with a skeletal aetiology and/or where dental compensation will not give an aesthetic or stable result. In some patients an anterior open bite is associated with a 'gummy' smile which can be difficult to reduce by orthodontics alone necessitating a surgical approach. The assessment and management of such cases is discussed in Chapter 20.

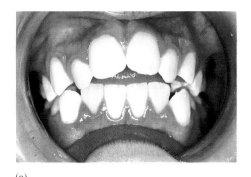
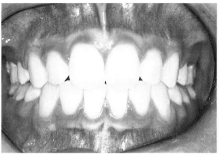

(a)   (b)

Fig. 12.12. Patient with an anterior open bite treated by extraction of all four first premolars to relieve crowding and fixed appliances: (a) pretreatment; (b) post-retention.

12.3.2. Management of patients with increased vertical skeletal proportions and reduced overbite

The specifics of treatment of patients with increased vertical skeletal proportions will obviously be influenced by the other aspects of their malocclusion (see appropriate chapters), but management requires careful planning to try and prevent an iatrogenic deterioration of the vertical excess. The following points should be borne in mind:

- Space closure appears to occur more readily in patients with increased vertical skeletal proportions.

- Avoid extruding the molars as this will result in an increase of the lower facial height. If headgear is required, a direction of pull above the occlusal plane is necessary, i.e. high-pull headgear. Cervical-pull headgear is contraindicated.

- If overbite reduction is required, this should be achieved by intrusion of the incisors rather than extrusion of the molars. For this reason anterior bite-planes should be avoided.

- Avoid upper arch expansion. When the upper arch is expanded the upper molars are tilted buccally which results in the palatal cusps being tipped downwards. If arch expansion is required, this is best achieved using a fixed appliance so that buccal root torque can be used to limit tipping downwards of the palatal cusps.

- Avoid Class II or Class III intermaxillary traction as this may extrude the molars.

12.4. POSTERIOR OPEN BITE

Posterior open bite occurs more rarely than anterior open bite and the aetiology is less well understood. In some cases an increase in the vertical skeletal proportions is a factor, although this is more commonly associated with an anterior open bite which also extends posteriorly. A lateral open bite is occasionally seen in association with early extraction of first permanent molars (Fig. 12.13), possibly occurring as a result of lateral tongue spread.

Posterior open bite is also seen in cases with submergence of buccal segment teeth. Submergence of deciduous molars is discussed in Chapter 3. There are two rare conditions which affect the eruption of the permanent buccal segment teeth:

- **Primary failure of eruption**: this condition almost exclusively affects molar teeth and is of unknown aetiology. Although bone resorption above the unerupted tooth proceeds normally, the tooth itself appears to lack any eruptive potential (Fig. 12.14). Extraction is the only treatment alternative. The aetiology is not understood.

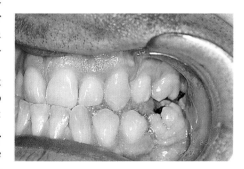

Fig. 12.13. Posterior open bite in a patient who had all four first permanent molars extracted in the mixed dentition.

Fig. 12.14. DPT radiographs showing failure of eruption of the upper left first permanent molar.

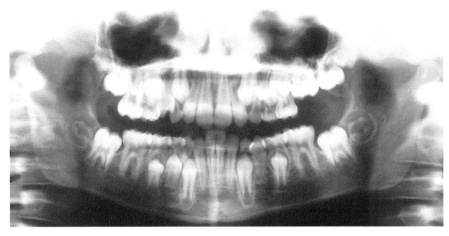

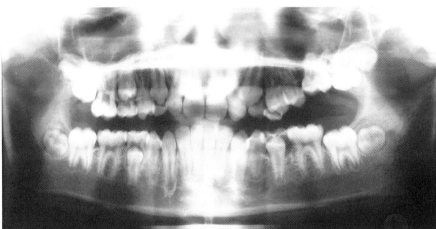

Fig. 12.15. DPT radiograph showing arrest of eruption of the lower left first permanent molar.

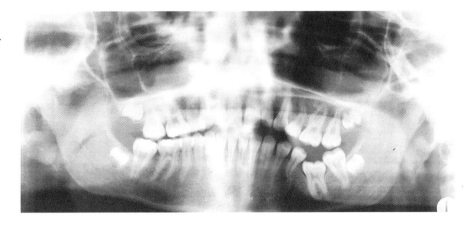

- **Arrest of eruption**: this also usually involves molar teeth. Affected teeth appear to erupt normally into occlusion, but then subsequently fail to keep pace with occlusal development. As growth of the rest of the dentition and alveolar processes continues, lack of movement of the affected tooth or teeth results in relative submergence (Fig. 12.15). The aetiology is not understood and again the usual treatment is extraction of the affected tooth or teeth.

More rarely, posterior open bite is seen in association with unilateral condylar hyperplasia, which also results in facial asymmetry. If this problem is suspected, a bone scan will be required. If the scan indicates excessive cell division in the condylar head region, a condylectomy alone, or in combination with surgery to correct the resultant deformity, may be required.

PRINCIPAL SOURCES AND FURTHER READING

Chate, R. A. C. (1994). The burden of proof: a critical review of orthodontic claims made by some general practitioners. *American Journal of Orthodontics and Dentofacial Orthopedics*, **106**, 96–105.
● An excellent discussion of the evidence on the postulated and actual effects of mouth breathing upon the dentition, plus much other information. Highly recommended.
Di Biase, D. (1992). The management of open bite. *Dental Practice*, November, 11–14.
● An excellent and very readable account of the aetiology and management of anterior open bite.
Linder-Aronson, S. (1970). Adenoids: their effect on mode of breathing and nasal airflow and their relationship to characteristics of the facial skeleton and dentition. *Acta Otolaryngologica (Supplement)*, **265**, 1.
Lopez-Gavito, G., Wallen, T. R., Little, R. M., and Joondeph, D. R. (1985). Anterior openbite malocclusion: a longitudinal 10-year postretention evaluation of orthodontically treated patients. *American Journal of Orthodontics*, **87**, 175–86.
Mizrahi, E. (1978). A review of anterior open bite. *British Journal of Orthodontics*, **5**, 21–7.
● A worthy review.
Oliver, R. G. (1980). Submerged permanent molars: four case reports. *British Dental Journal*, **160**, 128–30.
● The cases reported are classified into primary failure of eruption and arrest of eruption. The management of these two conditions is discussed.
Orton, H. S. (1990). *Functional appliances in orthodontic treatment*. Quintessence Books, London.
● A beautifully illustrated and informative book. The maxillary and buccal intrusion splints are described.
Vaden, J. L. (1998). Non-surgical treatment of the patient with vertical discrepancy. *American Journal of Orthodontics and Dentofacial Orthopedics*, **113**, 567–82.

13 Crossbites

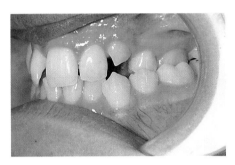

Fig. 13.1. A buccal crossbite.

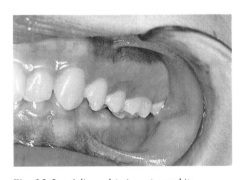

Fig. 13.2. A lingual (scissors) crossbite.

13.1. DEFINITIONS

- **Crossbite**: a discrepancy in the buccolingual relationship of the upper and lower teeth.

By convention the transverse relationship of the arches is described in terms of the position of the lower teeth relative to the upper teeth.

- **Buccal crossbite**: the buccal cusps of the lower teeth occlude buccal to the buccal cusps of the upper teeth (Fig. 13.1).
- **Lingual crossbite**: the buccal cusps of the lower teeth occlude lingual to the lingual cusps of the upper teeth. This is also known as a **scissors bite** (Fig. 13.2).
- **Displacement**: on closing from the rest position the mandible encounters a deflecting contact(s) and is displaced to the left or the right, and/or anteriorly, into maximum interdigitation (Fig. 13.3).

13.2. AETIOLOGY

A variety of factors acting either singly or in combination can lead to the development of a crossbite.

13.2.1. Local causes

The most common local cause is crowding where one or two teeth are displaced from the arch. For example, a crossbite of an upper lateral incisor often arises owing to lack of space between the upper central incisor and the deciduous canine, which forces the lateral incisor to erupt palatally and in linguo-occlusion with the opposing teeth. Posteriorly, early loss of a second deciduous molar in a crowded mouth may result in forward movement of the first permanent molar, forcing the second premolar to erupt palatally. Also, retention of a primary tooth can deflect the eruption of the permanent successor leading to a crossbite.

Fig. 13.3. Displacement on closure into crossbite.

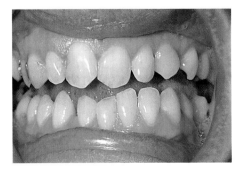
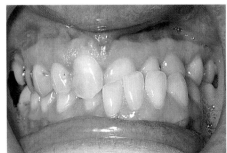

13.2.2. Skeletal

Generally, the greater the number of teeth in crossbite, the greater is the skeletal component of the aetiology. A crossbite of the buccal segments may be due purely to a mismatch in the relative width of the arches, or to an anteroposterior discrepancy, which results in a wider part of one arch occluding with a narrower part of the opposing jaw. For this reason buccal crossbites of an entire buccal segment are most commonly associated with Class III malocclusions (Fig. 13.4), and lingual crossbites are associated with Class II malocclusions. Anterior crossbites are associated with Class III skeletal patterns.

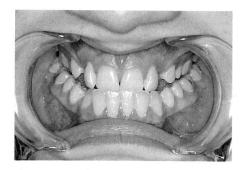

Fig. 13.4. A Class III malocclusion with buccal crossbite.

13.2.3. Soft tissues

A posterior crossbite is often associated with a digit-sucking habit, as the position of the tongue is lowered and a negative pressure is generated intra-orally.

13.2.4. Rarer causes

These include cleft lip and palate, where growth in the width of the upper arch is restrained by the scar tissue of the cleft repair. Trauma to, or pathology of, the temporomandibular joints can lead to restriction of growth of the mandible on one side, leading to asymmetry.

13.3. TYPES OF CROSSBITE

13.3.1. Anterior crossbite

An anterior crossbite is present when one or more of the upper incisors is in linguo-occlusion (i.e. in reverse overjet) relative to the lower arch (Fig. 13.5). Anterior crossbites involving only one or two incisors are considered in this chapter, whereas management of more than two incisors in crossbite is considered in Chapter 11 on Class III malocclusions. Anterior crossbites are frequently associated with displacement on closure (see Fig. 13.3).

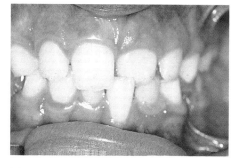

(a)

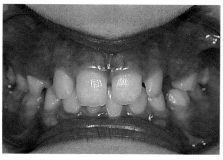

(b)

Fig. 13.5. Correction of an anterior crossbite. Using a removable appliance: (a) pretreatment. (note the gingival recession of the lower incisor in crossbite); (b) post-treatment.

13.3.2. Posterior crossbites

Crossbites of the premolar and molar region involving one or two teeth or an entire buccal segment can be subdivided as follows.

Unilateral buccal crossbite with displacement

This type of crossbite can affect only one or two teeth per quadrant, or the whole of the buccal segment. When a single tooth is affected, the problem usually arises because of the displacement of one or both teeth from the arch, leading to a deflecting contact on closure into the crossbite.

When the whole of the buccal segment is involved, the underlying aetiology is usually that the maxillary arch is of a similar width to the mandibular arch (i.e. it is too narrow) with the result that on closure from the rest position the buccal segment teeth meet cusp to cusp. In order to achieve a more comfortable and efficient intercuspation, the patient displaces their mandible to the left or right (see Chapter 5, Fig. 5.12). It is often difficult to detect this displacement on

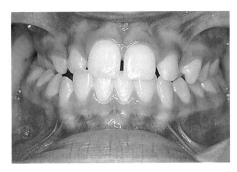

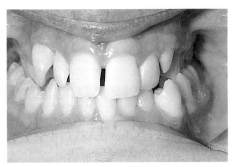

Fig. 13.6. A unilateral crossbite with associated centreline shift.

Fig. 13.7. A bilateral buccal crossbite.

closure as the patient soon learns to close straight into the position of maximal interdigitation. This type of crossbite may be associated with a centreline shift in the lower arch in the direction of the mandibular displacement (Fig. 13.6).

Unilateral buccal crossbite with no displacement

This category of crossbite is less common. It can arise as a result of deflection of two (or more) opposing teeth during eruption, but the greater the number of teeth in a segment that are involved, the greater is the likelihood that there is an underlying skeletal asymmetry.

Bilateral buccal crossbite

Bilateral crossbites (Fig. 13.7) are more likely to be associated with a skeletal discrepancy, either in the anteroposterior or transverse dimension, or in both.

Unilateral lingual crossbite

This type of crossbite is most commonly due to displacement of an individual tooth as a result of crowding or retention of the deciduous predecessor.

Bilateral lingual crossbite (scissors bite)

Again, this crossbite is typically associated with an underlying skeletal discrepancy, often a Class II malocclusion with the upper arch further forward relative to the lower so that the lower buccal teeth occlude with a wider segment of the upper arch.

13.4. MANAGEMENT

13.4.1. Rationale for treatment

Research has shown that displacing contacts *may* predispose towards temporomandibular joint dysfunction syndrome in a *susceptible* individual (see Chapter 1,

Section 1.7). Therefore a crossbite associated with a displacement is a functional indication for orthodontic treatment. Similarly, treatment for a bilateral crossbite without displacement should be approached with caution, as partial relapse may result in a unilateral crossbite with displacement. In addition, a bilateral crossbite is probably as efficient for chewing as the normal buccolingual relationship of the teeth. However, the same cannot be said of a lingual crossbite where the cusps of affected teeth do not meet together at all.

Anterior crossbites, as well as being frequently associated with displacement, can lead to movement of a lower incisor labially through the labial supporting tissues, resulting in gingival recession. In this case early treatment is advisable (see Fig. 13.5).

13.4.2. Treatment of anterior crossbite

The following factors should be considered:

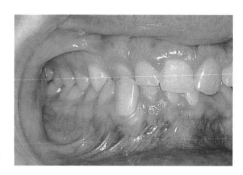

(a)

- What type of movement is required? If tipping movements will suffice, a removable appliance can be considered, however, if bodily or apical movement is required then fixed appliances are indicated.
- How much overbite is expected at the end of treatment? For treatment to be successful there must be some overbite present to retain the corrected incisor position. However, when planning treatment it should be remembered that proclination of an upper incisor will result in a reduction of overbite compared with the pretreatment position.
- Is there space available within the arch to accommodate the tooth/teeth to be moved? If not, are extractions required and if so which teeth?
- Is movement of the opposing tooth/teeth required? If reciprocal movement is required, a fixed appliance is indicated.

Provided that there is sufficient overbite and tilting movements will suffice, treatment can often be accomplished with a removable appliance. The appliance should incorporate the following features:

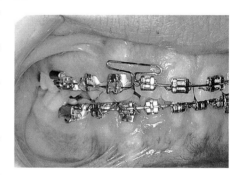

(b)

- good anterior retention to counteract the displacing effect of the active element (where two or more teeth are to be proclined, a screw appliance may circumvent this problem);
- buccal capping just thick enough to free the occlusion with the opposing arch (if the overbite is significantly increased a flat anterior bite-plane may be utilized instead);
- an active element, for example a Z-spring (see Chapter 16).
  Fixed appliances are indicated in the following cases:
- The apex of the incisor in crossbite is palatally positioned.
- If there will be insufficient overbite to retain the corrected incisor(s), consideration should be given to using fixed appliances to move the lower incisor(s) lingually at the same time as the upper incisor(s) is moved labially in order to try and increase overbite.
- Other features of a malocclusion necessitate the use of fixed appliances (Fig. 13.8).

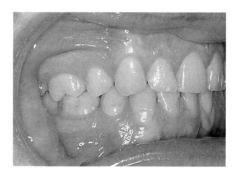

(c)

Fig. 13.8. A patient with a crossbite of the permanent canines on the right side who was treated by extraction of all four second premolars and fixed appliances:
(a) pretreatment; (b) fixed appliances;
(c) post-treatment.

If the upper arch is crowded, the upper lateral incisor often erupts in a palatal position relative to the arch. If the lateral incisor is markedly bodily displaced, relief of crowding by extraction of the displaced tooth itself may sometimes be an option, but it is wise to seek a specialist opinion before taking this step.

13.4.3. Treatment of posterior crossbite

It is important to consider the aetiology of this feature before embarking on treatment. For example, is the crossbite due to displacement of one tooth from the arch, in which case correction will involve aligning this tooth, or is reciprocal movement of two or more opposing teeth required? Also, if there is a skeletal component, will it be possible to compensate for this by tooth movement? The inclination of the affected teeth should also be evaluated. Upper arch expansion is more likely to be stable if the teeth to be moved were tilted palatally initially. As expansion will create additional space, it may be advisable to defer a decision regarding extractions until after the expansion phase has been completed.

Even when fixed appliances are used, expansion of the upper buccal segment teeth will result in some tipping down of the palatal cusps (Fig. 13.9). This has the effect of hinging the mandible downwards leading to an increase in lower face height, which may be undesirable in patients who already have an increased lower facial height and/or reduced overbite. If expansion is indicated in these

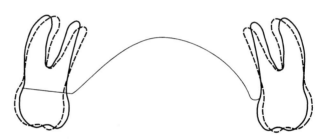

Fig. 13.9. Expansion of the upper arch results in the palatal cusps of the buccal segment teeth swinging down occlusally.

patients, fixed appliances are required to apply buccal root torque to the buccal segment teeth in order to try and resist this tendency, perhaps with high-pull headgear as well.

Unilateral buccal crossbite

Where this problem has arisen owing to the displacement of one tooth from the arch, for example an upper premolar tooth which has been crowded palatally, treatment will involve movement of the displaced tooth into the line of the arch, relieving crowding where and if necessary. If the displacement is marked, consideration can be given to extracting the displaced tooth itself or using fixed appliances to try and achieve bodily movement. Mild displacement of an upper premolar palatally can often be corrected using a T-spring on a removable appliance, but a screw type of appliance is preferable if buccal movement of a molar is required.

If correction of a crossbite requires movement of the opposing teeth in opposite directions, this can be achieved by the use of cross elastics (Fig. 13.10) attached to bands or bonded brackets on the teeth involved. If this is the only feature of a malocclusion requiring treatment, it is wise to leave the attachments *in situ* following correction, stopping the elastics for a month to review whether the corrected position is stable. If the crossbite relapses, the cross elastics can be re-instituted and an alternative means of retention considered.

A unilateral crossbite involving all the teeth in the buccal segment is usually associated with a displacement, and treatment is directed towards expanding the upper arch so that it fits around the lower arch at the end of treatment. If the

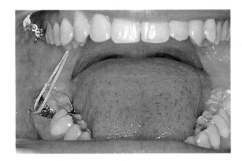

Fig. 13.10. Cross elastics.

upper buccal teeth are not already tilted buccally, this can be accomplished with an upper removable appliance incorporating a midline screw and buccal capping. Alternatively, a quadhelix appliance can be used (see below). As a degree of relapse can be anticipated, some overexpansion of the upper arch is advisable, but not to the degree where a lingual crossbite or fenestration of the buccal peri-odontal support results. Retention should be continued for approximately 3 months full time followed by 3 months nights only with the removable appliance, and the quadhelix should be made passive and recemented as a retainer for 3 to 6 months.

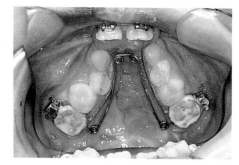

Fig. 13.11. Expansion of a repaired cleft maxilla with a quadhelix appliance.

Bilateral buccal crossbite

Unless the upper buccal segment teeth are tilted palatally to a significant degree, bilateral buccal crossbites are usually accepted. Rapid maxillary expansion can be used to try and expand the maxillary basal bone, but even with this technique a degree of relapse in the buccopalatal tooth position occurs following treatment, with the risk of development of a unilateral crossbite with displacement.

Bilateral buccal crossbites are common in patients with a repaired cleft of the palate. Expansion of the upper arch by stretching of the scar tissue is often indicated in these cases (see Chapter 21) and is readily achieved using a quadhelix appliance (Fig. 13.11).

Lingual crossbite

If a single tooth is affected, this is often the result of displacement due to crowding. If extraction of the displaced tooth itself is not indicated to relieve crowding, then pro-vided that space can be made available it is often possible to use an upper remov-able appliance to free the occlusion with the lower arch and move the affected upper tooth palatally with a buccal spring. More severe cases with a greater skeletal element usually need a combination of buccal movement of the affected lower teeth and palatal movement of the upper teeth with fixed appliances. Treatment is not straightforward and should only be tackled by the experienced orthodontist, partic-ularly as a scissors bite will often dislodge fixed attachments on the buccal aspect of the lower teeth until the crossbite is eliminated.

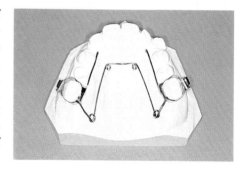

Fig.13.12. A quadhelix appliance.

13.4.4. The quadhelix appliance

The quadhelix is a very efficient fixed slow expansion appliance (Fig. 13.12). The quadhelix appliance can also be adjusted to give more expansion anteriorly or posteriorly as required, and when active treatment is complete it can be made passive and recemented to act as a retainer.

A quadhelix is fabricated in 1 mm stainless steel wire and attached to the teeth by bands cemented to a molar tooth on each side. Preformed types are available which slot into palatal attachments welded onto bands on the molars and can be readily removed by the operator for adjustment. However, the appliance can also be custom-made in a laboratory. The usual activation is about half a tooth width each side. Overexpansion can occur readily if the appliance is overactivated, and there-fore its use should be limited to those who are experienced with fixed appliances.

13.4.5. Rapid maxillary expansion

This upper appliance incorporates a screw similar to the type used for expansion in removable appliances except that it is soldered to bands, usually to both a pre-molar and molar tooth on both sides. The screw is turned twice daily, usually

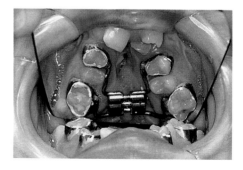

Fig.13.13. A rapid maxillary expansion appliance being used to expand a repaired cleft maxilla.

over an active treatment period of 2 weeks (Fig. 13.13). The large force generated is designed to open the midline suture and expand the upper arch by skeletal expansion rather than by movement of the teeth. For this reason its use is really limited to patients in their early teens before the suture fuses, or cleft palate patients where it can be utilized to expand the cleft segments by stretching the scar tissue.

Once expansion is complete the appliance is left *in situ* as a retainer, usually for several months. Bony infill of the expanded suture has been demonstrated but on removing the appliance approximately 50 per cent relapse due to soft tissue pressures can be anticipated, and for this reason some overexpansion is indicated.

This appliance should only be used by the experienced.

13.5. CLINICAL EFFECTIVENESS

The management of posterior crossbites is one of the few areas in orthodontics, which has been the subject of a systematic review. This process involves studying all the available literature on a subject and selecting only those randomized, controlled clinical trails, which have been carried out to the highest scientific standards (with no bias, adequate sample size, etc.). Disappointingly, only a few studies were suitable for inclusion. The authors concluded that removal of premature contacts of the deciduous teeth is effective in preventing a posterior crossbite being perpetuated into the mixed dentition. In those cases where it is not effective, an upper removable appliance can be used to expand the upper arch to reduce the risk of the crossbite continuing into the permanent dentition. The paucity of good quality research in this area meant that clear recommendations could not be made regarding treatment in the late mixed and permanent dentition. This does not mean that the management approaches discussed above are wrong. In fact they reflect currently accepted good practice, but further studies with appropriate sample sizes and methodology are required.

PRINCIPAL SOURCES AND FURTHER READING

Birnie, D. J. and McNamara, T. G. (1980). The quadhelix appliance. *British Journal of Orthodontics*, **7**, 115–20.
- The fabrication, management, and modifications of the quadhelix appliance are described in this paper.

Harrison, J. E. and Ashby, D. (1998). *Orthodontic treatment for posterior crossbites (Cocrane Review)*, The Cochrane Library, Issue 4. Update Software, Oxford.
- This is a systematic review of the effectiveness of different treatment modalities used in the correction of a posterior crossbite. Well worth the trouble taken to find it (try the Cochrane Collaboration on the Internet http://www.cochrane-oral.man.ac.uk)

Hermanson, H., Kurol, J., and Ronnerman, A. (1985). Treatment of unilateral posterior crossbites with quadhelix and removable plates. A retrospective study. *European Journal of Orthodontics*, **7**, 97–102.
- In this study it was found that the clinical results achieved were similar with the two types of appliance. However, the number of visits and chairside time were greater for the removable appliance. The authors calculated that the mean cost of treatment was 40 per cent greater for the removable appliance compared with the quadhelix.

Linder-Aronson, S. and Lindgren, J. (1979). The skeletal and dental effects of rapid maxillary expansion. *British Journal of Orthodontics*, **6**, 25–9.

14 Canines

14.1. FACTS AND FIGURES

Development of the upper and lower canines commences between 4 and 5 months of age. The upper canines erupt, on average, at 11–12 years of age. The lower canines erupt, on average, at 10–11 years of age.

In a Caucasian population (Gorlin *et al.* 1990): congenital absence of upper canines, 0.3 per cent; congenital absence of lower canines, 0.1 per cent; impaction of upper canines, 1–2 per cent, of which 8 per cent are bilateral; impaction of lower canines, 0.35 per cent; resorption of upper incisors due to impacted canine, 0.7 per cent of 10–13 year olds; transposition, exact prevalence not known (rare).

14.2. NORMAL DEVELOPMENT

The development of the maxillary canine commences around 4 to 5 months of age, high in the maxilla. Crown calcifiation is complete around 6 to 7 years of age. The permanent canine then migrates forwards and downwards to lie buccal and mesial to the apex of the deciduous canine before erupting down the distal aspect of the root of the upper lateral incisor. Pressure from the unerupted canine on the root of the lateral incisor leads to flaring of the incisor crowns, which resolves as the canine erupts.

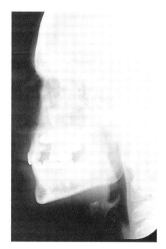

Fig. 14.1. Horizontally displaced maxillary canines.

14.3. AETIOLOGY OF MAXILLARY CANINE DISPLACEMENT

Canine displacement is generally classified into buccal or palatal displacement. More rarely, canines can be found lying horizontally above the apices of the teeth of the upper arch (Fig. 14.1) or displaced high adjacent to the nose (Fig. 14.2).

The following have been suggested as possible causative factors. However, the aetiology of canine displacement is still not fully understood.

- **Displacement of the crypt.** This is the probable aetiology behind the more marked displacements such as those shown in Figs 14.1 and 14.2.
- **Long path of eruption.**
- **Short-rooted or absent upper lateral incisor.** A 2.4-fold increase in the incidence of palatally displaced canines in patients with absent or short-rooted lateral incisors has been reported (Becker *et al.* 1981) (Fig. 14.3). It has been suggested that a lack of guidance during eruption is the reason behind this association. Because of the association of palatal displacement of an upper canine with missing or peg-shaped lateral incisors it is important to be particularly observant in patients with this anomaly.

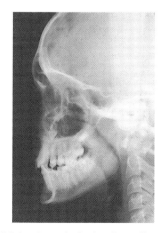

Fig. 14.2. Severely displaced maxillary canine.

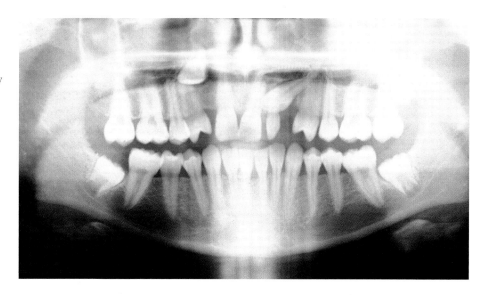

Fig. 14.3. DPT radiograph of patient with an absent upper right lateral incisor, a peg-shaped upper left lateral incisor, and displaced maxillary canines.

● **Crowding.** Jacoby (1983) found that 85 per cent of buccally displaced canines were associated with crowding, whereas 83 per cent of palatal displacements had sufficient space for eruption. If the upper arch is crowded, this often manifests as insufficient space for the canine, which is the last tooth anterior to the molar to erupt. In normal development the canine comes to lie buccal to the arch and in the presence of crowding will be deflected buccally.

● **Retention of the primary deciduous canine.** This usually results in mild displacement of the permanent tooth buccally. However, if the permanent canine itself is displaced, normal resorption of the deciduous canine will not occur. In this situation the retained deciduous tooth is an indicator, rather than the cause, of displacement.

● **Genetic factors.** It has been suggested that palatal displacement of the maxillary canine is an inherited trait with a pattern that suggests polygenic inheritance. The evidence cited for this includes:

  (a) the prevalence varies in different populations with a greater prevalence in Europeans than other racial groups;
  (b) affects females more commonly than males;
  (c) familial occurrence;
  (d) occurs bilaterally with a greater than expected frequency;
  (e) occurs in association with other dental anomalies (e.g. hypodontia, microdontia).

14.4. INTERCEPTION OF DISPLACED CANINES

Because of their high propensity for ectopic eruption, it is essential to palpate for unerupted canines when examining any child aged 9 years and older, as early detection of an abnormal eruption path gives the opportunity, if appropriate, for interceptive measures. It is also important to locate the position of the canines before undertaking the extraction of other permanent teeth. Canines, which are palpable in the normal developmental postion, buccal and slightly distal to the upper lateral incisor root, have a good prognosis for eruption.

Clinically, if a definite hollow and/or asymmetry is found on palpation, further investigation is warranted. On occasion, routine panoramic radiographic examination may demonstrate asymmetry in the position and development of the canines.

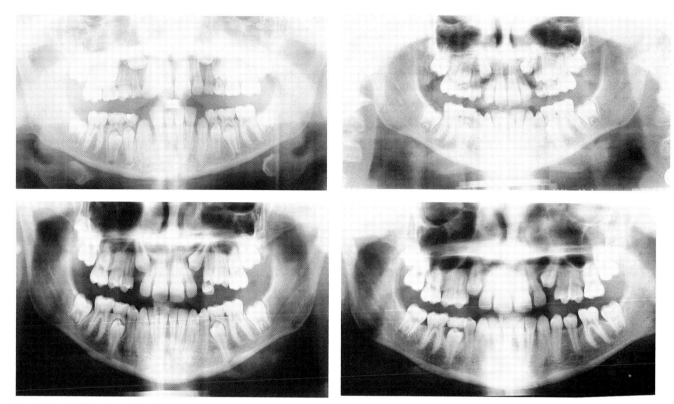

Fig. 14.4. DPT radiographs of a patient whose displaced maxillary permanent canines improved following the extraction of the upper deciduous canines.

It has been shown that extraction of a deciduous canine may result in improvement of the position of a displaced permanent canine, sufficient to allow normal eruption to occur (Fig. 14.4). As the success of this approach reduces with the degree of displacement it is advisable to seek the advice of a specialist before this step is undertaken in those cases where the canine is markedly displaced. The likelihood of the displaced canine position improving is also reduced in cases with crowding. It is prudent to warn the patient and their guardian that it may be necessary to expose the unerupted tooth and apply traction via an orthodontic appliance. This interceptive approach has also been used successfully for displaced mandibular canines.

14.5. ASSESSING MAXILLARY CANINE POSITION

The position of an unerupted canine should initially be assessed clinically, followed by radiographic examination if displacement is suspected.

Clinically

It is usually possible to obtain a good estimate of the likely location of an unerupted maxillary canine by palpation (in the buccal sulcus and palatally) and by the inclination of the lateral incisor (Fig. 14.5).

Radiographically

The radiographic assessment of a displaced canine should include the following:

- location of the position of both the canine crown and the root apex relative to adjacent teeth and the arch;

- the prognosis of adjacent teeth and the deciduous canine, if present;

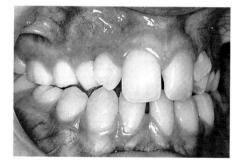

(a)

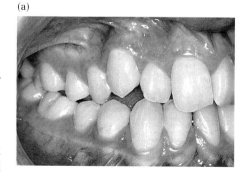

(b)

Fig. 14.5. (a) Patient aged 9 years showing distal inclination of the upper lateral incisor caused by the position of the unerupted canine; (b) the same patient aged 13 years showing the improvement that has occurred in the inclination of the lateral incisor following eruption of the permanent canine.

- the presence of resorption, particularly of the adjacent central and/or lateral incisors.

The views commonly used for assessing ectopic canines include the following.

- **Dental panoramic tomogram** (DPT), also known as an OPG or OPT. This film gives a good overall assessment of the development of the dentition and canine position. However, this view suggests that the canine is further away from the midline and at a slightly less acute angle to the occlusal plane, i.e. more favourably positioned for alignment, than is actually the case (Fig. 14.6(a)). This view should be supplemented with a periapical view.
- **Periapical.** This view is useful for assessing the prognosis of a retained deciduous canine and for detecting resorption (Fig. 14.6(b)).
- **Lateral cephalometric.** For accurate localization this view should be combined with an anteroposterior view (e.g. a DPT) (Fig. 14.6(c)).
- **Vertex occlusal.** This view is popular with oral surgeons, but involves a relatively high X-ray dose and irradiation of the orbit.

The principle of parallax can be used to determine the position of an unerupted tooth relative to its neighbours. To use parallax two radiographs are required with a change in the position of the X-ray tube between them. The object furthest away from the X-ray beam will appear to move in the same direction as the tube shift. Therefore, if the canine is more palatally positioned than the incisor roots it will move with the tube shift (Fig. 14.6 (b)). Conversely, if it is buccal it will move in the opposite direction to the tube shift. Examples of combinations of radiographs which can be used for parallax include two periapical radiographs (horizontal parallax) and a DPT and an upper anterior occlusal (vertical parallax).

14.6. MANAGEMENT OF BUCCAL DISPLACEMENT

The width of the maxillary canine is greater than the first premolar which in turn is greater than the deciduous canine.

Buccal displacement is usually associated with crowding, and therefore relief of crowding prior to eruption of the canine will usually effect some spontaneous improvement (Fig. 14.7). Buccal displacements are more likely to erupt than palatal displacements because of the thinner buccal mucosa and bone. Buccally displaced erupted canines are managed by relief of crowding, if indicated, and alignment. An upper removable appliance with a buccal canine retractor can be used where the canine tooth is mildly displaced, mesially inclined and tilting movements will suffice. Fixed appliances are indicated if the canine is upright or distally inclined and/or rotated. In such a case a sectional fixed appliance on the buccal segment teeth in that quadrant and the affected canine only may be useful to prevent 'round-tripping' the upper lateral incisor.

In severely crowded cases where the upper lateral incisor and first premolar are in contact and no additional space exists to accommodate the wider canine tooth, extraction of the canine itself may be indicated. In some patients the canine is so severely displaced that a good result is unlikely, necessitating removal of the canine tooth and the use of fixed appliances to close any residual spacing.

More rarely a buccally displaced canine tooth does not erupt or its eruption is so delayed that treatment for other aspects of the malocclusion is compromised. In these situations exposure of the impacted tooth may be indicated. To ensure an adequate width of attached gingiva either an apically repositioned or, preferably, a replaced flap should be used. In order to be able to apply traction to align the canine, either an attachment can be bonded or a band cemented to the tooth at the time of surgery. A gold chain or a stainless steel ligature can be attached to the bond or band and used to apply traction.

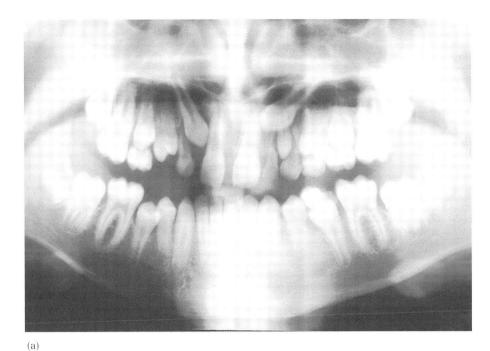

(a)

Fig. 14.6. The radiographs of a patient with displaced maxillary canines (note that the upper right lateral incisor is absent and the upper left lateral incisor is peg-shaped): (a) DPT radiograph; (b) periapical radiographs (note that both maxillary canines are palatally positioned as their position changes in the same direction as the tube shift); (c) lateral cephalometric radiograph.

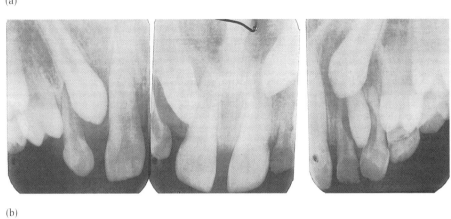

(b)

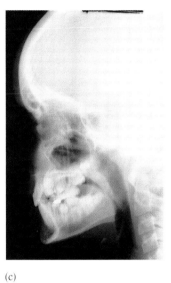

(c)

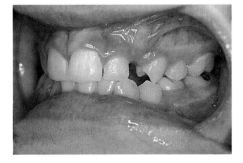

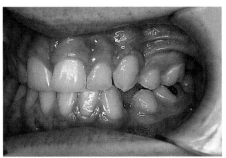

Fig. 14.7. Mildly buccally displaced maxillary canine which erupted spontaneously into a satisfactory position following relief of crowding.

14.7 MANAGEMENT OF PALATAL DISPLACEMENT

14.7.1. Factors affecting treatment decision

- Patient's opinion of appearance and motivation towards orthodontic treatment.
- Presence of spacing/crowding.
- Position of displaced canine: is it within range of orthodontic alignment?
- Malocclusion.
- Condition of retained deciduous canine, if present.
- Condition of adjacent teeth.

14.7.2. Treatment options

Surgical removal of canine

This option can be considered under the following conditions:

- The retained deciduous canine has an acceptable appearance and the patient is happy with the aesthetics and/or reluctant to embark on more complicated treatment (Fig. 14.8). The clinician must ensure that the patient understands that the primary canine will be lost eventually and a prosthetic replacement required. However, if the occlusion is unfavourable, for example a deep and increased overbite is present, this may affect the feasibility of bridgework later, necessitating the exploration of alternative options.
- The upper arch is very crowded and the upper first premolar is adjacent to the upper lateral incisor. Provided that the first premolar is not mesiopalatally rotated, the aesthetic result can be acceptable (Fig. 14.9).
- The canine is severely displaced. Depending upon the presence of crowding and the patient's wishes, either any residual spacing can be closed by forward movement of the upper buccal segments with fixed appliances, or a prosthetic replacement can be considered.

If space closure is not planned, it may be preferable to keep the unerupted canine under biannual radiographic observation until the fate of the third molars is decided. However, if any pathology, for example resorption of adjacent teeth or cyst formation, intervenes, removal should be arranged as soon as possible.

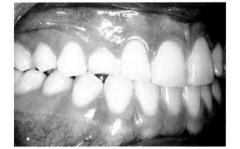

Fig. 14.8. This patient decided that the appearance of her retained deciduous canine was satisfactory and elected to have her unerupted displaced maxillary canine removed.

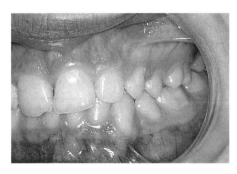

Fig. 14.9. Aesthetic result following removal of the displaced upper left permanent canine.

Surgical exposure and orthodontic alignment

Indications are as follows:

- well-motivated patient
- well-cared-for dentition
- favourable canine position
- space available (or can be created).

Whether orthodontic alignment is feasible or not depends upon the three-dimensional position of the unerupted canine:

- **Height.** The higher a canine is positioned relative to the occlusal plane the poorer is the prognosis. In addition, the access for surgical exposure will be more restricted. If the crown tip is at or above the apical third of the incisor roots, orthodontic alignment will be very difficult.

- **Anteroposterior position.** The nearer the canine crown is to the midline, the more difficult alignment will be. Most operators regard canines, which are more than halfway across the upper central incisor to be outside the limits of orthodontics.
- **Position of the apex.** The further away the canine apex is from normal, the poorer is the prognosis for successful alignment. If it is distal to the second premolar, other options should be considered.
- **Inclination.** The smaller the angle with the occlusal plane the greater is the need for traction.

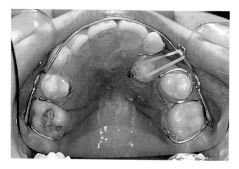

Fig. 14.10. Traction applied to an exposed canine using a removable appliance.

If these factors are favourable, the usual sequence of treatment is as follows:

(1) Make space available (although some operators are reluctant to embark on permanent extractions until after the tooth has been exposed and traction successfully started).
(2) Arrange exposure.
(3) Allow the tooth to erupt for 2 to 3 months.
(4) Commence traction.

With deeply buried canines there is a danger that the gingivae may cover the tooth again. If this is likely to be a problem, either an attachment plus the means of traction (for example a wire ligature or gold chain) can be bonded to the tooth at the time of exposure or about 2 days after pack removal.

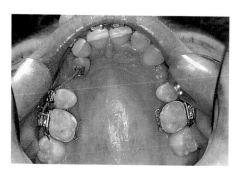

Fig. 14.11. A fixed appliance being used to move an exposed canine towards the line of the arch.

Traction can be applied using either a removable appliance (Fig. 14.10) or a fixed appliance (Fig. 14.11). To complete alignment a fixed appliance is necessary, as movement of the root apex buccally is required to complete positioning of the canine into a functional relationship with the lower arch.

Transplantation

Most orthodontists would agree that this option is best confined to those cases where there is no other alternative. If transplantation is attempted, it must be possible to remove the canine intact and there must be space available to accommodate the canine within the arch and occlusion. In some cases this will mean that some orthodontic treatment will be required prior to transplantation.

The main causes of failure of transplanted canines are replacement resorption and inflammatory resorption. Replacement resorption, or ankylosis, occurs when the root surface is damaged during the surgical procedure, and is promoted by rigid splinting of the transplanted tooth, which encourages healing by bony rather than fibrous union. Careful handling of the root surface and prevention of desiccation during surgery, followed by a method of splinting which allows functional movement of the canine during the immediate post-surgical phase, is now recommended. This can be achieved by use of an acid-etch composite splint for 1 to 2 weeks. Alternatively, a fixed appliance with a bracket on the canine can be employed, and is most suitable if space has to be created prior to transplantation.

Inflammatory resorption follows death of the pulpal tissues, and for this reason early pulp extirpation has been advocated by some authors.

Despite a better understanding of the factors leading to failure with transplantation, the long-term survival rates are not good in practice. The prognosis is improved if transplantation can be accomplished before root is 75 per cent formed. However, as this stage is reached around 12 years of age, early detection and planning is required to accomplish this.

14.8. RESORPTION

Unerupted and impacted canines can cause resorption of adjacent lateral incisor roots and may sometimes progress to cause resorption of the central incisor. Studies have indicated that incisor resorption is more common in females than males. Also, if the angulation of an ectopic canine to the midline on a DPT is greater than 25° then the risk increases by 50 per cent.

Swift intervention is essential, as resorption often proceeds at a rapid rate. If it is discovered on radiographic examination, specialist advice should be sought quickly. Extraction of the canine may be necessary to halt the resorption. However, if the resorption is severe it may be wiser to extract the affected incisor(s), thus allowing the canine to erupt (Fig. 14.12).

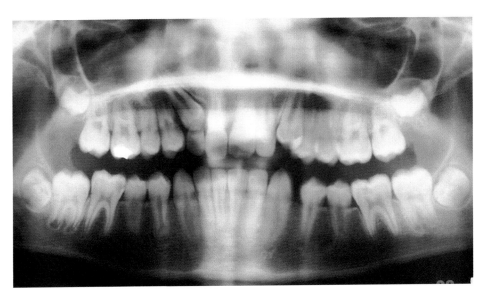

(a)

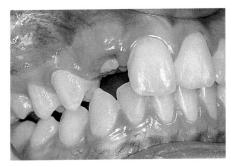

(b)

Fig. 14.12. (a) Resorption of the upper right lateral incisor by an unerupted maxillary canine; (b) following extraction of the lateral incisor the canine erupted adjacent to the central incisor.

14.9. TRANSPOSITION

Transposition is the term used to describe interchange in the position of two teeth. This anomaly is comparatively rare, but almost always affects the canine tooth. It affects the sexes equally and is more common in the maxilla. In the upper arch the canine and the first premolar are most commonly involved; however, transposition of the canine and lateral incisor is also seen (Fig. 14.13). In the mandible the canine and lateral incisor appear to be almost exclusively affected. The aetiology of this condition is not understood.

Management depends upon whether the transposition is complete (i.e. apical transposition is evident) or partial, the malocclusion, and the presence or absence of crowding. Possible treatment options include acceptance (particularly if transposition is complete), extraction of the most displaced tooth if the arch is crowded, or orthodontic alignment. In the last case, the relative positions of the root apices will be a major factor in deciding whether the affected teeth are corrected or aligned in their transposed arrangement.

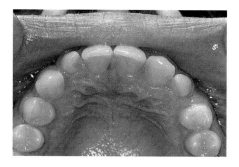

Fig. 14.13. Transposition of the upper left maxillary canine and lateral incisor.

PRINCIPAL SOURCES AND FURTHER READING

Becker, A., Smith, P., and Behar, R. (1981). The incidence of anomalous maxillary lateral incisors in relation to palatally-displaced cuspids. *Angle Orthodontist*, **51**, 24–9.
- The aetiology and management of displaced maxillary canines are considered in this very thorough paper.
Edmunds, D. H. and Beck, C. (1989). Root resorption in autotransplanted maxillary canine teeth. *International Endodontic Journal*, **22**, 29–38.
- The factors that lead to root resorption, and methods of reducing this sequela, are discussed.
Ericson, S. and Kurol, J. (1986). Longitudinal study and analysis of clinical supervision of maxillary canine eruption. *Community Dentistry and Oral Epidemiology*, **14**, 172–6.
Ericson, S. and Kurol, J. (1988). Early treatment of palatally erupting maxillary canines by extraction of the primary canines. *European Journal of Orthodontics*, **10**, 283–95.
- The first scientific evaluation of the widely held belief that extraction of a deciduous canine could improve the position of a displaced successor was given in this important paper.
Gorlin, R. J., Cohen, M. M., and Levin, L. S. (1990). *Syndromes of the head and neck* (3rd edn). Oxford University Press., Oxford.
- This excellent reference book includes, amongst a wealth of other information, data on the development and incidence of canine anomalies.
Jacoby, H. (1983). The etiology of maxillary canine impactions. *American Journal of Orthodontics*, **84**, 125–32.
- Evidence that leads the authors to conclude that palatal and buccal displacements have differing aetiologies is presented in this paper.
McSherry, P. F. (1998). The ectopic maxillary canine: A review. *British Journal of Orthodontics*, **25**, 209–16.
- Good review article in which the options for management of displaced canines are discussed.
Peck, S. M., Peck, L. and Kataja, M. (1994). The palatally displaced canine as a dental anomaly of genetic origin. *Angle Orthodontist*, **64**, 249–56.

15 Anchorage, tooth movement, and retention (B. Doubleday)

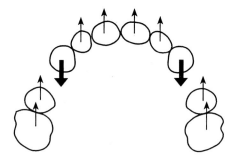

Fig. 15.1. Diagram showing the effect upon the anchor teeth of retracting upper canines with a fixed appliance.

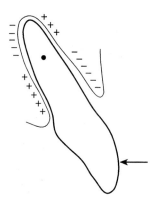

Fig. 15.2. Diagram showing the effect of a tipping force applied to the crown of a tooth (P = pressure   T = tension).

15.1. WHAT IS ANCHORAGE AND WHY IS IT IMPORTANT?

Anchorage has been defined as the source of resistance to the forces generated in reaction to the active components of an appliance. Anchorage is required to prevent unwanted tooth movements.

Anchorage is a difficult concept to grasp, but it may be helpful to consider it initially as the balance between the applied force and the available space. Whenever tooth movement is attempted there will be an equal and opposite reaction to the force(s) applied by the active components (Newton's third law of motion). This reaction force is spread over the teeth which are contacted by the appliance. For example, if both upper canines are being retracted with an upper fixed appliance, which has attachments on all the erupted teeth, an equal and opposite force to that being generated by the active canine retraction will also be acting on the remaining upper arch teeth which comprise the anchorage or resistance to that movement (Fig. 15.1). The amount of forward movement of the anchor teeth will depend upon their root surface area and the force applied (see Section 15.4). However, anchorage is not merely an anteroposterior phenomenon — unwanted tooth movements can also occur in the vertical and transverse dimensions.

The importance of anchorage is perhaps most keenly appreciated when it has been neglected. Anchorage loss may jeopardize a successful result because inappropriate movement of the anchor teeth results in insufficient space remaining to achieve the intended tooth movements. In some cases anchorage loss can result in a worsening of the occlusion, for example, during the canine retraction phase of appliance treatment for a Class II malocclusion, forward movement of the anchor teeth can result in an increase in overjet. However, in some situations loss of anchorage can be used to advantage, for example, in a class Class III malcclusion an increase in overjet can be advantageous. Therefore anchorage requirements need to be assessed at the time of treatment planning.

15.2. THE HISTOLOGICAL BASIS OF TOOTH MOVEMENT

When a point force is applied to the crown of a tooth, it will tilt around an axis approximately at the junction of the apical one-third and the coronal two-thirds of the root (however, this is variable depending upon the size of the force and local anatomy). As a result the force is concentrated at the coronal one-third of the socket wall in the direction of the force and at the root apex in the opposite direction, as shown in Fig. 15.2.

When an optimal force is applied, cell proliferation occurs within the periodontal ligament in areas of compression and osteoclasts (bone-resorbing cells) migrate in from the surrounding blood vessels. Direct resorption of the bone of the socket wall adjacent to the areas of pressure takes place within a few days. On the tension side the periodontal fibres are stretched, and proliferation of fibroblasts and osteoblasts (bone-forming cells) is followed by an increase in the length of the periodontal fibres which are subsequently remodelled. Osteoid is deposited on the bony socket wall on the tension side and is then calcified to form woven bone, which in turn is remodelled into mature bone. Thus the tooth moves through the alveolar bone under the influence of an applied force (see Table 15.1).

As these changes are mediated by cells derived from the blood supply, the latter is an important prerequisite for tooth movement to occur. Therefore a force which exceeds capillary pressure and reduces blood flow will not produce optimal movement.

If an excessive force is applied continuously, direct resorption of bone does not take place because compression of the blood vessels within the periodontal ligament results in a sterile necrosis (known as hyalinization because of its homogeneous, glass-like microscopic appearance) and initially a cessation of movement. After a delay of two to three weeks, indirect resorption takes place outwards from the marrow spaces of the adjacent alveolar bone (Fig. 15.3) and then the tooth moves. This is known as undermining resorption (see Table 15.1).

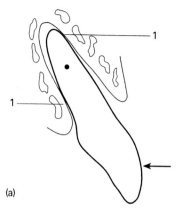

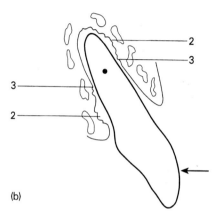

Fig. 15.3. Diagram showing the effect of applying an excessive force: (a) areas of hyalinization (1); (b) undermining resorption (2) and direct resorption in areas where force is less (3).

Table 15.1   Cellular reactions to the application of an orthodontic force

Optimal force
Pressure areas
1. Cellular proliferation within a few days
2. Osteoclasts migrate into the PDL from blood vessels
3. Resorption of bone and remodelling of PDL fibres
Tension areas
1. Stretching of PDL fibres
2. Cellular proliferation of fibroblasts and osteoblasts
3. Increase in length of PDL fibres
4. Deposition of osteoid
5. Remodelling and reattachment of PDL fibres, and calcification of osteoid into mature bone

Excessive force
Pressure areas
1. Capillary blood vessels are crushed resulting in death of cells in PDL (hyalinization)
2. In areas adjacent to the hyalinized sections of PDL cellular proliferation occurs
3. Resorption occurs deep to hyalinized area from cancellous bone outwards toward lamina dura of PDL (undermining resorption)
4. Tooth movement occurs
Tension areas
As for optimal force

PDL, periodontal ligament.

The optimum force for tooth movement is around 20–25 g/cm² of root surface area. The size of the force applied to an individual tooth will depend upon its root surface area and the type of tooth movement planned. In bodily tooth movement the applied force is spread over the whole of the root surface in the direction of translation (Fig. 15.4). Thus a larger force is required to achieve the threshold for movement. In contrast, intrusion requires light forces as the applied stress is concentrated at the apex of the tooth and the application of an excessive force runs the risk of occluding the blood supply to the pulpal tissues. Average forces for the

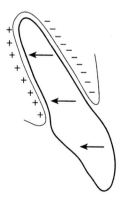

Fig. 15.4. Diagram showing distribution of the applied force with bodily movement (P = pressure   T = tension).

Table 15.2 A guide to force levels for tooth movement

Tipping movements	30–60 g
Bodily movements	100–150 g
Rotational movements	50–75 g
Extrusion	50–75 g
Intrusion	15–25 g

common tooth movements are given in Table 15.2, but it should be remembered that the optimal force for a given tooth will depend upon its root surface area.

The use of excessive force in orthodontic tooth movement is not advocated for a number of reasons, including the following:

- delay in tooth movement;
- the dispersal of an excessive force over the anchor teeth is more likely to reach the threshold for their movement, resulting in an increased risk of anchorage loss;
- a greater force leads to increased discomfort of the tooth being moved;
- increased tooth mobility (due to the removal of a greater amount of supporting bone);
- a greater risk of root resorption.

The success of orthodontic tooth movement also depends upon the duration of the applied force. It has been shown that the chemical mediators of tooth movement appear in the bloodstream within a few hours of a continuous force being applied and that clinical tooth movement will occur with a force duration of as little as 6 hours per day. However, for optimal tooth movement application of a continuous force, for 24 hours per day is preferable (but see Table 15.3 for the reasons for more rapid tooth movement in children). Irregularities in the bony socket wall mean that, even though overall an optimal force is applied, excessive forces can develop in small areas. To allow these areas to repair and to limit root resorption, reactivation of the force exerted by an appliance should be undertaken at intervals more than 3 weeks apart.

This discussion has outlined the response of cancellous bone to an orthodontic force. The greater density and reduced vascularity of cortical bone means that, if a force is applied which results in the tooth root contacting bone, resorption of the root rather than bone may result. In addition, although some remodelling of the alveolar process occurs during tooth movement, this is not limitless and it is quite possible to move a tooth root through the labial or palatal cortical plate. This may result in dehiscence of the root, with severe gingival recession and possibly loss of pulp vitality as well as root resorption.

By necessity this section has been a summary of the complex biochemical changes which occur as a result of pressure or tension applied to a tooth and its supporting structures. This interesting area is currently the subject of much research, and the reader is referred to the section on further reading.

Table 15.3 Reasons for more rapid tooth movement in children

- Physiological tooth movement is greatest when the teeth are erupting
- The periodontal ligament is more cellular, and therefore there are more cells available for resorption and remodelling
- The alveolar bone has a greater proportion of osteoblasts
- The cellular response in reaction to an applied force is quicker
- The width of the periodontal ligament is increased in newly erupted teeth, and so a greater force can be applied before constriction of the blood vessels occurs
- Growth can be utilized

15.3. TYPES OF ANCHORAGE

15.3.1. Intra-oral anchorage

Intra-oral anchorage has classically been subdivided as follows:

- **Simple anchorage**: active movement of one tooth versus several anchor teeth.
- **Compound anchorage**: teeth of greater resistance to movement are utilized as anchorage for the translation of teeth which have less resistance to movement.
- **Stationary anchorage**: this is a misnomer as it is extremely difficult to prevent movement of anchor teeth altogether.
- **Reciprocal anchorage**: two groups of teeth are pitted against each other, resulting in equal reciprocal movement of both. This concept is utilized in appliances to expand the upper arch. Activation of the expansion appliance results in a force acting equally but oppositely on the posterior teeth of both upper quadrants (Fig. 15.5).

In practice, it may be more helpful to consider intra-oral anchorage in terms of whether it is derived from teeth in the same arch, i.e. **intramaxillary** anchorage, or whether it is gained from the opposing arch, i.e. **intermaxillary** anchorage (see Section 15.6).

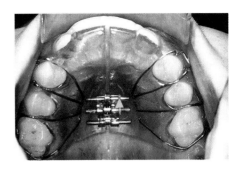

Fig. 15.5. An expansion appliance, showing the use of reciprocal anchorage.

15.3.2. Extra-oral anchorage

Extra-oral anchorage is achieved by the patient wearing headgear which applies a distal force upon the teeth. Essentially the patient's head is used for anchorage (see Section 15.7).

15.4. FACTORS AFFECTING ANCHORAGE

15.4.1. Type of tooth movement planned

A tipping force results in a concentration of the applied force at the apex and crestal bone margins of a tooth (see Fig. 15.2). In contrast, during bodily movement the force is spread over the root surface in the direction of movement (see Fig. 15.4), and so a greater force is required to achieve tooth movement and consequently a greater strain is placed on anchorage. However, this can be used to advantage as it is possible to increase the value of anchorage teeth by trying to ensure that they can only move bodily.

15.4.2. Root surface area of the teeth used for anchorage

Increasing the root surface area of the anchorage unit means that the reaction to an active orthodontic force is dissipated over a larger area. For this reason molar teeth are preferable to single-rooted teeth. Increasing the number of anchor teeth (e.g. by including second molars when bonding fixed appliances) also increases the root surface area resisting anchorage loss, but by the same token, movement of molar teeth places a greater strain on anchorage.

15.4.3. Skeletal pattern

It has been noted that, in patients with increased vertical skeletal dimensions and a backward pattern of growth rotation, mesial tooth movement and anchorage loss seem to occur more readily than in patients with reduced vertical skeletal proportions and a forward pattern of growth rotation (see Chapter 4, Figs 4.15 and 4.16). One possible explanation for this is the relative 'strength' of the facial musculature of the two facial types.

15.4.4. Occlusal interlock

A good buccal occlusion may act to resist tooth movement. This may or may not be an advantage, depending upon whether the tooth or teeth to be moved actively or the anchor teeth are affected.

15.4.5. Tendency for tooth movement in the arch

Anchorage loss is more rapid in the maxillary arch as upper teeth have a greater tendency for mesial drift.

15.5. ASSESSING ANCHORAGE REQUIREMENTS

When planning treatment, the type of tooth movement required (for example tipping or bodily movement) and the demands that this will place upon anchorage should be considered, together with the anticipated final position of both the molars and incisors. As a result of this process the particular malocclusion under consideration will fall into one of the following categories.

1. Excess space will remain following treatment. In this situation either the treatment plan should be re-examined or measures taken to try and 'burn up' anchorage.
2. The anchorage available should suffice. However, it is prudent to monitor anchorage throughout treatment.
3. No loss of anchorage can be tolerated. Therefore measures to reinforce anchorage should be instituted from the beginning of treatment.
4. Insufficient anchorage is available even with reinforcement during treatment. In this situation it is necessary to return to the aims of the treatment and to determine if these need to be modified. If not, additional extractions and/or extra-oral traction will be indicated.

15.6. REINFORCING ANCHORAGE

15.6.1. Intra-oral reinforcement of anchorage

Anchorage can be preserved intra-orally during treatment in the following ways.

Increasing the number of teeth in the anchor unit

This means including more teeth in the appliance to try to resist the unwanted effects of active tooth movement. For example, when fixed appliances are used, banding the second molars helps to increase anchorage.

Making movement of the anchor teeth more difficult

With fixed appliances it is possible to ensure that the anchor teeth can only move bodily. As bodily movement requires greater forces, the resistance of the anchorage unit is increased.

Intermaxillary anchorage

The anchorage available in one arch can be reinforced if the patient wears elastic traction to the opposing arch. For example, in a Class II malocclusion elastics from the upper canine region backwards to the lower first molars on both sides assist overjet reduction. This direction of elastic pull is described as Class II intermaxillary traction (Fig. 15.6). Class III traction is shown in Fig. 15.7.

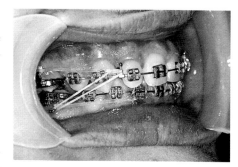

Fig. 15.6. Class II intermaxillary traction.

$$
\text{Class II traction} \quad \frac{6\diagup 3 \mid 3\diagdown 6}{6\ \ 3 \mid 3\ \ 6}
$$

$$
\text{Class III traction} \quad \frac{6\ \ 3 \mid 3\ \ 6}{6\diagdown 3 \mid 3\diagup 6}
$$

Elastic intermaxillary traction is difficult with removable appliances and is almost exclusively employed in fixed appliance treatments. Intra-oral elastics (see Chapter 17, Fig. 17.20) are available in a wide variety of sizes and weights.

However, intermaxillary traction is not without its disadvantages. Class II or Class III traction can lead to extrusion of the molar teeth, which has the effect of increasing the lower face height and reducing overbite. In patients with increased vertical proportions this will be counterproductive. Class II traction encourages forward movement of the lower molars, which may be advantageous if there is excess lower extraction space to close. However, the use of this type of traction where no lower arch space exists will have the effect of proclining the lower labial segment.

Intermaxillary traction can also be achieved with functional appliances (see Chapter 18).

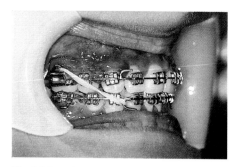

Fig. 15.7. Class III intermaxillary traction.

Palatal and lingual arches

An arch which connects contralateral molars either across the vault of the palate or around the lingual aspect of the lower arch will help to prevent movement of the molars and thus reinforce anchorage. The arches are usually attached to bands cemented to the molar teeth (Figs 15.8 and 15.9).

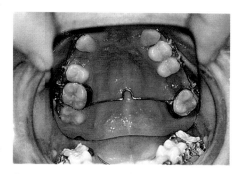

Fig. 15.8. Palatal arch.

Choice of appliance

Upper removable appliances actually afford more anchorage than fixed appliances because of their palatal coverage.

Implants

Implants act as a fixed structure and are useful for providing anchorage in patients with hypodontia or marked tooth loss.

15.6.2. Extra-oral reinforcement of anchorage

Extra-oral reinforcement of anchorage is discussed in Section 15.7.

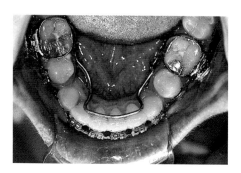

Fig. 15.9. Lingual arch.

15.7. EXTRA-ORAL ANCHORAGE AND TRACTION

15.7.1. General principles

In practice, the distinction between extra-oral anchorage (EOA) and extra-oral traction (EOT) is a matter of degree (Table 15.4), although confusingly the terms are often used interchangeably. Extra-oral anchorage is a method of increasing anchorage and therefore is designed to prevent forward movement of the anchor teeth. Extra-oral traction is a method of achieving tooth movement, most commonly in a distal direction. It is also sometimes used to try to move the maxilla distally and/or vertically, although in reality the net result is rather a restraint of maxillary growth. In order to achieve true (orthopaedic) maxillary movement, prolonged wear with forces in excess of 500 g over the years of active growth is required, followed by prolonged retention to reduce any rebound growth. Perhaps not surprisingly, most patients are unable to sustain this level of co-operation.

Table 15.4 Extra-oral traction and anchorage

	EOA	EOT
Purpose	Reinforcement of anchorage	Tooth movement
Force	200–250 g	400–500 g
Wear required	10–12 hours	14–16+ hours

In addition to magnitude and duration, the direction of the headgear force also needs to be considered, although this is of more consequence with extra-oral traction. A direction of force below the level of the occlusal plane (cervical-pull headgear) will tend to extrude the upper molar teeth and thus cause an increase in the vertical dimension of the lower face. While this may be an advantage in a patient with a reduced lower facial height, it is contraindicated in a patient with increased vertical proportions. In the latter case, a direction of pull above the occlusal plane (high-pull headgear) is usually preferable, as this will have the effect of intruding the upper buccal segment teeth and will also tend to restrain vertical maxillary development.

To achieve distal movement of the upper first permanent molars, a force directed slightly above the occlusal plane, through the centre of resistance of those teeth, is desirable. It is important to monitor the direction in which the teeth are being translated. For example, if it can be seen that the crowns of the teeth are being tilted distally, the direction of pull needs to be raised to counteract this.

The centre of resistance of the maxilla is estimated to lie at a point approximately above and between the premolar roots. If restraint of maxillary growth is to be attempted, the direction of headgear pull should be adjusted so that the force passes through this area.

Intrusion of the upper incisors can be attempted by applying headgear to the upper labial section of the archwire during fixed appliance treatments, but to avoid root resorption a force of less than 200 g is advisable.

A direction of force above the occlusal plane is also advisable when headgear is employed in conjunction with a removable appliance, to aid retention of the appliance.

15.7.2. Components of headgear

Headgear consists essentially of three parts.

Means of attachment to the teeth

This is achieved by using one of the following:

1. A face-bow (Fig. 15.10) which slots into tubes soldered onto the bridge of a removable appliance crib (see Chapter 16, Fig. 16.17), tubes which form an integral part of a molar band attachment (see Chapter 17, Fig. 17.29), or tubes which are incorporated in the design of a functional appliance.
2. J-hooks (Fig. 15.11) which can be directly attached onto the archwire in a fixed appliance or attached to hooks soldered onto the labial bow of a removable appliance.

Strap or headcap

A number of different types are available which are mainly described by the direction of pull that the headgear affords:

- **cervical pull** which consists of a neck strap (Fig. 15.12);
- **variable pull** which consists of a headcap with a variety of positions for the application of force (Fig. 15.13);
- **high pull** which is a headcap fitting over the back of the head (Fig. 15.14).

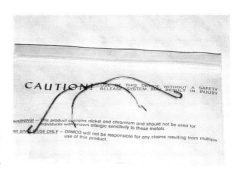

Fig. 15.10. A face-bow.

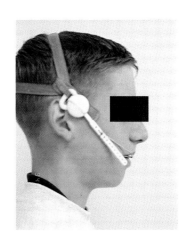

Fig. 15.11. J-hooks.

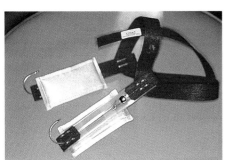
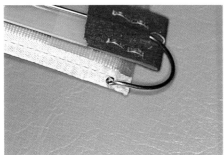

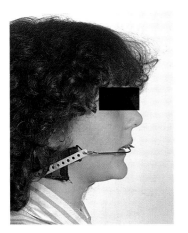

Fig. 15.12. Cervical-pull headgear with the force produced by an elastic strap. The headgear is attached to a face-bow and the patient is also wearing a rigid safety strap.

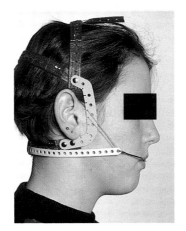

Fig. 15.13. Variable-pull headgear with force provided by elastic bands between the headgear and the face-bow. A rigid safety strap is also being used.

Fig. 15.14. High-pull headgear attached to a face-bow.

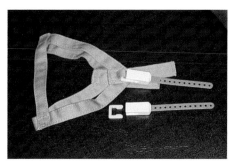

Fig. 15.15. Safety release headgear with a spring mechanism which breaks apart when excessive force is applied.

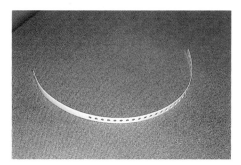

Fig. 15.16. Rigid safety strap.

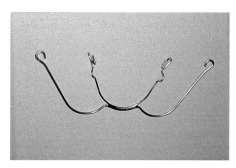

Fig. 15.17. Safety face-bow.

Elastic component or spring mechanism

This connects the two other elements and controls the magnitude of the force applied. Elastic force is produced either by an elastic strap (see Fig. 15.12) or by different sizes of extra-oral elastic bands (see Fig. 15.13). Spring mechanisms are shown in Figs 15.14 and 15.15.

15.7.3. Headgear safety

Tragically, several cases have been reported where severe ocular injuries, including blindness, have occurred owing to accidents with headgear. These incidents have mainly occurred with face-bows used in conjunction with some form of elastic force, where the face-bow has been pulled out of the mouth and recoiled back into the face or eyes. Various methods of increasing the safety of headgear have been introduced. One of the simplest designs is the rigid safety strap (Fig. 15.16; see also Figs 15.12 and 15.13) which, if correctly fitted, helps to prevent the face-bow from being dislodged. The spring mechanisms have also gained popularity as a safety release feature can be more easily be built into the headgear; if an excessive force is applied, the components come apart thus preventing recoil of the face-bow (see Figs 15.14 and 15.15)., Face-bows with the ends re-curved to form a guard over the sharp end of the intra-oral bow are available (Fig. 15.17). In addition a face-bow has been developed with a small catch to lock it into the molar tubes (Figs 15.18a and b), these are strongly recommended as they prevent the face-bow being pulled out.

Care is also required with J-hooks as the hook can be dislodged and cause serious injury. It is preferable to bend the hook round so that it forms a circle and is attached onto a hook soldered to the removable appliance or archwire. A relatively large headcap should be used with small heavy elastics so that the distance that the J-hook can travel is minimized.

It would now be considered neglilent to use headgear without safety features. Patients should be warned of the dangers and instructed that headgear should not be worn during any 'horseplay'. If the headgear dislodges during the night, patients should be advised to discontinue its use and to return for adjustment by the clinician.

15.7.4. Reverse headgear

This type of headgear is also known as a face-mask and is used to try and move teeth mesially to close up excess spacing or in Class III malocclusions in an attempt to move the maxilla forward (see Chapter 11, Fig. 11.15).

15.8. MONITORING ANCHORAGE DURING TREATMENT

15.8.1. Single-arch treatments

Monitoring anchorage during single-arch fixed or removable treatments is relatively straightforward, as it is possible to use the other arch as a reference. This can be done by recording the overjet and molar positions during treatment, preferably at each visit. The progress of the tooth or teeth being moved can be recorded most easily using dividers which can then be imprinted into the record card.

15.8.2. Upper and lower fixed appliance treatments

Where tooth movement is occurring in both arches simultaneously it is a little more difficult to determine where the teeth are spatially compared with their starting position. For example, in a Class II, division 1, malocclusion forward movement of the upper arch may occur owing to loss of anchorage, but if the lower labial incisor teeth have also been inadvertently proclined, due to enthusiastic use of Class II traction for example, loss of anchorage is more difficult to detect as the overjet measurement may be unchanged or even reduced. For this reason a lateral cephalometric radiograph should be taken prior to the placement of appliances, and then progress with tooth movement and growth can be evaluated by repeating the radiograph. If necessary, the treatment mechanics can then be modified. It is also advisable continually to bear in mind the final anticipated tooth positions, for example the desired buccal segment occlusion, and to record progress towards this goal at every visit.

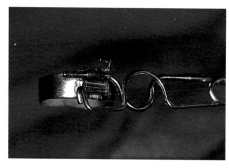

(a)

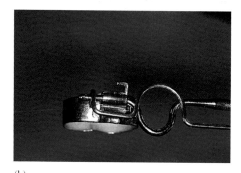

(b)

Fig. 15.18.   Locking face-bow: (a) open; (b) closed.

15.9. COMMON PROBLEMS WITH ANCHORAGE

The most common reasons for the occurrence of anchorage problems during treatment are as follows.

- Failure to appreciate fully the anchorage requirements of a particular malocclusion at the treatment planning stage. If this becomes apparent during treatment, it is probably wise to take up-to-date records and reassess the case. It may be necessary to institute extra-oral anchorage or, if problems are marked, extra-oral traction or even additional extractions. It is advisable to explain carefully to the patient and their parents the reasons for the change of treatment plan.

- Poor patient compliance. It is important during any orthodontic treatment to monitor carefully patient compliance with the appliance, ideally at every visit. The major problem with removable appliance treatment is to ensure that the patient wears the appliance full-time. If compliance is particularly poor, forward movement of the anchor molars owing to mesial drift can occur, leading to loss of anchorage. With fixed appliances, breakages and failure to wear headgear or elastic traction are the most common problems leading to anchorage loss. Sometimes encouragement and an explanation of the effect of the patient's actions upon the success of treatment may be sufficient. However, for a proportion of patients this does not have the desired effect, which emphasizes the need for careful patient selection. Unfortunately, escalating treatment to overcome anchorage loss is often poorly received by this group of patients, and a compromise result may have to be accepted.

15.10. RETENTION

Relapse has been defined by the British Standards Institute as the return, following correction, of the features of the original malocclusion.

   After a course of orthodontic treatment a period of retention is usually necessary. This allows the recently formed osteoid and bone to mature and gives time for reorganization of new periodontal fibres. Retention should not be relegated to being an afterthought at the end of treatment; it should be considered at the planning stage and explained to the patient as an integral part of the overall management package. In addition, it is advisable to identify those cases where the prognosis for a stable result has to be guarded and a decision made whether to embark on treatment at all.

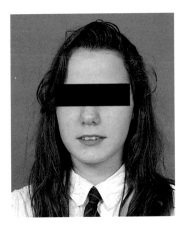

Fig. 15.19.   Potentially competent lips.

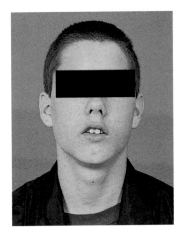

Fig. 15.20.   Grossly incompetent lips.

15.10.1. Factors to be considered when planning retention

Soft tissues

Where possible, appliance therapy should aim to place the teeth in a position of soft tissue balance following treatment. Sadly, no amount of retention will stabilize an inherently unstable result.

If the lips are incompetent prior to treatment, the method by which a patient achieves an anterior oral seal should be assessed and the probable effect of treatment upon lip competence determined. For example, in a Class II division 1, malocclusion, the lower lip should ideally rest in front of the retracted upper incisors at the end of treatment. This is more likely to be achieved in the patient shown in Fig. 15.19 than in the patient shown in Fig. 15.20, who has grossly incompetent lips which will not act in front of the incisors even if the overjet is reduced.

In patients with advanced periodontal disease, normal soft tissue pressures may lead to drifting of the teeth. In these cases, permanent retention is usually required following treatment to prevent relapse (see Chapter 19).

Facial growth

The probable direction of any future growth and its effect should be estimated and taken into consideration at the time of treatment planning. Class III malocclusions and the extremes of the vertical range, i.e. anterior open bites and deep overbites, are most commonly adversely affected by further growth. In these cases it is wise to overcorrect the incisor relationship and, if possible, to continue retention until the end of the teens when the growth rate slows or to defer treatment until this time. In severe class Class III cases particularly it may be appropriate to wait until the slow rate of adult growth has been reached before deciding whether extraction of teeth and orthodontic 'camouflage' or surgical correction would be the best treatment.

Although lower incisor crowding is multifactorial, late facial growth has been implicated. Crowding of the lower labial segment is common, even following orthodontic treatment. One study in the USA found that lower incisor crowding increased in around 66 per cent of a sample of 450 post-orthodontic patients. Given these statistics, it is not surprising that, particularly in the USA, there is a growing trend towards permanent retention of the lower labial segment, for example with a bonded retainer.

Supporting tissues

During active tooth movement the periodontal ligament fibres are placed under tension. If the force is removed, the tension in these fibres could result in the tooth's springing back against the newly formed immature bone which is more readily resorbed, resulting in relapse. The rate of turnover of the different groups of periodontal ligament fibres varies. The fibres which run between the socket wall and the cementum are remodelled with the bony changes; however, the supracrestal fibres take over six 6 months to be reorganized. Therefore some retention is advisable to allow the supporting tissues to adapt. However, de-rotation is particularly prone to relapse. This is related to the slow turnover of the free gingival fibres, which remain under tension for months or even years after rotational movements. One method of overcoming this is pericision or circumferential supracrestal fibrotomy, in which a scapel blade is run around the gingival crevice to cut through the supracrestal fibres. Alternatively, rotated teeth can be overcorrected, but relapse is unpredictable and some teeth remain stubbornly overcorrected. In any case prolonged retention, for example with a bonded retainer, is advisable.

An upper midline diastema present after eruption of the permanent canines also has a strong tendency to reopen after closure. It has been suggested that this is due to discontinuity of the transeptal fibres between the central incisors. If the diastema is associated with radiographic and clinical evidence of insertion of the fraenal fibres through the midline suture to the incisive papilla, a fraenectomy during space closure is advisable. Again, prolonged retention is usually required.

Occlusal factors

Achievement of a satisfactory inter-incisal relationship will aid retention: for example establishment of an adequate overbite is essential to retain an anterior tooth (or teeth) which has been proclined from being in crossbite (Fig. 15.21) and correction of the inter-incisal angle is necessary to prevent relapse of a deep overbite (Chapter 10, Fig. 10.11). In contrast, a poor buccal segment interdigitation, particularly associated with a displacement on closure, can contribute to relapse.

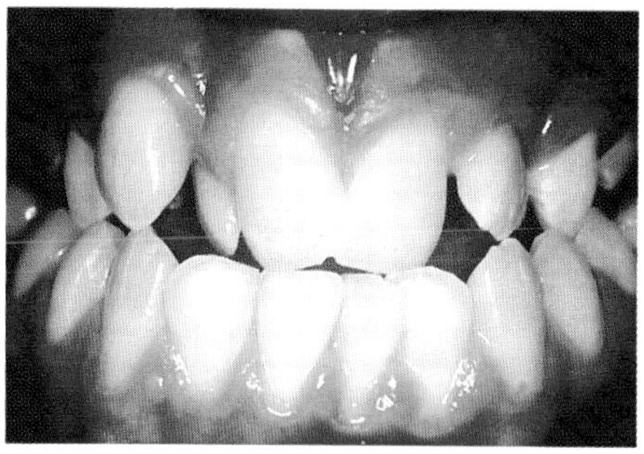

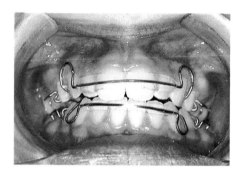

Fig. 15.21. If the anterior teeth are proclined to correct the crossbite, lack of overbite will lead to relapse.

15.10.2. Retention regimes

To minimize relapse it is advisable to commence retention immediately after the end of active appliance therapy. It is difficult to lay down rigid rules for retention, as each case should be assessed individually. Therefore the following regimes are for guidance only.

Tilting movements into the line of the arch

Following a course of removable appliance therapy to align one or two teeth, 3 months full-time wear of the passive appliance will usually suffice. If the teeth have been proclined from a crossbite position and there is sufficient overbite, 3 months of night-only wear is usually adequate.

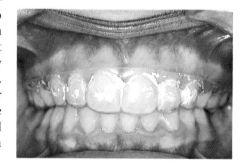

Fig. 15.22. Upper and lower removable retainers.

Bodily movements

After correction of more severe malocclusions with a fixed appliance it is common practice to fit removable Hawley retainers (Fig. 15.22) or vacuum-formed thermoplastic retainers (Fig. 15.23) for 3 to six 6 months of full-time wear followed by 6 months of night-only wear. Alternatively, many operators fit bonded retainers on the lingual aspect of the lower incisors and canines (Fig. 15.24). These are often left *in situ* until the fate of the third molars is determined. Bonded retainers lie passively against the teeth and are retained using light-cured acid-etch retained composite. They may be fabricated from flexible multistrand wire and bonded to each tooth or formed from more rigid solid stainless steel wire and bonded at either end to the canine teeth only. Pre-formed bonded retainers with pads for bonding to the palatal surfaces of the upper central incisors can be effective in holding a median diastema closed. Micro-magnets have also been used in this situation.

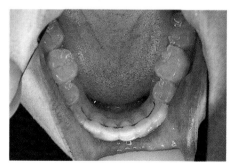

Fig. 15.23. Vacuum-formed thermoplastic upper removable retainer.

Opening space for prosthetic replacement of missing teeth

This has been considered separately for the following reasons:

1. If a removable partial denture cum retainer is to be used following active tooth movement, C-clasps or stops should be placed mesial and distal to the pontic tooth to help prevent relapse.
2. It has been shown that if acid-etch retained bridgework is placed immediately after the end of active tooth movement there is a higher rate of bond failure. Therefore it is advisable to retain with a removable retainer for at least 9 months.

De-rotation

Prolonged retention is wise after correction of rotations. This is perhaps most easily accomplished with a bonded lingual/palatal retainer (see Fig. 15.24).

Fig. 15.24. Bonded retainer.

'Orthopaedic' movement

After growth modification with a functional appliance or with the use of headgear, it is advisable to continue retention with the appliance, at least for nights only, until the growth rate has slowed to the low levels of adulthood, in the late teens.

15.11. SUMMARY

Anchorage is the balance between the tooth movements desired to achieve correction of a malocclusion and the undesirable movement of any other teeth. The strain placed upon anchorage depends upon the type of tooth movement to be carried out and the applied force(s). Anchorage can be increased by maximizing the number of teeth (and root surface area) resisting the active tooth movement, either within the same arch (intramaxillary anchorage) or in the opposing arch (intermaxillary anchorage). Extra-oral forces can also be utilized with headgear. It is important to map out anchorage requirements at the planning stage and monitor throughout treatment.

Retention is usually necesssary to overcome the elastic recoil of the periodontal supporting fibres and to allow remodelling of the alveolar bone. Retention requirements should be planned prior to the start of treatment.

PRINCIPAL SOURCES AND FURTHER READING

Bowden, D. E. J. (1978). Theoretical considerations of headgear therapy: a literature review. *British Journal of Orthodontics*, **5**, 145–52.

Bowden, D. E. J. (1978). Theoretical considerations of headgear therapy: a literature review. Clinical response and usage. *British Journal of Orthodontics*, **5**, 173–81.

● These two papers provide an authoritative review of the principles of headgear.

Firouz, M., Zernik, J., and Nanda, R. (1992). Dental and orthopedic effects of high-pull headgear in treatment of Class II, division 1, malocclusion. *American Journal of Orthodontics and Dentofacial Orthopedics*, **102**, 197–205.

Hill, P. A. (1998). Bone remodelling. *British Journal of Orthodontics*, **25**, 101–7

Kaplan, H. (1988). The logic of modern retention procedures. *American Journal of Orthodontics and Dentofacial Orthopedics*, **93**, 325–40.

Little, R. M., Reidel, R. A., and Årtun, J. (1988). An evaluation of changes in mandibular anterior alignment from 10 to 20 years postretention. *American Journal of Orthodontics and Dentofacial Orthopedics*, **93**, 423–8.

Meghji, S. (1992). Bone remodelling. *British Dental Journal*, **172**, 235–42.

Melrose, C. and Millett, D. T. (1998). Toward a perspective on orthodontic retention? *American Journal of Orthodontics and Dentofacial Orthopedics*, **113**, 507–14.

Nanda, R. S. and Nanda, S. K. (1992). Considerations of dentofacial growth in long-term retention and stability. Is active retention needed? *American Journal of Orthodontics and Dentofacial Orthopedics*, **101**, 297–302.

Postlethwaite, K. (1989). The range and effectiveness of safety headgear products. *European Journal of Orthodontics*, **11**, 228–34.

Proffit, W. R. (2000). *Contemporary Orthodontics* (3rd edn). Mosby, St Louis, MO.

Samuels, R. H. (1996) A review of orthodontic face-bow injuries and safety equipment. *American Journal of Orthodontics and Dentofacial Orthopedics*, **110**, 269–72.

Samuels, R. H. (1997) A new locking face-bow *Journal of Clinical Orthodontics*, **31**, 24–7.

Sandy, J. R. (1992). Tooth eruption and orthodontic movement. *British Dental Journal*, **172**, 141–9.

● An erudite paper detailing the cellular and biochemical theories of the mechanisms involved in tooth movement.

Seel, B. D. S. (1980). Extra-oral hazards of extra-oral traction. *British Journal of Orthodontics*, **7**, 53–5.

16 Removable appliances

This chapter concerns those appliances that are fabricated mainly in acrylic and wire, and (as the name suggests) can be removed from the mouth. Most removable appliances are made for the upper arch. Functional appliances are made of the same materials, but work primarily by exerting intermaxillary traction and so are considered separately in Chapter 18.

16.1. INDICATIONS FOR THE USE OF REMOVABLE APPLIANCES

Although widely utilized in the past as the sole appliance to treat a malocclusion, with the increasing availability and acceptance of fixed appliances the limitations of the removable appliance have become more apparent. The removable appliance is only capable of producing tilting movements of individual teeth, which can be used to advantage where simple movements are required to correct a mild malocclusion but can lead to a compromise result if employed where more complex tooth movements are indicated. As a result the role of the removable appliance is changing, and it is becoming more widely used to transmit forces to blocks of teeth and as an adjunct to fixed appliance treatment. Removable appliances provide a useful means of applying extra-oral traction to segments of teeth, or an entire arch, to help achieve intrusive and/or distal movement. Examples of these types of appliance include the *en masse* appliance, which is described in Section 16.4.6 or the maxillary and buccal segment intrusion splints discussed in Chapter 12. Removable appliances are also employed for arch expansion, which is another example of their usefulness in moving blocks of teeth.

Removable appliances are particularly helpful where a flat anterior bite-plane or buccal capping is required to influence development of the buccal segment teeth and/or to free the occlusion with the lower arch. They are used passively as space maintainers following permanent tooth extractions and also as retaining appliances following fixed appliance treatment, as wear can gradually be reduced, allowing the occlusion to 'settle in'. The advantages and disadvantages of removable appliances are summarized in Table 16.1.

Table 16.1 Advantages and disadvantages of removable appliances

Advantages	Disadvantages
Can be removed for tooth-brushing	Appliance can be left out
Palatal coverage increases anchorage	Only tilting movements possible
Easy to adjust	Good technician required
Can be used for overbite reduction in a growing child avoiding a lower appliance	Affects speech
Acrylic can be thickened to form flat anterior bite plane or buccal capping	Intermaxillary traction not practicable
Useful as passive retainer or space maintainer	Lower removable appliances are difficult to tolerate
Can be used to transmit forces to blocks of teeth	Inefficient for multiple individual tooth movements

On occasion it may be helpful to 'test out' the cooperation of patients whose motivation for more complex treatment is uncertain by fitting a removable appliance and reviewing progress before deciding whether to proceed.

Lower removable appliances are generally poorly tolerated by patients. This is due in part to their encroachment upon tongue space, but also the lingual tilt of the lower molars makes retentive clasping difficult.

16.2. DESIGNING REMOVABLE APPLIANCES

16.2.1. General principles

The design of an appliance should never be delegated to a laboratory (to do this is equivalent to driving a car blindfolded with the passenger giving directions) as they are only able to utilize the information provided by the plaster casts. Success depends upon designing an appliance that is easy for the patient to insert and wear, and is relevant to the occlusal aims of treatment.

16.2.2. Steps in designing a removable appliance

Four components need to be considered for every removable appliance:
Active component(s)
Retaining the appliance
Anchorage
Baseplate.

This gives the acronym ARAB, which may help to jog the memory. A detailed consideration of each of these components is given in the sections below.

Generally, extractions should be deferred until after an appliance is fitted. The rationale for this is twofold:

1. If the extractions are carried out first, there is a real risk that the teeth posterior to the extraction site will drift forward, resulting in an appliance that does not fit well or even does not fit at all. This is most noticeable when upper first permanent molars have been extracted or there is a conspicuous delay before the appliance is fitted.
2. Occasionally a patient decides after an appliance is fitted that they do not wish to continue with treatment. It is obviously preferable if this change of mind occurs before any extractions have been undertaken.

Rarely, it is necessary to carry out extractions first, for example when a displaced tooth will interfere with the design of the appliance. However, even in these cases it is preferable to take impressions for the fabrication of the appliance before the extractions and to instruct the technician to remove the tooth concerned from the model. The appliance should then be fitted as soon as practicable after the teeth are extracted.

16.3. ACTIVE COMPONENTS

16.3.1. Springs

Springs are the most commonly used active component. Their design can readily be adapted to the needs of a particular clinical situation and they are inexpensive. However, a skilled technician will make the difference between a spring that works efficiently with the minimum of adjustment on fitting and one that requires the clinician to try to compensate for its inadequacies at every visit.

The expression for the force F exerted by an orthodontic spring is the only formula remembered by the author and on this basis is recommended to the reader as being worthwhile:

$$F \propto \frac{dr^4}{l^3}$$

where d is the deflection of the spring on activation, r is the radius of the wire, and l is the length of the spring. Thus even small changes in the diameter or length of wire used in the construction of a spring will have a profound impact upon the force delivered. It is obviously desirable to deliver a light (physiological) force (Chapter 15) over a long activation range, but there are practical restrictions upon the length and diameter of wire used to construct a spring. The span of a spring is usually constrained by the size of the arch or the depth of the sulcus. However, incorporating a coil into the design of a spring increases the length of wire and therefore results in the application of a smaller force for a given deflection. A spring with a coil will work more efficiently if it is activated in the direction that the wire has been wound so that the coil unwinds as the tooth moves.

In practice the smallest diameter of wire that can be used for spring construction is 0.5 mm. However, wire of this diameter is liable to distortion or breakage and therefore the spring has to be strengthened by being sleeved in tubing (e.g. the Roberts retractor) or protected with acrylic (e.g. the palatal finger spring).

The effect of wire diameter upon the force delivered by a spring can be appreciated by considering the amount of activation required to deliver a force in the region of 30–50 g for the same design of buccal canine retraction spring (Fig. 16.1) fabricated using wires of two different diameters. For a spring composed of 0.5 mm wire an activation of about 3 mm will be required. For the same spring composed of 0.7 mm wire an activation of 1 mm is required. It can readily be appreciated that the 0.7 mm spring gives little margin for error — an activation of 1.5 mm would give an excessive force, but an activation of 0.5 mm would deliver insufficient force.

The stability ratio of a spring is readily appreciated when trying to adjust a buccal canine retraction spring. In mechanical terms it is:

$$\frac{\text{Stiffness in the direction of unwanted displacement}}{\text{Stiffness in the intended direction of tooth movement}} = \text{stability ratio}$$

In practice, springs which have a high stability ratio, for example, the palatal finger spring are straightforward to adjust, whereas those with a low stability ratio are difficult to position precisely on the tooth to be moved.

16.3.2. Screws

Screws are less versatile than springs, as the direction of tooth movement is determined by the position of the screw in the appliance. They are also bulky and expensive. However, a screw appliance may be useful when it is desirable to utilize the teeth to be moved for additional clasping to retain the appliance. This is helpful when a number of teeth are to be moved together (for example in an appliance to expand the upper arch (Fig. 16.2)) or in the mixed dentition where retaining an appliance is always difficult.

There are basically two types of screw. The most commonly used type consists of two halves on a threaded central cylinder (Fig. 16.3) turned by means of a key which separates the two halves by a predetermined distance, usually about 0.2 mm for each quarter turn. The other variety is the spring-loaded piston screw (Fig. 16.4) which is activated by moving the whole screw assembly forwards by means of a screwdriver.

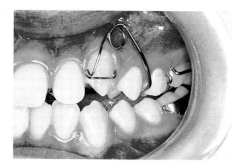

Fig. 16.1. Buccal canine retractor.

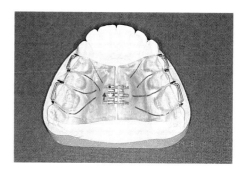

Fig. 16.2. Screw appliance to expand the upper arch.

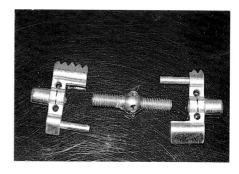

Fig. 16.3. Components of a screw.

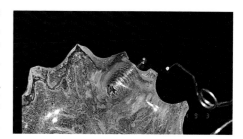

Fig. 16.4. Spring-loaded piston screw (Landin screw).

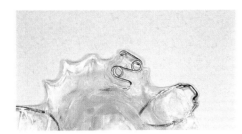

Fig. 16.5. Z-spring.

Double cantilever

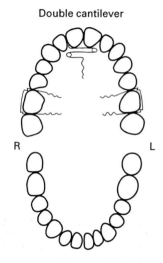

Fig. 16.6. Double-cantilever spring.

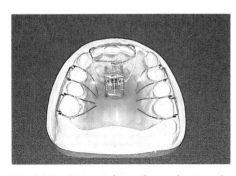

Fig. 16.7. Screw appliance for proclination of
the incisors.

Activation of a screw is limited by the width of the periodontal ligament, as to exceed this would result in crushing of the ligament cells and cessation of tooth movement (see Chapter 15).

16.3.3. Elastics

Special intra-oral elastics are manufactured for orthodontic use (see Chapter 17, Fig. 17.20). These elastics are usually classified by their size, ranging from 1/8 inch to 3/4 inch, and the force that they are designed to deliver, usually 2 oz, 3.5 oz or 4.5 oz. Selection of the appropriate size and force is based upon the root surface area of the teeth to be moved and the distance over which the elastic is to be stretched. The elastics should be changed every day.

16.4 COMMONLY USED COMPONENTS

16.4.1. Labial movement of the incisors

Z-spring (Fig. 16.5)

This is actually a small double-cantilever spring fabricated in 0.5 mm wire. It has the advantage that the direction of movement can be altered. Good anterior retention is required to resist the displacing effect of this spring.

Activation is by pulling the spring about 1–2 mm away from the baseplate at an angle of approximately 45° in the direction of desired movement (so that the spring is not caught on the incisal edge as the appliance is inserted).

Double-cantilever spring (Fig. 16.6)

This spring is designed for moving more than one tooth labially and is made in 0.7 or 0.8 mm wire depending upon its length.

Activation is in the same way as for the Z-spring.

Crossed-cantilever springs

This design is used for proclining more than one tooth and also allows variation in the direction of individual tooth movement.

Activation is the same as for the Z-spring.

Screw appliance (Fig. 16.7)

This design is helpful where retention is limited, as the incisors to be moved can also be clasped for additional retention. However, a screw appliance tends to be bulky, which limits its application to the movement of at least three incisors.

Activation is by giving the screw one-quarter turn every three to four days.

Landin screw (Fig. 16.4)

The piston or Landin screw is used for proclining one incisor, but the direction of tooth movement is determined by the technician's placement of the screw in the acrylic. Now rarely used.

Activation is by turning the screw with a watchmaker's screwdriver (or flat plastic instrument) in the direction of movement (about 1 mm).

16.4.2. Palatal movement (retraction) of the incisors

Removable appliances are only indicated for overjet reduction if the upper incisors are proclined and the overjet not significantly increased.

Labial bow (0.7 mm wire)

A conventional labial bow is really too stiff for active overjet reduction. Although splitting the bow increases its flexibility, it also increases its liability to distortion and to causing tissue trauma. Other designs are preferable.

Roberts retractor (Fig. 16.8)

This spring is made of 0.5 mm wire which is sheathed with tubing distal to the coils. While useful for retracting proclined incisors, it is difficult to repair and requires an adequate depth of sulcus. A separate retaining appliance is advisable after overjet reduction.

Activation is by bending the arms of the spring towards the incisors.

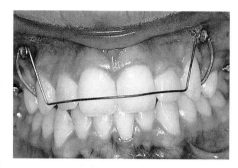

Fig. 16.8. Roberts retractor.

Strap spring (Fig. 16.9)

The spring is also known as a self-straightening arch. It is fabricated by winding 0.5 mm wire onto a heavier labial bow with one end attached to the U-loop of the bow and the other free-sliding. It has the advantage that the same appliance can be used for canine retraction, overjet reduction, and retention, as the strap spring can easily be added and removed. Some orthodontists recommend using two strap springs to prevent flattening of the arch, whilst others feel that this is unnecessary. Certainly, it is easier to adjust and insert one strap spring than two.

Activation is by tightening the base labial bow, and not the strap spring itself. It is important to ensure that the free-sliding end is indeed free-sliding. If it is not, then it is usually necessary to replace the strap spring.

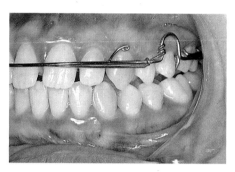

Fig. 16.9. Strap spring appliance (the palatal finger spring on the canine was removed at this visit). Note that the labial bow has been soldered to the bridge of the Adams clasp.

Elastics

Using elastics to reduce an overjet is popular with patients as they are less visible than a metal spring. An appliance used for canine retraction can be converted for overjet reduction with elastics by dividing the labial bow and fashioning hooks adjacent to the upper canines. Alternatively, a purpose-designed appliance can be made. For most patients a 3.5 oz, 5/8 inch elastic is required. This method of overjet reduction should be avoided in cases with very proclined incisors as the elastics tend to slide up the teeth and retract the gingivae instead.

Whatever the means of overjet reduction, if a bite-plane has been used for overbite reduction this must be trimmed away behind the incisors as they are retracted. Adjustment should be made from the fitting surface, as well as antero-posteriorly (Fig. 16.10). Contact needs to be maintained with the lower incisors to prevent their re-eruption, and the bite-plane should only be trimmed away completely during the final phases of overjet reduction.

16.4.3. Mesial/distal movement of incisors

Palatal finger spring

See the section below on the canine palatal finger spring.

Activation (half a tooth width) as for the canine palatal finger spring.

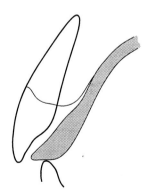

Fig. 16.10. Diagram showing how a flat anterior bite-plane should be trimmed during overjet reduction to give space for retraction of the upper incisors and their associated gingivae. The bite-plane should be maintained to prevent re-eruption of the lower incisors and only removed towards the end of overjet reduction.

16.4.4. Retraction of canines

It is sometimes tempting to start retraction of a canine before it has erupted sufficiently. Placement of an active spring on the inclined mesial cusp of a canine tooth will at best delay further eruption and may intrude the tooth.

Palatal finger spring (Fig. 16.11)

This design of spring has better vertical stability than a buccal retractor — this is readily appreciated when trying to adjust a buccal spring. It is wise to ask the technician to box out the acrylic overlying the spring and to place a guard wire to prevent distortion. To make adjustment of a spring as straightforward as possible the coil should be positioned midway between the starting position of the tooth and the intended finishing location. Where possible, a palatal finger spring should be used in conjunction with a labial bow, as this will help to guide the tooth around the arch and prevent flaring of the tooth buccally.

Before activation is attempted the spring should be adjusted so that it is lying at the level of the gingival margin with a point of application at 90° to the intended direction of movement. The spring can be activated at any point between the coil and where it emerges from underneath the guard wire, but placing the bend nearer to the tip of the spring moves the point of application more buccally. As a rule of thumb an optimal force for canine retraction is delivered by an activation of just under half a tooth width.

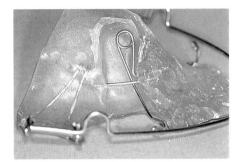

Fig. 16.11. Palatal finger spring. Note that the spring is boxed in with acrylic and a guard wire is present to help prevent distortion.

Buccal canine retractor — 0.5 mm tubed

Where a canine needs to be moved palatally a buccally approaching spring is required. The author's preferred design is shown in Fig. 16.1.

Activation is by winding up the coil or by adjusting the anterior leg. However, this has the effect of lowering the point of application of the spring, and a compensatory adjustment of the more posterior leg is needed to correct this.

Buccal canine retractor — 0.7 mm

There are several permutations of the 0.7 mm buccal canine retractor. A similar design to the 0.5 mm retractor in Fig. 16.1 or the type shown in Fig. 16.12 can be used. This type of spring is known colloquially as a 'cut and bend' spring, as this is the manner by which it is activated.

Activation will depend upon the design of spring used, but to be effective it must curve around and engage the mesial aspect of the tooth. The disadvantage of a retractor formed in 0.7 mm wire is that an activation of about 1 mm is required to deliver an optimal force for canine retraction, and this is difficult to achieve precisely in practice.

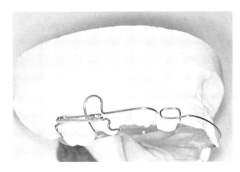

Fig. 16.12. 'Cut and bend' buccal canine retractor.

16.4.5. Buccal movement of premolars and molars

T-spring

This spring is used for the buccal movement of a single premolar or molar tooth (Fig. 16.13). Good retention is required to resist the displacing effect of the spring.

Activation is by pulling the spring away from the acrylic at an angle of 45°.

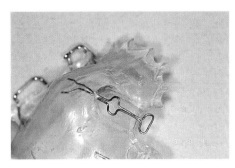

Fig. 16.13. T–spring.

Screw appliance

This design is applicable if it is required to move more than one tooth buccally, for example correction of a crossbite by upper arch expansion (see Fig. 16.2).

Activation: the patient should give the screw a one-quarter turn twice a week (for example on a Wednesday and a Saturday). If opened too far, the screw will come apart; therefore patients should be warned that if the screw portion becomes loose they should turn it back one turn and not advance the screw again.

16.4.6. Mesial/distal movement of premolars and molars

Palatal finger spring

See the section on the canine palatal finger spring.

Nudger appliance (Fig. 16.14)

This appliance is used in conjunction with headgear to bands on the first molar teeth. It is usually used to achieve distal movement of the molar teeth when it is intended to go onto fixed appliances to complete alignment. The appliance incorporates palatal finger springs to retract the first permanent molars. The appliance is worn full-time and the patient asked to wear the headgear for 12 to 16 hours per day. The palatal finger springs are only lightly activated with the aim of minimiszing forward movement of the molars when the headgear is not worn. This appliance is also very useful if unilateral distal movement is required. In this case the contralateral molar can be clasped to aid retention. If overbite reduction is required then a bite-plane can be included in the appliance. It is advisable to fit the bands on the molar teeth and then take an impression to fabricate the appliance.

Activation: the palatal finger springs are activated 1–2 mm.

Screw appliance

This is similar to the design used for buccal movement of one or two molars or premolars, except that the screw is positioned to open anteroposteriorly.

En masse appliance

The *en masse* appliance is used for distal movement of the upper buccal segments with headgear. There are several variants, but essentially the appliance comprises extra-oral traction, either as an integral part of the appliance or by tubes soldered to the bridge of the cribs, which allow the insertion of a face-bow and a means of expansion to maintain arch coordination.

Activation: the active force is provided by the headgear and at least 14–16 hours wear per day is required. If the appliance incorporates a midline screw this should be given a one-quarter turn per week. A coffin spring is activated by pulling apart the two halves of the appliance. (Sometimes appliances with a coffin spring arrive from the laboratory without the acrylic being divided — it is advisable to cut the acrylic down the middle before attempting to activate the coffin spring!)

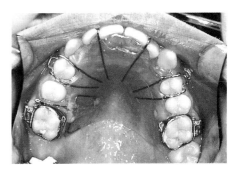

Fig. 16.14. Nudger appliance for unilateral movement of the upper right first permanent molar.

16.4.7. Palatal movement of an individual tooth

Self-supporting buccal spring

As for the buccal canine retractor.

Activation is the same as for the buccal canine retractor, bearing in mind the root surface area of the tooth to be moved (i.e. less activation for a lateral incisor).

16.5. RETAINING THE APPLIANCE

16.5.1. Adams clasp

This crib was designed to engage the undercuts present on a fully erupted first permanent molar at the junctions of the mesial and distal surfaces with the buccal aspect of the tooth (Fig. 16.15). The crib is usually fabricated in hard 0.7 mm stainless steel wire and should engage about 1 mm of undercut. In practice this means that in children the arrowheads will lie at or just below the gingival margin. However, in adults with some gingival recession the arrowheads should lie part way down the crown of the tooth (Fig. 16.16).

This crib can also be used for retention on premolars, canines, central incisors, and deciduous molars. However, it is advisable to use 0.6 mm wire for these teeth. When second permanent molars have to be utilized for retention soon after their eruption it is wise to omit the distobuccal arrowhead, as little undercut exists and if included it may irritate the cheek.

The reason for the popularity of the Adams crib is its versatility as it can be easily adapted:

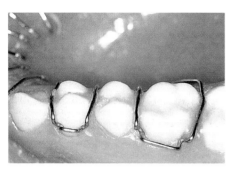

Fig. 16.15. Adams clasp.

- Extra-oral traction tubes, labial bows, or buccal springs can be soldered onto the bridge of the clasp (Fig. 16.17; see also Fig. 16.9).
- Hooks or coils can be fabricated in the bridge of the clasp during construction (Fig. 16.18).
- Double cribs can be constructed (see Fig. 16.12).

Adjustment: the crib can be adjusted in two places. Bends in the middle of the flyover will move the arrowhead down and in towards the tooth. Adjustments near the arrowhead will result in more movement towards the tooth and will have less effect in the vertical plane (Fig. 16.19).

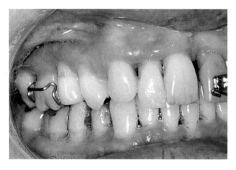

Fig. 16.16. Ideally the Adams clasp should engage about 1 mm of undercut. Therefore in adults with some gingival recession the arrowheads will probably lie part way down the crown of the tooth.

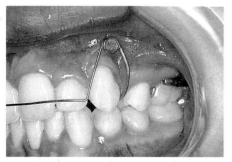

Fig. 16.17. A tube for an extra-oral face-bow has been soldered to the bridge of this clasp.

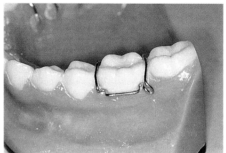

Fig. 16.18. A loop which provides a hook for placement of elastic traction has been incorporated into this Adams crib.

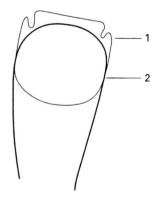

1 Arrowhead moves horizontally in towards tooth

2 Arrowhead moves in towards tooth and also vertically towards gingival crevice

Fig. 16.19. Adjustment of an Adams clasp.

16.5.2. Other methods of retention

Southend clasp (Fig. 16.20)

This clasp is designed to utilize the undercut beneath the contact point between two incisors. It is usually fabricated in 0.7 mm hard stainless steel wire.

Adjustment: retention is increased by bending the arrowhead in towards the teeth.

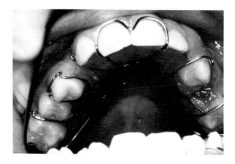

Fig. 16.20. Southend clasp

Ball-ended clasps (see Fig. 18.12)

These clasps are designed to engage the undercut interproximally. This design affords minimal retention and can have the effect of prising the teeth apart.

Adjustment: the ball is bent in towards the contact point between the teeth.

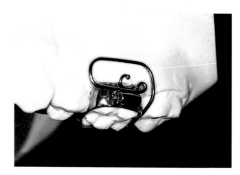

Fig. 16.21. Plint clasp.

Plint clasp (Fig. 16.21)

This clasp is used to engage under the tube assembly on a molar band.

Adjustment: by moving the clasp under the molar tube.

Labial bows (Fig. 16.22)

A labial bow is useful for anterior retention, particularly if mesial or distal tooth movement is planned, as it will help to guide tooth movement along the arch and prevent buccal flaring. Fitted labial bows provide particularly good retention and are often employed in retaining appliances following fixed appliance treatment.

Adjustment: this will depend upon the exact design of an individual bow. However, the most commonly used type with U-loops is adjusted by squeezing together the legs of the U-loop and then adjusting the height of the labial bow by a bend at the anterior leg to compensate (Fig. 16.23).

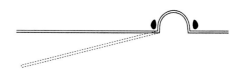

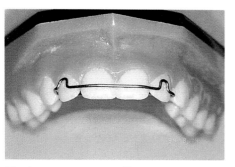

Fig. 16.22. Two types of labial bow.

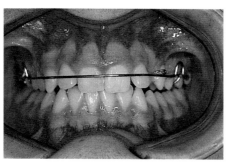

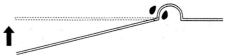

Fig. 16.23. Diagram illustrating how to tighten a labial bow. The first adjustment is to squeeze together the two legs of the U-loop. This causes the anterior section of the bow to move occlusally and therefore a second adjustment is required to lift it back to the desired horizontal position.

16.6. BASEPLATE

The other individual components of a removable appliance are connected by means of an acrylic baseplate, which can be a passive or active component of the appliance.

16.6.1. Self-cure or heat-cure acrylic

Heat-curing of polymethylmethacrylate increases the degree of polymerization of the material and optimizes its properties, but is technically more demanding to produce. It is common practice to make the majority of appliances in self-cure acrylic, retaining heat-cure acrylic for those situations where additional strength is desirable, for example some functional appliances.

16.6.2. Anterior bite-plane

Increasing the thickness of acrylic behind the upper incisors forms a bite-plane onto which the lower incisors occlude. A bite-plane is prescribed when either the overbite needs to be reduced by eruption of the lower buccal segment teeth or elimination of possible occlusal interferences is necessary to allow tooth movement to occur.

Anterior bite-planes are usually flat. Inclined bite-planes may lead to proclination or retroclination of the lower incisors, depending upon their angulation, and therefore should be avoided.

When prescribing a flat anterior bite-plane the following information needs to be given to the technician:

- How far posteriorly the bite-plane should extend. This is most easily conveyed by noting the overjet.
- The depth of the bite-plane. To increase the likelihood that the patient will wear the appliance, the bite-plane should result in a separation of only 1–2 mm between the upper and lower molars. The depth is prescribed in terms of the height of the bite-plane against the upper incisors, for example 'half height of the upper incisor'.

In a proportion of cases more than 1–2 mm of overbite reduction is required, and therefore it will be necessary to add to the height of the bite-plane during treatment.

16.6.3. Buccal capping

Buccal capping is prescribed when occlusal interferences need to be eliminated to allow tooth movement to be completed and reduction of the overbite is undesirable. Buccal capping is produced by carrying the acrylic over the occlusal surface of the buccal segment teeth (Fig. 16.24) and has the effect of propping the incisors apart. The acrylic should be as thin as practicably possible to aid patient tolerance. To assist adjustment of posterior clasping, the buccal capping can be extended only halfway across the buccal segment teeth. During treatment it is not uncommon for the bite-plane to fracture away and it is wise to warn patients of this, advising them to return if a sharp edge results. However, if as a result a tooth is left free of the acrylic and is liable to over-erupt, a new appliance will be necessary (as additions to buccal capping are rarely successful).

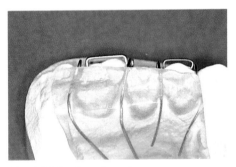

Fig. 16.24. Buccal capping.

16.7. FITTING A REMOVABLE APPLIANCE

It is always useful to explain again to the patient (and their parent/guardian) the overall treatment plan and the role of the appliance that is to be fitted. It is also prudent to delay any permanent extractions until after an appliance has been fitted and the patient's ability to achieve full-time wear has been demonstrated.

Table 16.2 Instruments which are useful for fitting and adjusting removable appliances

- Adams pliers (no. 64)
- Spring-forming pliers (no. 65)
- Maun's wire cutters
- Pair of autoclavable dividers
- Steel rule (these are generally cheaper from ironmongers than from dental supply companies)
- A straight handpiece and an acrylic bur (preferably tungsten carbide)
- A pair of robust hollow-chop pliers is a useful addition, but not essential

Fitting an appliance can be approached in the following way (see also Table 16.2):

1. Check that you have the correct appliance for the patient in the chair (everyone will make this mistake at some stage) and that your prescription has been followed.

2. Show the appliance to the patient and explain how it works. It is advisable to stress to the patient that they should not remove the appliance by the springs.

3. Check the fitting surface for any roughness.

4. Try in the appliance. If it does not fit check the following:
   - Have any teeth erupted since the impression was taken? If necessary, adjust the acrylic.
   - Have any teeth moved since the impression was recorded? This usually occurs if any extractions have been recently carried out. Occasionally, to salvage the situation, it is necessary to bend the cribs forward to compensate for anterior movement of the molars.
   - Has there been a significant delay between taking the impression and fitting the appliance?

5. Adjust the retention until the appliance just clicks into place.

6. If the appliance has a bite-plane or buccal capping, this will need to be trimmed so that it is active but not too bulky.

7. The active element(s) to be used in the first stage of treatment should be gently activated, provided that extractions are not required to make space available into which the teeth are to be moved.

8. Give the patient a mirror and demonstrate how to insert and remove the appliance. Then let them practice.

9. Go through the instructions with the patient (and parent or guardian), stressing the importance of full-time wear. A sheet outlining the important points and containing details of what do in the event of problems is advisable, but unfortunately is not always read (Table 16.3). Medicolegally it is prudent to note in the patient's records if instructions have been given.

10. Arrange the next appointment.

If a working model is available, it is wise to store this with the patient's study models as it may prove helpful if the appliance has to be repaired

Table 16.3 Sample instructions to patients for removable appliances

- Your appliance should be worn all the time, including meals and in bed at night
- Your appliance should only be removed for tooth cleaning and during vigorous sports (when it should be stored in a strong container)
- It is usual to experience some discomfort and a little difficulty with speech initially, but this should pass in a few days as you become accustomed to wearing the appliance
- It is important to avoid hard or sticky foods and chewing gum
- If you cannot wear your appliance as instructed or if it becomes damaged or causes pain, please contact (...) immediately.

16.8. MONITORING PROGRESS

Ideally, patients wearing active removable appliances should be seen every 3 to 4 weeks. Activation of an appliance more frequently than this will increase the risk of anchorage loss and root resorption (see Chapter 15). The exception to this guideline is the screw appliance where only a small amount of activation is possible at a time and therefore more frequent small activations are required. Passive appliances can be seen less frequently, but it is advisable to check, and if necessary adjust, the retention of the clasps every 3 months.

During active treatment it is important to establish that the patient is wearing the appliance as instructed. A more accurate answer may given in response to the question 'How much are you managing to wear your brace?' rather than 'Are you wearing your brace full-time?' Indications of a lack of compliance include the following:

- the appliance shows little evidence of wear and tear;
- the patient lisps (ask the patient to count from 65 to 70 with, and without, their appliance);
- no marks in the patient's mouth around the gingival margins palatally or across the palate;
- frequent breakages.

16.8.1. At each visit

If wear is satisfactory the following should be checked at each visit:

- The treatment plan: this may seem facetious, but it is all too easy to lose sight of the precise aims of treatment. Referring back to the original plan will ensure that each step is carried out methodically and will act as a reminder of how long treatment has been under way, so that progress can be monitored.
- The patient's oral hygiene.
- Loss of anchorage by recording overjet and buccal segment relationship.
- Tooth movement since the last visit: a good tip is to use dividers which can be imprinted into the records.
- Retention of the appliance by asking the patient and adjusting the clasps or labial bow (see Section 16.5) as indicated.
- Whether the active elements of the appliance need adjustment (see Section 16.4).

- Whether the bite-plane or buccal capping need to be increased and/or adjusted.
- Record what action needs to be undertaken at the next visit.

16.8.2. Common problems during treatment

Slow rate of tooth movement

Normally tooth movement should proceed at approximately 1 mm per month in children, and less in adults. If progress is slow, check the following.

- Is the patient wearing the appliance full-time? If the appliance is not being worn as much as required, the implications of this need to be discussed with the patient and the parent. If poor cooperation continues, resulting in a lack of progress, consideration will have to be given to abandoning treatment.
- Are the springs correctly positioned? If not, explain again to the patient the purpose of the spring and show them how to insert the appliance correctly.
- Are the springs underactive, overactive, or distorted? If the springs were correctly adjusted at the patient's last visit (see Section 16.4), check that the patient is not using them to remove the appliance or putting it in their pocket during meals.
- Is tooth movement obstructed by the acrylic or wires of the appliance? If this is the case, these should be removed or adjusted.
- Is tooth movement prevented by occlusion with the opposing arch? It may be necessary to increase the bite-plane or buccal capping to free the occlusion.

Frequent breakage of the appliance

The main reasons for this are as follows:

- The appliance is not being worn full-time.
- The patient has a habit of clicking the appliance in and out (see below).
- The patient is eating inappropriate foods whilst wearing the appliance. Success lies in dissuading the patient from eating hard and/or sticky foods altogether. Partial success is a patient who removes their appliance to eat hard or sticky foods!

Appliance quickly becomes loose fitting

The most common cause of this is a patient who is clicking the appliance in and out. This habit can also lead to intrusion of the teeth, which are clasped by the appliance and to frequent breakages. The patient's close family are often very grateful if the habit is stopped, as the clicking noise that it generates can be very irritating.

Excessive tilting of tooth being moved

Removable appliances are only capable of tilting movements. However, this is exaggerated by the following:

- The further that the spring is from the centre of resistance of the tooth the greater is the degree of tilting. Therefore a spring should be adjusted so that it is as near the gingival margin as possible without causing gingival trauma.

● Excessive force is being applied to the tooth, as this has the effect of moving the centre of resistance more apically.

Anchorage loss

This can be increased by the following:

● Part-time appliance wear, thus allowing the anchor teeth to drift forwards.
● The forces being applied by the active elements exceed the anchorage resistance of the appliance. Care is required to ensure that the springs, etc. are not being overactivated or that too much active tooth movement is being attempted at a time.

If anchorage loss is a problem see Chapter 15.

Palatal inflammation

This can occur for two reasons:

1. Poor oral hygiene. In the majority of cases the extent of the inflammation exactly matches the coverage of the appliance and is caused by a mixed fungal and bacterial infection (Fig. 16.25). This may occur in conjunction with angular cheilitis. Management of this condition must address the underlying problem, which is usually poor oral hygiene. However, in marked cases it may be wise to supplement this with an antifungal agent (e.g. nystatin, amphotericin, or miconazole gel) which is applied to the fitting surface of the appliance four times daily. If associated with angular cheilitis, miconazole cream may be helpful.

2. Entrapment of the gingivae behind the upper incisors during overjet reduction between the incisors themselves and the acrylic of the bite-plane (Fig. 16.26). A mistake commonly made during overjet reduction is to trim away the fitting surface of the appliance to allow for palatal movement of the incisors only, forgetting that space should also be created for retraction of the palatal gingivae. To prevent this from occurring, it is necessary to achieve good overbite reduction in the initial stages of appliance therapy and trim the acrylic as shown in Fig. 16.10 during overjet reduction.

Lack of overbite reduction

Lack of progress with overbite reduction can be a problem in patients who are not actively growing vertically, such as adults or those with a horizontal direction of mandibular growth. In these cases it may be necessary to proceed onto fixed appliances. In children, the most common reason for lack of progress with overbite reduction is that the appliance is not being worn during meals. Patients should be advised that their treatment will be quicker and more successful if they wear their appliance for eating, and that adaptation will be enhanced if they start with softer foods.

16.9. LOWER REMOVABLE APPLIANCES

Lower removable appliances are rarely used because they are poorly tolerated by patients. Not only do they encroach upon tongue space, but retention is a problem owing to the lingual tilt of the lower molars and the displacing action of the tongue. In addition, it is difficult to incorporate lingual springs and there is

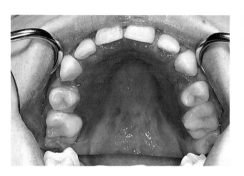

Fig. 16.25. Inflammation of the palate corresponding to the coverage of a removable appliance.

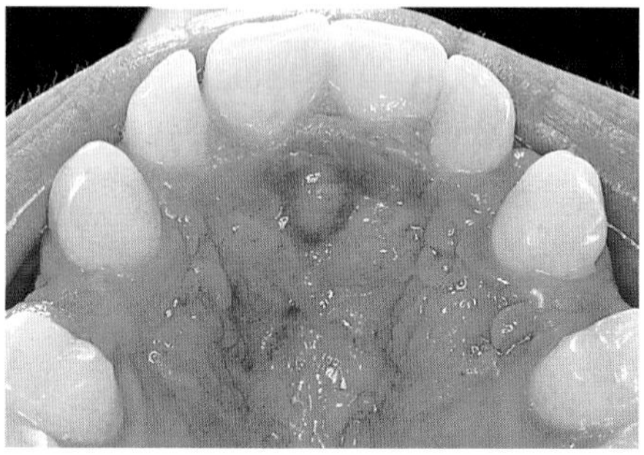

Fig. 16.26. Inadequate trimming of the fitting surface under the anterior bite-plane during overjet has resulted in entrapment of the gingivae between the acrylic and the teeth.

limited depth of sulcus for buccal springs. Various designs have been suggested to overcome these shortcomings, but where tooth movement in the lower arch is required a fixed appliance is usually more efficient. Therefore the most commonly used design of lower removable appliance is the retainer.

16.10. APPLIANCE REPAIRS

Before arranging for a removable appliance to be repaired the following should be considered:

- How was the appliance broken? If a breakage has been caused by the patient failing to follow instructions, it is important to be sure any cooperation problems have been overcome before proceeding with the repair.
- Would it be more cost-effective to make a new appliance, perhaps incorporating the next stage of the treatment planned?
- Occasionally it is possible to adapt what remains of the spring or another component of the appliance to continue the desired movement. For example, a long labial bow can be cut and adapted to form a buccal retractor.
- Is the working model available, or is an up-to-date impression required to facilitate the repair?
- How will the tooth movements which have been achieved be retained while the repair is being carried out? Often there is no alternative but to try and carry out the repair in the shortest possible time.

PRINCIPAL SOURCES AND FURTHER READING

Houston, W. J. B. and Isaacson, K. G. (1980). *Orthodontic treatment with removable appliances* (2nd edn). Wright, Bristol.

Houston, W. J. B. and Waters, N. E. (1977). The design of buccal canine retraction springs for removable orthodontic appliances. *British Journal of Orthodontics*, **4**, 191–5.

Kerr, W. J. S., Buchanan, I. B., and McColl, J. H. (1993). Use of the PAR Index in assessing the effectiveness of removable orthodontic appliances. *British Journal of Orthodontics*, **20**, 351–7.

- This study found that when removable appliances were used in selected cases, 89 per cent showed an improved or a greatly improved result (as indicated by the PAR Index).

Lloyd, T. G. and Stephens, C. D. (1979). Spontaneous changes in molar occlusion after extraction of all first premolars: a study of Class II division 1 cases treated with removable appliances. *British Journal of Orthodontics*, **6**, 91–4.

17 Fixed appliances

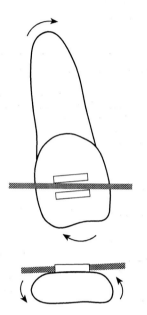

Fig. 17.1. Generation of a force couple by the interaction between the bracket slot and the archwire.

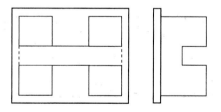

Fig. 17.2. Diagrammatic representation of an edgewise bracket.

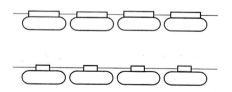

Fig. 17.3. Narrower brackets increase the span of wire between brackets, thus increasing the flexibility of the archwire. However, wider brackets allow greater rotational and mesiodistal control, as the force couple generated has a greater moment.

17.1. PRINCIPLES OF FIXED APPLIANCES

Fixed appliances are attached to the teeth and are thus are capable of a greater range of tooth movements than is possible with a removable appliance. Not only does the attachment on the tooth surface (called a bracket) allow the tooth to be moved vertically or tilted, but also a force couple can be generated by the interaction between the bracket and an archwire running through the bracket (Fig 17.1). Thus rotational and apical movements are also possible. The interplay between the archwire and the bracket slot determines the type and direction of movement achieved. A bewildering variety of different types of bracket are now manufactured, and the choice of archwire materials and configurations is extensive. Therefore, for clarity, we shall consider the edgewise type of bracket (Fig. 17.2) in this section; other bracket systems are described briefly in Section 17.6.

The edgewise bracket is rectangular in shape and is typically described by the width of the bracket slot, usually 0.018 or 0.022 inch. The depth of the slot is commonly between 0.025 and 0.032 inch. Modifying the shape of the bracket can affect tooth movement. For example, a narrow bracket (Fig. 17.3) results in a greater span of archwire between the brackets which increases the flexibility of the archwire. In contrast, a wider bracket reduces the interbracket archwire span, but is more efficient for de-rotation and mesiodistal control. Nowadays a wide variety of bracket designs are available. In most modern appliance systems each bracket is a different width corresponding to the type of tooth for which it is intended; for example, lower incisors have the narrowest brackets (see photographs of fixed appliances shown later in the chapter).

A round wire in a rectangular edgewise type of slot will give a degree of control of mesiodistal tilt, vertical height, and rotational position. The closer the fit of the archwire in the bracket, the greater is the control gained. However, with a round wire only tipping movements in a buccolingual direction are possible (Fig. 17.4). When a rectangular wire is used in a rectangular slot, a force couple can be generated by the interaction between the walls of the slot and the sides of the archwire and buccolingual apical movement produced (Fig. 17.5). However, some tipping movements will take place before the rectangular wires engage the sides of the bracket slot, with the degree of 'slop' depending on the differences between the dimensions of the archwire and the bracket slot (Fig. 17.6).

Thus fixed appliances can be used in conjunction with rectangular archwires to achieve tooth movement in all three spatial planes. In orthodontics these are described by the types of bend that are required in an archwire to produce each type of movement (Fig. 17.7):

- **First-order bends** are made in the plane of the archwire to compensate for differing tooth widths.
- **Second-order bends** are made in the vertical plane to achieve correct mesiodistal angulation or tilt of the tooth.

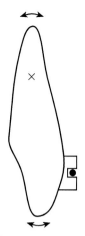

Fig. 17.4. When a round wire is used in a rectangular slot, buccolingual forces tip the tooth around a fulcrum in the root.

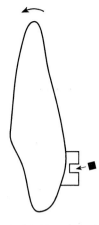

Fig. 17.5. When a rectangular wire is used with a rectangular slot more control of buccolingual root movement is achieved, allowing bodily and torquing movements to be accomplished.

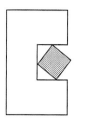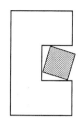

Fig. 17.6. When an archwire closely fits the dimensions of the bracket slot there is less latitude before it binds and therefore interacts with the bracket. With a smaller rectangular archwire, more tilting and rotation can occur before it binds with the walls of the bracket slot. This latitude is known as 'slop'.

- **Third-order bends** are applicable to rectangular archwires only. They are made by twisting the plane of the wire so that when it is inserted into the rectangular bracket slot a buccolingual force is exerted on the tooth apex. This type of movement is also known as torque.

In the original edgewise appliance (see below) these bends were placed in the archwire during treatment so that the teeth were moved into their correct positions. Modern bracket systems have average values for tip (Fig. 17.8) and torque built into the bracket slot itself, and the bracket bases are of differing thicknesses to produce an average buccolingual crown position (known ingeniously as in–out). These 'pre-adjusted' systems have the advantage that the amount of wire bending required is reduced. However, they do not eliminate the need for archwire adjustments because average values do not always suffice. The disadvantage to these pre-adjusted systems is that a larger inventory of brackets is required as each individual tooth has different requirements in terms of tip, in–out, and torque. Pre-adjusted systems are discussed in more detail in Section 17.6.

Whilst it is possible to achieve a more sophisticated range of tooth movement with fixed appliances than with removable appliances, the opportunity for problems to arise is increased. Fixed appliances are also more demanding of anchorage, and therefore adequate training should be sought before embarking on treatment with fixed appliances.

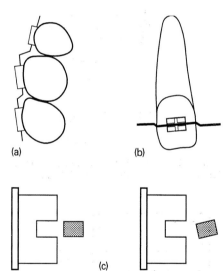

Fig. 17.7. (a) A first-order bend; (b) a second-order bend; (c) a third-order bend.

17.2. INDICATIONS FOR THE USE OF FIXED APPLIANCES

- **Correction of mild to moderate skeletal discrepancies** As fixed appliances can be used to achieve bodily movement it is possible, within limits, to compensate for skeletal discrepancies and treat a greater range of malocclusions.

- **Intrusion/extrusion of teeth** Vertical movement of individual teeth, or tooth segments, requires some form of attachment on the tooth surface onto which the force can act.

- **Correction of rotations**

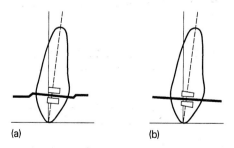

Fig. 17.8. Diagram (a) an edgewise bracket with a second-order bend placed in the archwire to achieve the desired amount of tip. Diagram (b) a pre-adjusted bracket with tip built into the bracket slot.

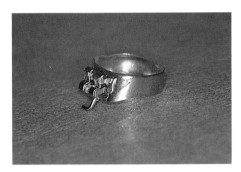

Fig. 17.9. A lower first permanent molar band. Note the gingivally positioned hook, which is useful for applying elastic traction.

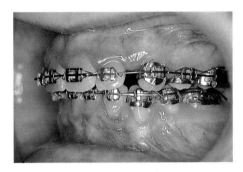

Fig. 17.10. Fixed appliance case where bands have been used for the canines, premolars and molar teeth. The impact of bands upon the aesthetics of the appliance can be readily appreciated.

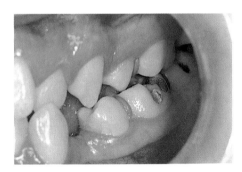

Fig. 17.11. Separating elastics have been placed between the contact points of the second premolars and first permanent molars prior to placement of bands on the latter.

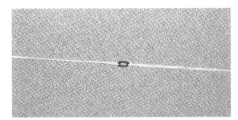

Fig. 17.12. A separating elastic being stretched between two pieces of floss. One side of the elastic is then worked through the contact point so that it encircles the contact point.

- **Overbite reduction by intrusion of incisors**
- **Multiple tooth movements required in one arch**
- **Active closure of extraction spaces, or spaces due to hypodontia** Fixed appliances can be used to achieve bodily space closure and ensure a good contact point between the teeth.

Fixed appliances are *not* indicated as an alternative to poor cooperation with removable appliances. Indeed, if a successful result is to be achieved with the minimum of deleterious side-effects, treatment with fixed appliances should only be embarked upon in patients who are willing to:

- maintain a high level of oral hygiene;
- avoid hard or sticky foods and the consumption of sugar-containing foodstuffs between meals;
- cooperate fully with wearing headgear or elastic traction, if required;
- attend regularly to have the appliance adjusted.

17.3. COMPONENTS OF FIXED APPLIANCES

Tooth movement with fixed appliances is achieved by the interaction between the attachment or bracket on the tooth surface and the archwire which is tied into the bracket. Brackets can be carried on a band which is cemented to the tooth or attached directly to the tooth surface by means of an adhesive (known colloquially as bonds).

17.3.1. Bands

These are rings encircling the tooth to which buccal, and as required, lingual, attachments are soldered or welded (Fig. 17.9). Prior to the introduction of the acid-etch technique, bands were the only means of attaching a bracket to a tooth. With the development of modern bonding techniques, directly bonded attachments became popular. However, many operators still use bands for molar teeth because a band will remain *in situ* if cement failure occurs, whereas a debonded molar attachment (through which the end of the archwire passes) may traumatize a patient's cheek. In addition, a molar band is more secure where headgear is to be used.

Bands can be used on teeth other than molars, most commonly following the failure of a bonded attachment or where de-rotation or correction of a crossbite dictate the need for both lingual and buccal attachments. However, this must be balanced against the poorer aesthetics of a band (Fig. 17.10).

Prior to placement of a band it may be necessary to separate the adjacent tooth contacts. The most widely used method involves placing a small elastic doughnut around the contact point (Fig. 17.11), which is left *in situ* for 2 to 7 days and removed prior to band placement. These separating elastics are inserted by being stretched, with either special pliers or floss (Fig. 17.12), and working one side through the contact point.

Band selection is aided by trying to guess the approximate size of the tooth from the patient's study models. A snug fit is essential to help prevent the band from becoming loose during treatment. The edges of the band should be flush with the marginal ridges with the bracket in the midpoint of the clinical crown at 90° to the long axis of the tooth (or crown, depending upon the type of bracket). Most orthodontists use glass ionomer cement for band cementation.

17.3.2. Bonds

Bonded attachments were introduced with the advent of the acid-etch technique and the modern composite (see Section 17.3.3). Adhesion to the base of metal brackets is gained by mechanical interlock (Fig. 17.13). More recently, ceramic brackets have been introduced (Fig. 17.14), but despite the obvious aesthetic advantages their use has been limited by a number of disadvantages which are currently the subject of considerable research. Ceramic brackets were originally marketed with a silane coupler designed to provide chemical adhesion between the bracket and the bonding composite. This was unfortunately so successful that enamel fracture occasionally occurred during debonding, because the bond between the bracket and the adhesive was so strong. Manufacturers have tried to overcome this problem in a variety of ways, for example using mechanical rather than chemical retention, with varying success. Ceramic brackets are brittle and are prone to fracture in clinical usage. Fracturing away of the wings of the bracket makes tying in the archwire difficult, and in addition the brackets tend to break up during removal of the appliance. The hardness of ceramic brackets can lead to wear of opposing teeth; therefore using ceramic brackets for lower incisors is inadvisable. The hard ceramic can also notch the archwire, which makes sliding the teeth along the wire difficult.

Edgewise brackets are subdivided according to the width of the bracket slot in inches. Two systems are widely used, 0.018 and 0.022. The depth of the slot varies between 0.025 and 0.032.

17.3.3. Orthodontic adhesives

The most popular cement for cementing bands is glass ionomer (Fig. 17.15), mainly because of its fluoride-releasing potential and affinity to stainless steel and enamel. Glass ionomers can also be used for retaining bonded attachments, but unfortunately the bracket failure rate with this material is greater than that with composite. Much current research work is directed towards hybrid compomer materials which it is hoped will combine the advantages of composites and glass ionomer adhesives.

Use of the acid-etch technique with a composite produces clinically acceptable bonded attachment failure rates of the order of 5–10 per cent for both self- and light-cured materials. Although conventional self-cured composites can be used for bonding, a modification has been manufactured specifically for orthodontics to circumvent the problem of air bubbles, which would obviously compromise bond retention. No-mix orthodontic composites (Fig. 17.16) comprise an activator, which is painted onto both the bracket base and the tooth surface (after etching). Following this, a small amount of the composite itself is applied to the bracket, which is then placed on the tooth surface under pressure. Squeezing the sandwich of composite and catalyst into a thin layer mixes the two components, and the material usually sets within a few minutes.

Whatever material is used, any excess should be cleared from the perimeter of the bracket before the final set to reduce plaque retention around the bonded attachment.

17.3.4. Auxiliaries

Very small elastic bands, often described as elastomeric modules (Fig. 17.17), or wire ligatures (Fig. 17.18) are used to secure the archwire into the archwire slot (Fig. 17.19). Elastic modules are quicker to place and are usually more comfortable for the patient, but wire ligatures are often preferred, particularly in the

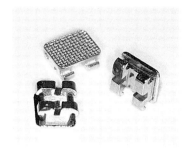

Fig. 17.13. Brackets for bonding showing a mesh base which increases the surface area for mechanical attachment of the composite.

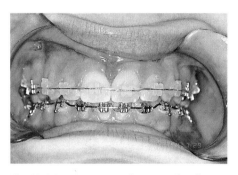

Fig. 17.14. A patient with ceramic brackets on the upper anterior teeth.

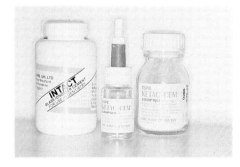

Fig. 17.15. Glass ionomer cement.

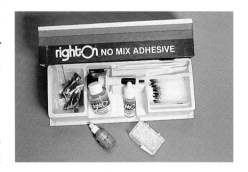

Fig. 17.16. No-mix composite for orthodontic bonding.

Fig. 17.17. Coloured elastomeric modules used to secure the archwire into the bracket slot.

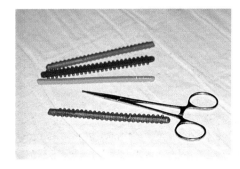

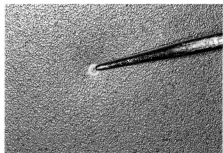

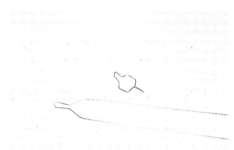

Fig. 17.18. Metal ligatures for securing the archwire into the bracket slot.

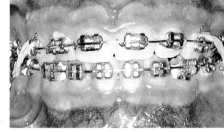

Fig. 17.19. This patient's upper archwire has been tied into place with wire ligatures in the upper arch and with elastomeric modules in the lower arch.

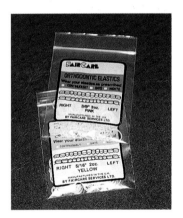

Fig. 17.20. Intra-oral elastics.

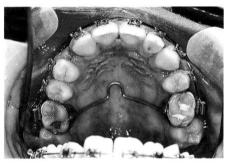

Fig. 17.21. A palatal arch, which is used to help provide additional anchorage in the upper arch by helping to resist forward movement of the maxillary molars.

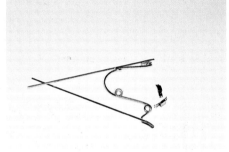

Fig. 17.22. A proprietary removable quadhelix. The distal aspect of the arms of the helix slot into the lingual sheaths (also shown) which are welded onto the palatal surface of bands on the upper molars.

later stages of treatment, as they can be tightened to maximize contact between the wire and the bracket.

Intra-oral elastics for traction are commonly available in 2 oz, 3.5 oz and 4.5 oz strengths and a variety of sizes, ranging from 1/8 inch to 3/4 inch (Fig. 17.20). For most purposes they should be changed every day. Class II and Class III elastic traction is discussed in Section 15.6. Latex-free varieties are now available.

Palatal or lingual arches can be used to reinforce anchorage, to achieve expansion (the quadhelix appliance), or molar de-rotation. They can be made in the laboratory from an impression of the teeth (Fig. 17.21). Proprietary forms of most of the commonly used designs are also available, and these have the additional advantage that they are removable, thus facilitating adjustment (Fig. 17.22).

Springs are an integral part of the Begg technique (see Section 17.6.2).

17.3.5 Archwires

Once an operator has chosen to use a particular type of bracket, the amount and type of force applied to an individual tooth can be controlled by varying the cross-sectional diameter and form of the archwire, and/or the material of its construction. In the initial stages of treatment a wire which is flexible with good resistance to permanent deformation is desirable, so that displaced teeth can be aligned without the application of excessive forces. In contrast, in the later stages of treatment rigid archwires are required to engage the archwire slot fully and to provide fine control over tooth position while resisting the unwanted effects of other forces, such as elastic traction.

The physical properties of an archwire material which are of interest to the orthodontist are as follows.

- **Springback** This is the ability of a wire to return to its original shape after a force is applied. High values of springback mean that it is possible to tie in a displaced tooth without permanent distortion.
- **Stiffness** The amount of force required to deflect or bend a wire. The greater the diameter of an archwire the greater the stiffness.
- **Formability** This is the ease with which a wire can be bent to the desired shape, for example the placement of a coil in a spring, without fracture.
- **Resilience** This is the stored energy available after deflection of an archwire without permanent deformation.
- **Biocompatibility**
- **Joinability** This is whether the material can be soldered or welded.
- **Frictional characteristics** If tooth movement is to proceed quickly a wire with low surface friction is preferable.

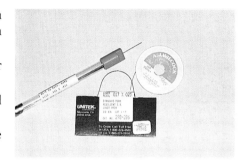

Fig. 17.23. The most popular archwire material is stainless steel which is available in straight lengths, as a coil on a spool, or pre-formed into archwires.

Table 17.1 Properties of some of the more commonly used archwire materials

	SS	NiTi	TMA	CoCr*
Springback	Low	High	Medium	Low
Stiffness	High	Low	Medium	High
Formability	Good	Poor	Good	Good
Resilience	Low	High	Medium	Low
Biocompatibility	Good	?	Good	Good
Friction	Low	Medium	High	Medium

SS, stainless steel; NiTi, nickel titanium; TMA, β-titanium; CoCr, cobalt chromium.
*CoCr wires can be manipulated in the softened state and then heat-treated to increase resistance to deformation.

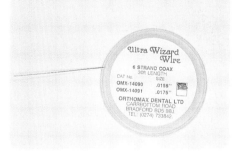

(a)

The most popular wire is stainless steel (Fig. 17.23), because it is relatively inexpensive, easily formed and exhibits good stiffness. Because of these characteristics, stainless steel is particularly useful in the later stages of treatment. More flexible stainless steel wires have been developed which consist of three or more strands of fine stainless steel wire twisted or braided together. These are known as multistrand or twistflex wire (Fig. 17.24) and they are more flexible than a solid stainless steel wire of comparable diameter. However, whilst relatively inexpensive, multistrand wires can exert too high a force, and be distorted if tied into a markedly displaced tooth.

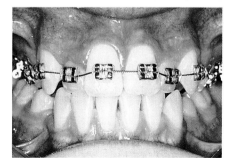

(b)

Fig. 17.24. Multistrand wire (a) wound onto a coil and (b) as an initial archwire to align the upper arch.

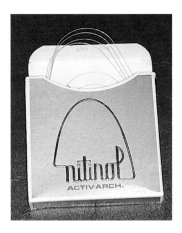

Fig. 17.25.   Nickel titanium wire.

Alternatively, other alloys which have a greater resistance to deformation and greater flexibility can be used. Of these, nickel titanium (Fig. 17.25) is the most popular. Archwires made of nickel titanium are capable of applying a light force without deformation, even when deflected several millimetres, but this alloy is more expensive than stainless steel. By virtue of their flexibility, nickel titanium wires provide less control against the unwanted side-effects of auxiliary forces. Cobalt chromium has the advantage that it can be readily formed, and then the stiffness and rigidity of the archwire can be improved by heat-treatment. β-titanium, popularly known as TMA (tungsten molybdenum alloy), has properties midway between stainless steel and nickel titanium; it has been estimated that a β-titanium wire exerts approximately half the force of a stainless steel wire of comparable diameter. It is often employed in the later stages of treatment, being particularly useful when the operator wishes to torque individual teeth.

Archwires are described according to their dimensions. An archwire described as 0.016 inches (0.4 mm) is a round archwire, and an 0.016 × 0.022 inches (0.4 × 0.55 mm), is a rectangular archwire.

Archwires are available in straight lengths, as coils, or as preformed archwires (see Fig. 17.23). The latter variant is more costly to buy but saves chairside time. There are a wide variety of archform shapes; however, regardless of what design is chosen, some adjustment of the archwire to match the pretreatment archform of the patient will be required (see Section 17.4).

The force exerted by a particular archwire material is given by the formula

$$F \propto \frac{dr^4}{l^3}$$

where d is the distance that the spring/wire is deflected, r is the radius of the wire, and l is the length of the wire.

Thus it can be appreciated that increasing the diameter of the archwire will significantly affect the force applied to the teeth, and increasing the length or span of wire between the brackets will inversely affect the applied force. As mentioned earlier, the distance between the brackets can be increased by reducing the width of the brackets, but the interbracket span can also be increased by the placement of loops in the archwire. Prior to the introduction of the newer more flexible alloys, multilooped stainless steel archwires were commonly used in the initial stages of treatment. Loops are still utilized in retraction archwires (see Section 17.5) and where a combination of a rigid archwire (to resist unwanted forces) with localized flexibility is required.

17.4. TREATMENT PLANNING FOR FIXED APPLIANCES

By virtue of their coverage of the palate, removable appliances inherently provide more anchorage than fixed appliances. It is important to remember that, with a fixed appliance, movement of one tooth or a segment of teeth in one direction will result in an equal but opposite force acting on the remaining teeth included in the appliance. In addition, apical movement will place a greater strain on anchorage. For these reasons it is necessary to pay particular attention to anchorage when planning treatment involving fixed appliances and, if necessary, this can be reinforced with headgear and/or a palatal or lingual arch (see Chapter 15).

The importance of keeping the teeth within the zone of soft tissue balance has been discussed in Chapter 7. Therefore care is required to ensure that the archform, particularly of the lower arch, present at the beginning of treatment is largely preserved. It is wise to check the dimensions of any archwire against a model of the lower arch, taken before the start of treatment (Fig. 17.26), bearing in mind that the upper arch will of necessity be slightly broader. Of course, there

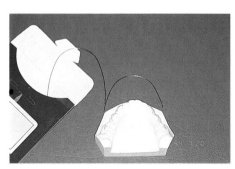

Fig. 17.26.   The amount of adjustment required to a pre-formed lower archwire, as taken from the packet, to ensure that it conforms to the patient's pretreatment archform and width.

are exceptions, as discussed in Chapter 7. However, these should be foreseen at the time of treatment planning and, if necessary, the implications for retention of the final result discussed fully with the patient at that time.

17.5. PRACTICAL PROCEDURES

Accurate bracket placement is crucial to achieving success with fixed appliances. The 'correct' position of the bracket on the facial surface will depend upon the bracket system used. Some fixed appliance systems require the operator to position the bracket at different heights on each tooth to compensate for differing crown lengths. Others, notably the pre-adjusted systems, require the bracket to be placed in the middle of the tooth along the long axis of the clinical crown. Bracket placement is particularly important with these pre-adjusted systems, as the values for tip and torque are calculated for the midpoint of the facial surface of the tooth. Incorrect bracket positioning will lead to incorrect tooth position and ultimately affect the functional and aesthetic result; therefore errors in bracket placement should be corrected as early as possible in the treatment. Alternatively, adjustments can be made to each archwire to compensate, but over the course of a treatment this can be time-consuming.

As mentioned in Section 17.3.5, when a fixed appliance is first placed a flexible archwire is advisable to avoid applying excessive forces to displaced teeth, which can be painful for the patient and result in bond failure. Commonly, either a pre-formed nickel titanium archwire or a multistranded stainless steel archwire is used to achieve initial alignment. Alternatively, loops can be placed in a stainless steel archwire, as mentioned in Section 17.3.5, to increase the span of wire between brackets and thus increase flexibility. This approach is useful if a rigid archwire is desirable in other areas of the arch.

It is important to move on from these initial aligning archwires as soon as alignment is achieved, as by virtue of their flexibility they do not afford much control of tooth position. However, it is equally important to ensure that full bracket engagement has been achieved before proceeding to a more rigid archwire. In the edgewise or pre-adjusted appliance systems it is usual to progress through round archwires of increasing diameter to achieve progressively better intra-arch alignment. If tooth alignment alone is required, for example in a Class I malocclusion with rotations, a stiff round archwire which nearly fills the bracket slot will suffice. However, correction of inter-arch relationships and space closure is usually best carried out using rectangular wires for apical control. The exact archwire sequence will depend upon the dimensions of the archwire slot and operator preference.

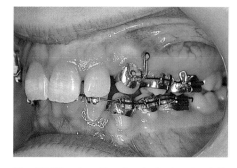

Fig. 17.27. A sectional archwire to retract /3.

Mesiodistal tooth movement can be achieved by one of the following:

1. Moving teeth with the archwire: this is achieved by incorporating loops into the archwire which, when activated, move a section of the archwire and the attached teeth as shown in Fig. 17.27.
2. Sliding teeth along the archwire (Fig. 17.28), usually under the influence of elastic force: this approach requires greater force to overcome friction between the bracket and the wire, and therefore places a greater strain on anchorage. This type of movement is known as 'sliding mechanics' and is more applicable to pre-adjusted appliances where a straight archwire is used. In the edgewise appliance the first-, second-, and third-order bends necessary in the archwire make sliding teeth along it difficult.

Fig. 17.29 shows the steps involved in the treatment of a maximum anchorage Class II division 1 malocclusion with fixed appliances.

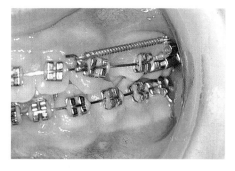

Fig. 17.28. Sliding teeth along the archwire using a nickel titanium coil spring.

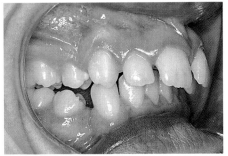

(a)

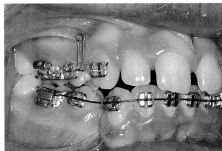

(B)

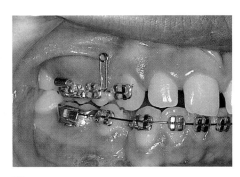

(C)

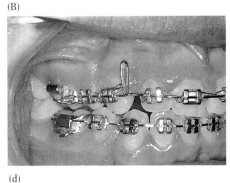

(d)

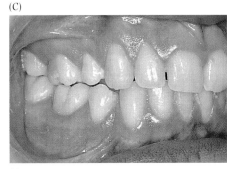

(e)

Fig. 17.29. (a) The right buccal view of a 12-year-old patient with a Class II division 1 malocclusion and previous extraction of all first premolars. It was decided to gain space for reduction of the overjet by using headgear to 6/6. (b) Retraction of 3/3 with a sectional archwire, whilst a lower fixed appliance is used to align the lower arch and reduce the overbite. (c) The molars and canines are now Class I, with the overbite reduced. (d) Retraction of 21/12 with a looped archwire to reduce the overjet. (e) At the completion of treatment.

Adjustments to the appliance need to be made on a regular basis, usually every 6 weeks. Once space closure is complete and incisor position corrected, some operators will place a more flexible full-sized archwire, often in conjunction with vertical elastic traction, to help 'sock-in' the buccal occlusion.

The subject of retention is covered in more detail in the chapter on retention. However, in order to try and overcome the greater tendency for relapse of rotational or apical movements, some orthodontists overcorrect these aspects of a malocclusion.

17.6. FIXED APPLIANCE SYSTEMS

17.6.1. Pre-adjusted appliances

Because of their advantages these systems are now universally accepted. The need for first-, second-, and third-order bends in the archwire during treatment is considerably reduced because the brackets are manufactured with the slot cut in such a way that these movements are built in. Therefore plain preformed archwires can be used so that the teeth are moved progressively from the very start of treatment to their ideal position. Hence they are also known as the straight wire appliance.

As individual tooth positions are built into the bracket, it is necessary to produce a bracket for each tooth, but the time saved in wire bending and the superior results achieved more than compensate for the increased cost of purchasing a greater inventory of brackets. However, a pre-adjusted bracket system will not eliminate the need for wire bending as only average values are built into the appliance, and often additional individual bends need to be placed in the archwire.

Not surprisingly, there are many different opinions as to the correct position of each tooth, and many manufacturers keen to join a lucrative market. The result is an almost bewildering array of pre-adjusted systems, all with slightly differing

Table 17.2 Typical pre-adjusted values for tip and torque (at mid-point of facial surface)

	Torque (deg)	Tip (deg)
Maxilla		
Central incisor	7	5
Lateral incisor	3	9
Canine	7	11
First premolar	−7	2
Second premolar	−7	2
First molar	−9	5
Second molar	−9	5
Mandible		
Central incisor	−1	2
Lateral incisor	−1	2
Canine	−11	5
First premolar	−17	2
Second premolar	−22	2
First molar	−26	2
Second molar	−31	2

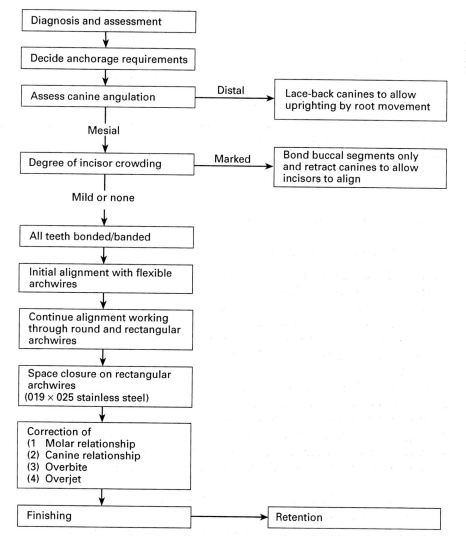

Fig. 17.30. A flow diagram showing the sequence of treatment with a 022 pre-adjusted bracket system.

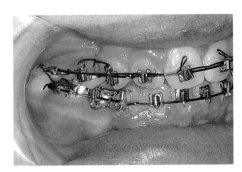

Fig. 17.31. This shows the problems posed for toothbrushing by the Begg appliance.

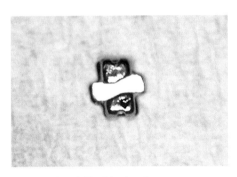

Fig. 17.32. A Tip Edge bracket.

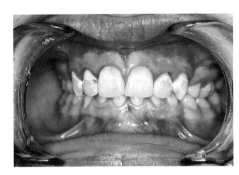

Fig. 17.33. Picture showing severe decalcification following fixed appliance treatment (naturally this patient was not treated by the author!)

degrees of torque and tip. Of these perhaps the best known are the Andrews' prescription, developed by Andrews, the father of the straight wire appliance (see Table 17.2) and the Roth system.

Fig. 17.30 is a flow diagram illustrating one approach to using a pre-adjusted appliance system.

17.6.2. Begg appliance

Named after its originator, the Begg appliance (Fig. 17.31) is based on the use of round wire which fits fairly loosely into a channel at the top of the bracket. Apical and rotational movement is achieved by means of auxiliary springs or by loops placed in the archwire. Begg used 'differential force systems' to accomplish tooth movement, claiming that the intra-oral forces were adjusted so that they were optimal for movement of the anterior segment teeth whilst ensuring that the posterior segment teeth acted as an anchorage unit. The Begg appliance was often used in conjunction with extractions to provide intra-oral anchorage, so that reliance was not placed on the patient wearing headgear. However, patient compliance with wearing elastics for the duration of treatment was required instead.

Apart from the problems experienced by patients cleaning around the auxiliary springs favoured in the Begg technique, the main drawback to this appliance is that it is difficult to position the teeth precisely at the end of treatment.

17.6.3 Tip Edge appliance

This appliance was designed with the aim of combining the advantages of both the straight wire and the Begg systems. Orthodontists disagree as to the extent to which the Tip Edge technique achieves this. The Tip Edge bracket (Fig. 17.32), allows tipping of the tooth in the initial stages of treatment when round archwires are employed, as in the Begg technique, but when full-sized rectangular archwires are used in the latter stages, the built-in pre-adjustments help to give a better degree of control of final tooth positioning.

17.7. DECALCIFICATION AND FIXED APPLIANCES

Placement of a fixed attachment upon a tooth surface leads to plaque accumulation. In addition, if a diet rich in sugar is consumed, this results in demineralization of the enamel surrounding the bracket and occasionally frank cavitation. The incidence of decalcification (Fig. 17.33) with fixed appliances has been variously reported as between 15 and 85 per cent. As any decalcification is undesirable, considerable interest has focused on ways of reducing this problem. The main approaches that have been used are as follows:

1. Fluoride mouth rinses for the duration of treatment. The problem with this approach is that the individuals most at risk of decalcification are those least likely to comply fully with a rinsing regime.

2. Local fluoride release from fluoride-containing cements and bonding adhesives. Variable results have been reported for those composites which have been marketed for their fluoride-releasing potential. Glass ionomer cements have been shown to be effective at reducing the incidence of decalcification around bands, whilst achieving equal or better retention results than conventional cements. Although glass ionomer cements appear effective at reducing decalcification around bonded attachments, this is at the expense of poorer retention rates (see Section 17.3.3).

3. Dietary advice. This important aspect of preventive advice should not be forgotten. Patients are often advised to avoid chewy sweets during treatment, but the importance of avoiding sugared beverages and fizzy drinks, particularly between meals, should not be overlooked.

17.8. STARTING WITH FIXED APPLIANCES

It is extremely unwise to embark on treatment with fixed appliances without first gaining some expertise in their use. This is best achieved by a longitudinal course in the form of an apprenticeship with a skilled operator. It is mandatory that this is supplemented by a thorough appreciation of orthodontic diagnosis and treatment planning, so that the novice orthodontist realizes his or her limitations and is selective in the type of case tackled. The 2 or 3 day courses comprising a practical typodont with a small theoretical element are always heavily oversubscribed, but most serve to put off the general dental practioner (perhaps not unintentionally). They do not provide an adequate basis for launching into fixed appliances, unless a more experienced orthodontist is readily available for advice.

Some orthodontic supply companies offer the practioner a kit containing brackets, bands, and a few archwires in return for an impression and a fee. Of course, this is an expensive alternative and, in addition, bands selected from an impression are unlikely to be a good fit. Those interested in gaining further orthodontic skills are advised to gain adequate experience on a longitudinal basis and to buy an adequate stock of pliers, bands, and brackets to make fixed appliance treatment rewarding and successful for both the practitioner and patient.

PRINCIPAL SOURCES AND FURTHER READING

Howels, D. J. (1986). The straight-wire appliance. *Dental Update*, **13**, 367–76.
● The background to, and use of, the first pre-adjusted system.
Williams, J. K., Isaacson, K. G., and Cook, P. A. (1995). *Fixed orthodontic appliances. Principles and practices.* Butterworth Heinemann, London.
● An excellent book, which should be read by anyone using fixed appliances.
Kapila, S. and Sachdeva, R. (1989). Mechanical properties and and clinical applications of orthodontic wires. *American Journal of Orthodontics and Dentofacial Orthopedics*, **96**, 100–9.
● An excellent, and readable, account of archwire materials.
Kusy, R. P. (1997). A review of contemporary archwires: their properties and characteristics. *Angle Orthodontist*, **67**, 197–207.
Millett, D. T. and Gordon, P. H. (1994). A 5-year clinical review of bond failure with a no-mix adhesive (Right-on). *European Journal of Orthodontics*, **16**, 203–11.
● This paper provides scientific justification for all the old wives' tales about bond failure rates.
Rock, P. (1995). A practical introduction to fixed appliances: the straight wire appliance. *Dental Update*, **22**, 18–21, 61–5.
O'Higgins, E. A. *et al.* (1999). The influence of maxillary incisor inclination on arch length. *British Journal of Orthodontics*, **26**, 97–102.
● A fascinating article — a 'must read' for those practitioners using fixed appliances.
Shaw, W. C. (ed.) (1993). *Orthodontics and occlusal management.* Wright, Bristol.
● Chapter 15 on fixed appliances is well written and informative and is complemented by the chapter on common treatment procedures.

18 Functional appliances (N. E. Carter)

18.1. INTRODUCTION

The functional appliances are a group of orthodontic appliances which are quite distinct in the way that they work. In general they have no active components such as springs or elastics, but instead harness forces generated by the masticatory and facial musculature (they are often called myofunctional appliances). This is achieved by constructing the appliance such that it holds the mandible in a postured position away from its position of rest, and, whilst there are many designs of functional appliance, they all engage both dental arches and cause mandibular posturing with displacement of the condyles within the glenoid fossae. Functional appliances of all types are most effective during active growth.

The purpose of functional appliances is to alter the anteroposterior occlusion between the two dental arches, and they cannot on their own treat irregularities of arch alignment such as crowding. The temporomandibular joints primarily permit opening and protrusion of the mandible, and the vast majority of functional appliances are made to a forward postured working bite. Thus they are mostly used in the treatment of Class II malocclusions, particularly Class II division 1 where the overjet is increased.

Before discussing functional appliances in detail, Fig. 18.1 gives an overview of this type of functional appliance in clinical use. This patient has a Class II division 1 malocclusion of the type for which functional appliances are very suitable, and for which they have been used for many years.

There are a number of important features to note which will be discussed further later in the chapter. First, the patient is still growing and the signs are that her pattern of facial growth is likely to be favourable. Although the skeletal pattern is Class II, the vertical relationships are close to average and the direction of mandibular growth is likely to be a mild forward rotation (see Chapter 4) which is favourable to the correction of a Class II malocclusion. Second, the soft tissue morphology is favourable despite the lips being incompetent, with the lower lip resting behind the upper incisors. The lower lip line is above the level of the upper incisal edges, and after the overjet has been reduced the lower lip will rest labially to the upper incisors, so helping to resist any tendency for relapse of the overjet. Third, the arches are well aligned — functional appliances have no mechanism for treating irregularities of alignment of the teeth.

The appliance holds the mandible in a forward postured position, in this case with the incisors edge to edge (Fig. 18.1(f)). The facial musculature is thus stretched, and applies a posterior force to the upper arch and an anterior force to the lower arch. The lower incisors have acrylic capping to prevent excessive labial tilting of the lower incisors, and this also serves as a bite-plane to reduce the overbite (Chapter 10). The appliance must be worn for at least 14–16 hours each day, but once the overjet has been reduced fully the amount of daily wear can gradually be reduced to sleeping hours only. The patient should continue to wear the appliance overnight in this way as a retainer, at least until the period of rapid pubertal growth is complete. Figures 18.1(g) and 18.1(h) show the dental and facial changes which occurred during treatment.

A functional appliance can be used as the first part of a two-stage treatment, in which the overjet is reduced, followed by a second phase of treatment with fixed appliances to deal with crowding or other irregularities of dental alignment.

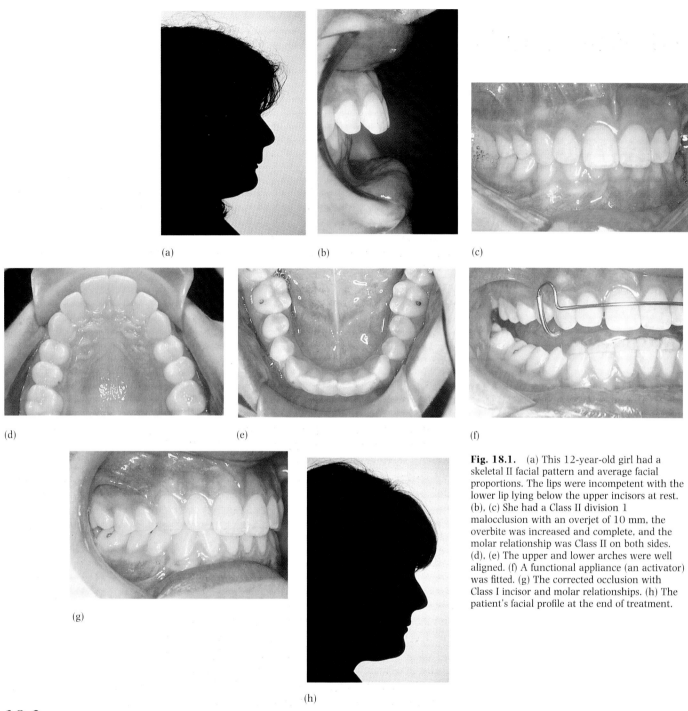

Fig. 18.1. (a) This 12-year-old girl had a skeletal II facial pattern and average facial proportions. The lips were incompetent with the lower lip lying below the upper incisors at rest. (b), (c) She had a Class II division 1 malocclusion with an overjet of 10 mm, the overbite was increased and complete, and the molar relationship was Class II on both sides. (d), (e) The upper and lower arches were well aligned. (f) A functional appliance (an activator) was fitted. (g) The corrected occlusion with Class I incisor and molar relationships. (h) The patient's facial profile at the end of treatment.

18.2. MODE OF ACTION

The way that functional appliances work is not fully understood, but they are thought to achieve their effect by the posturing of the mandible causing stretching of the facial musculature. This generates forces which are delivered primarily to the teeth, and there is no doubt that a posteriorly directed force acts upon the upper arch and an anteriorly directed force must therefore act upon the lower. However, it is the clinical impression of many orthodontists that there are more widespread effects upon the facial skeleton as well as upon the dentition. The sites where functional appliances might induce facial changes are the maxillary complex, the mandible, and the glenoid fossa.

The extent of these changes has become something of a controversy within orthodontics. There are those who claim that functional appliances alter the environment of the growing facial skeleton enough to bring about significant changes in the growth pattern. The alternative point of view is that growth of the facial skeleton is under close genetic control and therefore orthodontic appliances can have little effect other than to move the teeth within the alveolar bone. The truth probably lies somewhere in between. However, one important principle is clear: functional appliances only work in growing children and have their greatest effect when growth is most rapid.

Much research effort is directed at trying to determine what impact functional appliances have upon facial growth, but studies in this field face problems and limitations. The main types of research have been animal experiments and cephalometric studies of human subjects.

Animal studies allow greater control of the experimental conditions than is possible with human clinical studies. For example, variables such as the genetic background of the animals can be controlled and operative techniques can be standardized. Precise measurements of the jaws can be made after sacrifice, and studies at a cellular level can demonstrate changes indicative of active growth, for instance in the mandibular condyle. These studies have involved various species but primates are most relevant to the human situation. However, primate studies are very expensive and therefore the numbers of animals involved are small. There are also the obvious limitations that species other than the human are being investigated and that the regime of appliance wear is different. Appliances to produce mandibular posturing in animals have usually been fixed, unlike the functional appliances for humans which are removable and are worn only part-time. Animal facial morphology is very different and the facial skeletal discrepancies seen in humans are almost unknown in animals; therefore the appliances are usually making normal occlusions become abnormal. Thus the changes seen in animals do not compare directly with humans and the results must be applied to human clinical practice with caution.

Human studies of necessity are non-invasive, and cephalometric radiography has proved to be a useful tool in the measurement of human facial growth. However, it does have significant limitations in terms of technique error, which are discussed in Chapter 6. Measurements are made from landmarks identified on the radiographs, and it is not always possible to select a landmark which is both easy to identify reliably and truly representative of the structure being measured. The measurement errors which are inherent within the technique may be as large as the changes which are being examined, and there is also considerable variation among patients in their responses to appliances. These difficulties do not invalidate cephalometry as a research tool but, if the findings of a cephalometric study are to have any real meaning, proper experimental design and the inclusion of sufficiently large numbers of patients are essential.

Many reported studies are retrospective, that is subjects are selected for inclusion in the study after completion of the orthodontic treatment. These tend to have an element of bias as, for various reasons, studies have often only included patients who have achieved a successful result from the treatment being examined, but very few have also looked at those in whom the treatment failed. Thus the study sample may be biased in that these successful patients may have inherently favourable growth patterns while the unsuccessful ones, which perhaps were not included in the study, were those with unfavourable growth. The changes induced by the treatment need to be distinguished from those which occur during normal growth, and in theory this can be done by comparing the group of treated patients with an untreated control group which is matched for age, sex, and malocclusion. In practice this is also difficult, as very few patients with malocclusions of any severity decline treatment and yet have serial orthodontic records taken over a period of years.

Prospective randomly allocated clinical trials give much better evidence by eliminating selection bias. In these studies, subjects are selected for inclusion before the treatment begins and are allocated randomly to one of the treatment methods being examined. Such studies have to be large to allow for patients abandoning the treatment being studied or being lost to follow-up, and they have to extend over several years to allow the long-term effects of treatment to be assessed. Several prospective clinical studies of functional appliances are currently under way but so far only preliminary results have been reported.

In summary, the question of the precise mode of action functional appliances is not easily resolved and it continues to be controversial. At present, the evidence of the better scientific studies suggests the following changes when a forward postured functional appliance is used:

- **Dento-alveolar changes** There is no doubt that functional appliances move the upper teeth posteriorly. Anterior movement of the lower arch may also occur but is a less consistent finding.

- **Changes in maxillary growth** There is restriction of forward growth of the maxilla, similar to the effect of headgear. However, this change may not be permanent as there is evidence that 'catch-up' growth of the maxilla occurs after treatment.

- **Changes in mandibular growth** There is evidence that functional appliances may induce on average an extra 1–2 mm of growth of the mandible. However, there appears to be considerable variation in this response, and it is possible that some patients exhibit significant acceleration of mandibular growth during functional appliance treatment, although such effects may be only be transitory, and others do not. The direction of mandibular growth may also be improved by functional appliance therapy. Unfortunately, at present, reliable prediction of patient response is not possible, but on average the changes are modest.

- **Changes in the glenoid fossae** Remodelling of the glenoid fossa more anteriorly has been seen in animal experiments and there is some evidence that it may occur in humans. If this does happen, the temporomandibular joint and the mandible would become repositioned slightly further forward.

18.3. INDICATIONS FOR FUNCTIONAL APPLIANCES

All patients must meet the following general criteria for a functional appliance to be appropriate:

- The patient must still be growing, preferably approaching a phase of rapid growth.

- The pattern and direction of facial growth should be reasonably favourable. While functional appliances may have a small effect on growth, this must be regarded as being limited and it is not possible to make a dramatic improvement upon a very unfavourable growth pattern.

- The patient must be well motivated. These appliances are bulky and must be worn for a substantial amount of time. This requires a considerable effort and commitment by the patient and the family, particularly in the early stages of treatment.

The **timing of treatment** needs careful consideration. These appliances only work in patients who are growing, and their effect is greatest when growth is most rapid. The timing of dental development correlates poorly with that of skeletal growth and the pubertal growth spurt, and some children establish the permanent dentition at a relatively early age while others are still in the late mixed dentition at puberty. It is common practice to fit functional appliances in the mixed dentition stage, but some designs of functional appliance become difficult to manage when many primary teeth are mobile and exfoliating. The appliance should be worn until the end of the pubertal growth spurt, and if treatment is started early in a young child it is likely to be very lengthy. The patient's enthusiasm for treatment may well wane in these circumstances. However, in many cases the advantages of early treatment may be felt to outweigh the disadvantages, such as where the overjet is very large and causing concern because of teasing or risk of trauma to the upper incisors.

Therefore it can be quite difficult in some cases to decide when to begin treatment, particularly when the functional appliance is to be used in conjunction with other treatment such as for crowding. It is useful to record the patient's standing height over a period before and during treatment, as this gives some indication of the rate of growth. Although it is not possible to predict the onset of the pubertal growth spurt precisely, this information may help to determine when the treatment should start.

18.3.1. Class II division 1

Functional appliances are most often used in Class II division 1 malocclusions. They are particularly appropriate where the arches are well aligned as they contain no mechanism for aligning irregular arches (Fig. 18.1). It is possible to use a functional appliance where there is crowding within the arches, but these cases are often more easily treated in other ways. Where a functional appliance is to be used, arch alignment is carried out either before or after the functional appliance phase of treatment.

The functional appliance may be fitted during the mixed dentition stage to achieve anteroposterior correction of the malocclusion, and the crowding treated later in a second phase of treatment after the first premolar teeth have erupted. This usually requires extractions and either removable or fixed appliances to align the arches. This sequence of treatment has the advantage of achieving early overjet reduction, but overall treatment time is often long. There is also a risk of some relapse of the overjet when the functional appliance has been stopped to make way for the appliances needed to align the arches. It may be necessary to reinsert a functional appliance as a retainer after the teeth have been aligned, but this must be done before the growth spurt is finished.

Fig. 18.2. (a)–(c) Class II division 1 malocclusion with lower arch crowding; (d) a combination of removable and fixed appliances to align the arches prior to fitting the functional appliance; (e) activator appliance modified to fit over the fixed appliance; (f) the occlusion at the end of treatment.

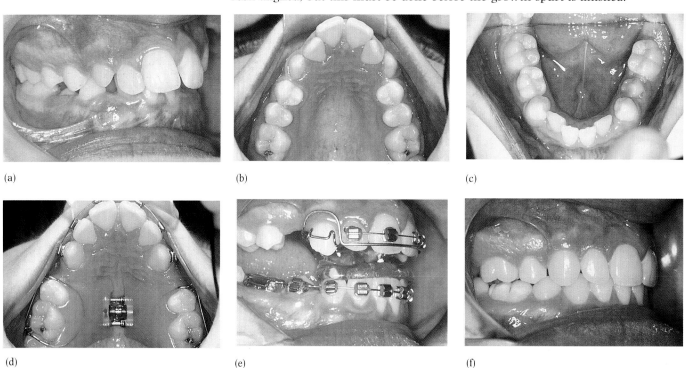

(a)   (b)   (c)

(d)   (e)   (f)

Where the premolars erupt before the pubertal growth spurt takes place, the sequence of treatment can be reversed. The crowding is relieved by extracting premolar teeth, and then the arches are aligned using fixed or removable appliances, or a combination of the two, but making no attempt to correct the incisor or molar relationships (Fig. 18.2). The functional appliance is fitted when the arches have been aligned, and some designs can be made to fit over a fixed appliance. It should be worn until the growth spurt is complete, and can serve as a retainer after the brackets have been removed.

The degree of overbite should be considered when selecting the design of functional appliance. Lower incisor capping acts as an anterior bite-plane to reduce an increased overbite, limiting lower incisor eruption and allowing molar eruption. Conversely, where the overbite is reduced, a design which incorporates molar capping, such as the twin-block appliance (see Section 18.5.6), will help to prevent an anterior open-bite from developing.

18.3.2. Class II division 2

Treatment of a Class II division 2 malocclusion can be prolonged and difficult because correction of the incisor relationship requires reduction of the overbite and reduction of the inter-incisal angle to ensure stability of the result (Chapter 10). This can be done with fixed appliances, but the treatment is extensive as it involves correcting the retroclination of the upper incisors by moving their apices palatally, thus reducing the inter-incisal angle.

An alternative approach is to correct the upper incisor angulation by moving their crowns labially, which is often straightforward using a removable appliance. The resulting increased overjet and the deep overbite can then be corrected using a functional appliance. This method is particularly appropriate where the lower arch is well aligned. The retroclined upper incisors are often crowded, but this resolves as they are tilted labially into a larger arc. The malocclusion has then been changed from Class II division 2 to a Class II division 1 with aligned arches, which is ideal for treatment with a functional appliance (Fig. 18.3).

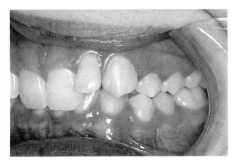
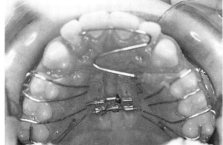

(a) (b)

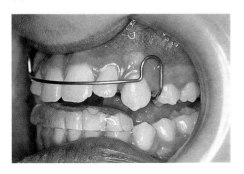
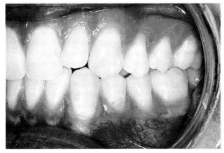

(c) (d)

Fig. 18.3. (a) Class II division 2 malocclusion with well-aligned lower arch; (b) upper removable appliance to expand the arch and procline the upper incisors; (c) activator appliance in place; (d) some overcorrection was achieved.

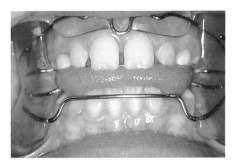

Fig. 18.4. Frankel appliance for Class III correction.

18.3.3. Class III

The problem faced by functional appliances designed to correct Class III malocclusion is that only minimal posterior posturing of the mandible is possible. Thus they are limited in the degree of activation which can be achieved, and the working bite is usually open rather than forced posteriorly. The pattern of mandibular growth is also less likely to be favourable for correction of a Class III malocclusion. One of the more popular designs of Class III functional appliances is a variant of the Frankel appliance, the FR3 (Fig. 18.4). This includes wires lying labial to the lower incisors and palatal to the upper incisor which, together with the acrylic shield in the upper labial sulcus, induce slight lingual movement of the lower incisors and labial movement of the upper incisors. Thus the effect is a dento-alveolar correction of the Class III incisor relationship, and at present there is no evidence that functional appliances achieve any clinically significant skeletal correction in Class III cases.

18.4. MANAGEMENT OF FUNCTIONAL APPLIANCES

It is essential that adequate records, comprising study models and panoramic and lateral skull radiographs, are taken before treatment begins. Photographs and a note of the patient's standing height are also useful.

Well-extended upper and lower impressions are needed together with a working bite. The exact nature of the bite depends on the type of functional appliance to be used, but all of them require the mandible to be postured forward, usually by no more than about 8 mm or to edge-to-edge, whichever is less. The upper and lower centrelines should be coincident, and a degree of opening is usually necessary, with the exact amount depending upon the overbite and design of appliance to be used.

When the appliance is fitted, the patient should find it comfortable, if strange, to start with. These appliances are demanding to wear and the patient needs to be well motivated. With this type of treatment, almost more than any other, the orthodontist must enthuse the patient and family. The appliance should be worn for at least 14 hours out of every 24, and preferably more. Clinical experience has shown that, while some patients may achieve some improvement with less wear than this, many do not, and it certainly seems that the more the appliance is worn each day, the faster will be the response. As with all orthodontic appliances, the patient will find that the first few days after fitting are the most difficult, and they will need time to become accustomed to wearing it. Initially, it should be worn for a few hours each day as a training period, gradually increasing the amount of wear over the first week or two until the minimum of 14 hours is being achieved. For most children this time is found between coming home from school and getting up next morning. Appliance wear does not need to be continuous as long as the total time is achieved, and most designs of functional appliance have to be removed for meals. Children can increase the amount of wear by taking the functional appliance to school, provided that they can be trusted to take care of it when it is out of the mouth. It is helpful to give patients a time chart so that they can record for themselves how they are getting on.

The patient should be seen after 2 weeks to ensure that the appliance is comfortable and to encourage adequate wear. During active treatment, review appointments should be every 6 to 8 weeks. Progress is assessed by measuring the overjet and observing correction of the buccal segment relationship, ensuring that the mandible is fully retruded and that the patient is not posturing forwards.

The fit of the appliance should be checked and adjusted — for obvious reasons it must be as comfortable as possible. It is important to check that the appliance is not causing unwanted interference with the eruption of permanent teeth, and it should be trimmed as appropriate. The activation of the appliance should be checked, and in cases where the initial overjet was large it may be necessary to reactivate or replace it. Finally, it is worth recording the standing height, as slow progress with the appliance may be because the patient is not in a rapid growth phase.

One of the main tasks at review appointments is to encourage and motivate the patient, and this is made much easier if the patient and family can see an improvement for themselves. The patient's time chart should be looked at and discussed — it is important to remember to take an interest in this. The rate of response will vary, but if progress is slow or non-existent the problem should be talked through with the patient and parent. If growth in height is rapid this should be pointed out forcibly, as the overjet should be reducing rapidly and there is no second chance once the growth spurt has finished.

When the overjet has been reduced fully, or preferably overcorrected slightly, the amount of time that the appliance is worn each day can be reduced progressively to 12 hours, then 10 hours, and finally down to sleeping hours only. This reduction should be very gradual, over about a year, and the overjet and buccal segment correction must be monitored to ensure that they remain stable. The patient should continue to wear the appliance at night until they are well through the pubertal growth spurt, as clinical experience has shown that gradual relapse may occur during the late stages of growth if the appliance is withdrawn too soon. Wearing the appliance in bed at night is not a problem for most teenagers.

18.5. TYPES OF APPLIANCE

There are many designs of functional appliance, but they all share the common feature that the mandible is held in a postured position. One of the earliest designs was Pierre Robin's *monobloc* which was designed to hold the mandible forward in infants with extreme mandibular retrognathism (Pierre Robin syndrome). Andresen originally developed his appliance as a retainer for use after fixed appliances had been removed and found that it continued to reduce increased overjets.

Six popular designs of functional appliance will be described briefly here, but there are many adaptations and most orthodontists have developed their own variants. Some designs are worn with headgear which further helps the Class II correction.

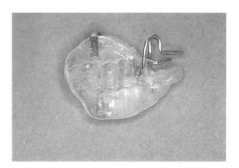

18.5.1. The Andresen activator

There are many variations upon Andresen's original design. An Andresen activator is shown in Fig. 18.5. It is a monoblock design, that is to say it comprises upper and lower acrylic appliances fused together. The original design had a solid palate, but that shown has been made with an open palate to reduce its bulk. The lower incisors are capped to minimize the tendency for them to procline during overjet reduction, and which also serves as a bite-plane to reduce the overbite. The capping resists tipping of the teeth so that any labial movement will have to be bodily translation and is therefore minimized. The labial bow lies passively against the upper incisors, and the palatal wire is again intended to minimize palatal tilting of the upper incisors.

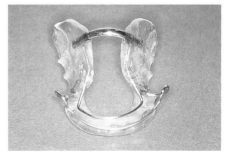

Fig. 18.5. Andresen activator used to treat the patient shown in Fig. 18.1.

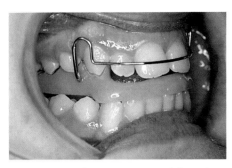

Fig. 18.6. Andresen activator with buccal capping to prevent excessive reduction of overbite.

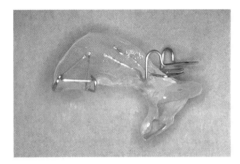

Fig. 18.7. Medium opening activator.

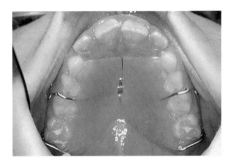

Fig. 18.8. Expansion appliance fitted prior to the functional appliance.

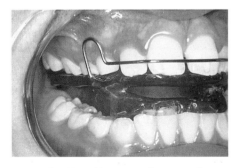

Fig. 18.9. Harvold activator (courtesy of Mr T. G. Bennett).

The interdental acrylic in the buccal segments has been trimmed to make a series of inclined planes which guide the eruption of the upper molars and premolars buccally and distally. The distal movement is intended to help correct the Class II buccal segment relationship. The buccal movement is needed because, as the buccal segment relationship corrects, the upper posterior teeth occlude against a wider part of the lower arch. With lower incisor eruption restricted by the capping, eruption of the molars brings about reduction of the overbite. Where the overbite is normal at the start of treatment, the molar capping should be trimmed to allow expansion but not eruption, so that the molars cannot erupt more than the incisors and cause an anterior open bite to develop (Fig. 18.6).

The appliance has no clasps; the intention is that the looseness in the mouth causes the patient to bite into it. Many patients find this difficult to tolerate in the early stages of treatment, finding that the appliance often comes out during the night, and a common modification is to clasp the upper first molars although this prevents spontaneous expansion.

18.5.2. The medium opening activator

The acrylic in this variant of the activator has been kept to a minimum to make it better tolerated (Fig. 18.7). The lower acrylic extends lingually the labial segment only, and the upper and lower parts are joined by two stout acrylic posts, leaving a breathing hole anteriorly. The appliance has clasps in the upper buccal segments. There is no molar capping, and this design is thus not suitable where the initial overbite is normal or reduced.

Where the upper molars are clasped, there can be no spontaneous expansion of the upper arch while the activator is being worn. Therefore it is necessary to fit an expansion appliance first, such as that shown in Fig. 18.8. This gives the patient an easy introduction to appliance wear, and it may also include springs to improve the alignment of the upper incisors. In cases where a fixed appliance has been used to align the arches before fitting the functional appliance, the medium opening activator design can be modified to fit around fixed attachments (Fig. 18.2).

18.5.3. The Harvold activator

The most obvious differences between the Harvold and Andresen activators are that the Harvold appliance is made to a widely open working bite so as to gain maximum effect from stretching the muscles and has occlusal shelves which contact the upper but not the lower posterior teeth (Fig. 18.9). As the lower posterior teeth erupt they move forwards slightly, and the theory is that using occlusal shelves to prevent eruption of the upper posterior teeth and encourage eruption of the lower posterior teeth helps to correct the molar relationship from Class II to Class I. However, where the overbite is normal and does not need to be reduced, the shelves should contact both upper and lower posterior teeth. The appliance has no clasps and can be used in conjunction with fixed appliances.

18.5.4. The bionator

The bionator was originally designed to modify tongue behaviour on the basis that the tongue was the main cause of increased overjet. It is now recognized that this is only very rarely the case, if at all, but the bionator design has proved to a be a useful functional appliance with a minimal bulk of acrylic which makes it easy to wear. A heavy wire loop takes the place of the palatal acrylic and buccal extensions of the labial bow hold the cheeks out of contact with the buccal segment teeth to allow some arch expansion (Fig. 18.10). It is usually made to an edge-to-edge working bite which is opened up as little as possible. The original bionator design has no lower incisor capping but does have posterior capping, which potentially causes problems with excessive proclination of the lower incisors and with management of a deep overbite. The appliance can be modified to include lower incisor capping and omit posterior capping, and in this form it becomes another variant of the activator.

18.5.5. The Frankel appliance

Frankel originally called this the function regulator (FR). It looks very different, having acrylic shields in the buccal sulci and little or no acrylic lingually, but in common with all functional appliances it induces mandibular posturing. The buccal shields are intended to cause expansion of the arches by holding the cheeks away from the teeth and also to enlarge the alveolar process by stretching the periosteum in the depth of the sulcus, thus causing bone to be laid down on the buccal aspect. There is little evidence to support this theory, but the appliance is very effective for anteroposterior correction.

Frankel described three main variants of the appliance. The FR1 (Fig. 18.11) is for treatment of Class II division 1 malocclusions and incorporates lip pads labial to the lower incisors to allow forward development of the mandibular alveolar process. Where the lower lip is trapped behind the upper incisors, the lip pads help the lower lip to unfurl and function in front of the upper incisors. Overbite control is less easy because of the lack of lower incisor capping, but variants have been described which incorporate capping.

The FR2 has in addition a palatal wire to procline the upper incisors and is intended for Class II division 2 malocclusions.

The FR3 (Fig. 18.4) is for treatment of Class III malocclusions, having acrylic shields labial to the upper incisors which, together with a palatal arch, procline them, and a lower labial bow which retroclines the lower incisors. Thus the FR3 achieves only a dento-alveolar correction of the incisor relationship, but it is the best of the functional appliance designs for Class III malocclusions. There is little evidence that any skeletal correction is achieved.

Frankel appliances are complex and must be made to a very high standard if they are to be tolerated — an ill-fitting Frankel appliance is extremely uncomfortable, particularly where the acrylic shields extend deeply into the buccal sulci. However, a keen patient with a well-fitting appliance can wear it virtually full-time, except for eating, and induce rapid changes. The complex design makes the appliance expensive to make and vulnerable to distortion of the wires, and it can be difficult or impossible to correct a distorted or damaged appliance.

18.5.6. The twin-block appliance

The unique feature of this appliance is that it is constructed in two parts, as separate upper and lower appliances (Fig. 18.12). Forward mandibular posturing is achieved by incorporating buccal blocks with interlocking inclined planes, with the lower blocks engaging in front of the upper ones. The appliance is often used with headgear to the upper arch. The two-part construction makes it well tolerated, even during eating, and many operators instruct the patient to wear their twin blocks full time. It will therefore often produce rapid changes.

This appliance's main difficulty is management of deep overbite, because of the buccal blocks. As the overjet reduces, lateral open bites develop which are then closed by progressively trimming the blocks in such a way as to allow the posterior teeth to erupt but at the same time maintain the forward posturing.

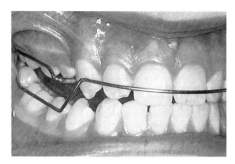

Fig. 18.10. Bionator appliance (courtesy of Mr T. G. Bennett).

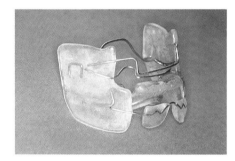

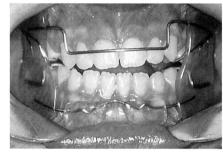

Fig. 18.11. Frankel appliance for correction of Class II division 1 malocclusion.

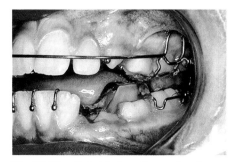

Fig. 18.12. Twin-block appliance, showing the lower buccal block engaging anteriorly to the upper buccal block.

This can be very fiddly and as a result many operators find the appliance most useful where the overbite is normal or reduced, rather than increased.

PRINCIPAL SOURCES AND FURTHER READING

Barton, S. and Cook, P. A.. (1997). Predicting functional appliance treatment outcome in Class II malocclusions — a review. *American Journal of Orthodontics and Dentofacial Orthopedics*, **112**, 282–6.
- A concise summary of the evidence about the use and effects of functional appliances.

Clark, W. J. (1988). Twin block technique. A functional orthopedic appliance system. *American Journal of Orthodontics and Dentofacial Orthopedics*, **93**, 1–18.
- The twin block appliance described by its originator.

Isaacson, K. G., Reed, R. T., and Stephens, C. D. (1990). *Functional orthodontic appliances*. Blackwell, Oxford.
- The use and effects of functional appliances, including an extensive literature review.

Mills, J. R. E. (1983). Clinical control of craniofacial growth: a skeptic's viewpoint. In *Clinical alterations of the growing face*. (ed. J. A. McNamara, K. A. Ribbons, and R. P. Howe), Monograph 14,. Center for Human Growth and Development, University of Michigan.
- An exhaustive appraisal of the evidence concerning the effects of functional appliances.

Orton, H. S. (1990). *Functional appliances in orthodontic treatment*. Quintessence, London.
- A manual of laboratory construction of the appliances.

19 Adult orthodontics

As dental awareness is growing and orthodontic appliances are now becoming more socially acceptable, a increasing number of adult patients are seeking orthodontic treatment. At the same time, a greater proportion of the general public are keeping their teeth for longer, which is resulting in an increasing demand for orthodontic treatment to facilitate restorative and periodontal care.

19.1. DIFFICULTIES POSED BY ORTHODONTIC TREATMENT FOR ADULTS

Orthodontic treatment is usually carried out in children around the time of the pubertal growth spurt and/or soon after eruption of the permanent dentition. Both spontaneous and dynamic tooth movement are accomplished more readily at this age, and active growth facilitates the correction of skeletal discrepancies. In contrast, if orthodontic treatment is delayed until adulthood treatment may be complicated by the following:

- **Negligible growth** Although recent studies indicate that growth does continue throughout adulthood, this is at a much diminished rate compared with childhood. This means that the threshold for surgery is lower in adult patients with skeletal discrepancies or increased overbite.

- **Reduced tissue blood supply and cell turnover** As a result the response to orthodontic force is more sluggish (in children the initial reaction to orthodontic force occurs within 24 hours, whereas in adults it can take up to 3 weeks) and tissue reorganization following tooth movement takes longer.

- **Reduced periodontal attachment** The incidence and severity of periodontal attachment loss increases with age, and the load upon a reduced periodontium can be further exacerbated by tooth loss. In some cases the teeth are less able to resist soft tissue and occlusal forces, leading to migration and drifting of particularly the incisors. Where orthodontic treatment is planned for teeth with reduced periodontal support, the forces applied to the teeth need to be decreased accordingly, and patients with gingival recession should be counselled that orthodontic treatment may accelerate this problem.

- **Missing and heavily restored teeth** Tooth loss may lead to migration and/or tilting of the adjacent teeth and to over-eruption of the opposing teeth, thus contributing to disruption of the occlusion. In addition, atrophy of the alveolar bone following extraction can lead to 'necking' (Fig. 19.1). Inadequate restorations with poor contact points, deficient occlusal stops, or premature contacts may also lead to occlusal disharmonies and/or mandibular displacement. The choice of teeth for extraction in adults is often determined by the prognosis of individual teeth.

- **Adults are less able to adapt to discrepancies in the occlusion** Therefore even more care is required to ensure that a good functional occlusion is achieved at the end of treatment.

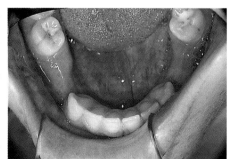

Fig. 19.1. Necking.

19.2. PRACTICAL ORTHODONTIC MANAGEMENT IN ADULTS

A thorough orthodontic assessment (Chapter 5) should be carried out prior to planning treatment, and this should include a careful examination of the condition of the teeth, both periodontally and restoratively. In some adults this may involve taking full-mouth radiographs. If the patient has several missing teeth it is important to observe the path of closure of the mandible on the hinge axis, looking particularly for displacements. As with children, good dental care is a prerequisite to orthodontic treatment, but in the adult it is even more important that any periodontal disease is controlled before orthodontic appliances are placed. In many adult patients assessment and treatment planning should be carried out jointly with other disciplines, particularly if periodontal disease is present and/or restorative work is necessary.

Management of Class I, Class II, and Class III malocclusions in the adult will generally run along the lines discussed in Chapters 8–11. However, owing to the lack of growth there is a lower threshold for surgery in the management of skeletal discrepancies and increased overbite. Treatment planning in the adult, including anchorage requirements, may be compromised by previous tooth loss and the condition of the remaining teeth, and in some cases a compromise may have to be accepted as a result.

Where possible, overbite reduction should be achieved by intrusion, as extrusion of the molars tends to relapse once appliances are removed. On occasion, limited crown reduction can be considered when over-eruption has occurred. Rarely, this may involve elective devitalization to prevent pulpal problems, followed by crowning when treatment is complete. Alternatively, surgery may be required.

Lighter forces should be used in the adult, particularly initially and where periodontal support is reduced. A slower rate of tooth movement can be expected in the older patient, particularly initially. Spontaneous tooth movement and space closure is also much reduced in the adult dentition. Distal movement of the upper buccal segments is not really an option in the mature dentition, although extraoral anchorage can be used provided that the patient is prepared to accept it. Despite the increased acceptance of orthodontics, adult patients are usually keen for appliances to be as unobtrusive as possible. Tooth-coloured brackets (Fig. 19.2) lingual or minibrackets can be used, and these improve the aesthetics of a fixed appliance. Crowned or heavily restored teeth often pose a problem for bonded attachments. Silane coupling agents can be used in conjunction with a composite orthodontic adhesive for bonding to porcelain veneers or crowns, but the retention rates are often disappointing. If much of the labial surface is involved in a metal restoration, there may be no alternative but to use a band around the tooth. Patients should be warned prior to starting treatment if there is a risk of a restoration being dislodged when the appliance is removed, and if complex restorative treatment is required this is often best delayed until after the orthodontic phase is complete.

Because of the slower rate of tissue reorganization, retention following orthodontic treatment in the adult may need to be prolonged or even permanent.

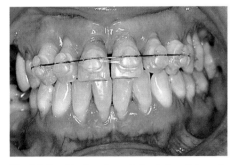

Fig. 19.2. Tooth-coloured plastic bracket used to align this patient's upper labial segment.

19.3. ORTHODONTICS AS AN ADJUNCT TO RESTORATIVE WORK

As the proportion of the population with some natural teeth increases, so does the need for joint management of adults with 'mutilated' dentitions due to tooth loss and periodontal disease. Where collaboration between orthodontist and restorative dentist is required in the management of a case, it is preferable to see the patient jointly to formulate a integrated treatment plan. The following are examples of problems that benefit from a joint restorative–orthodontic approach:

- **Redistribution/closing of space** Following unplanned tooth loss, space closure or movement of a proposed abutment tooth into the middle of an edentulous span may be indicated to facilitate fabrication of a durable prosthesis.
- **Uprighting of tilted bridge abutments** If, following the loss of a permanent tooth, the adjacent teeth tilt into the space, replacement of the missing unit with bridgework may be complicated by a lack of parallelism of the abutment teeth. One possible option is to upright the adjacent teeth prior to bridgework.
- **Intrusion of over-erupted teeth** Intrusion of over-erupted teeth may be required prior to restorative work in the opposing arch.
- **Extrusion of fractured teeth** This is usually required where the fracture line extends below the gingival margin. Although extrusion brings the margin supragingivally and facilitates placement of a crown or restoration, it must be remembered that extrusion will also adversely affect the crown-to-root ratio.

Where a combined approach is indicated, it is often wise to allow a period of stabilization between the phases of treatment of differing specialities.

19.4. MIGRATION OF PERIODONTALLY INVOLVED INCISORS

Migration of periodontally compromised incisors is an increasingly common problem and therefore is considered separately in this section.

19.4.1. Aetiology

Patients with loss of periodontal attachment may experience labial drifting of the teeth, most commonly the upper incisors, although other teeth can be affected. This may be due to a number of factors, and one or more may be operating in an individual case:

- Reduced bony support means that the teeth are less able to withstand adverse soft tissue and occlusal forces, and tooth movement occurs.
- Periodontal inflammation leads to extrusion of the teeth, bringing them into traumatic occlusion. If the periodontal support is also reduced, the teeth may drift as a result (Fig. 19.3).
- If a premature contact which results in a forward slide of the mandible on closure occurs in a patient with periodontally involved upper incisors, proclination of the upper labial segment may occur as a result.
- Lack of posterior support due to tooth loss places undue pressures on the incisors, leading particularly to proclination of the upper incisors.

19.4.2. Management

Initial management has to include stabilization of the periodontal condition and an assessment of the prognosis of the affected teeth. If the prognosis is satisfactory and orthodontic alignment is planned, the most difficult aspect is often overbite reduction. If the overbite is not markedly increased, a removable bite-plane appliance can be used (Fig. 19.4), but it should be remembered that this will

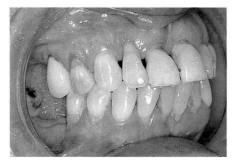
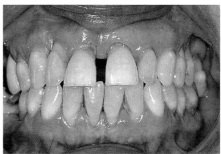
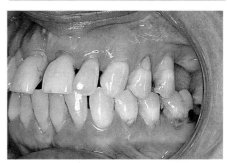

Fig. 19.3. Periodontal disease and lack of posterior support contributed to the proclination and spacing of this patient's upper labial segment (see also Fig. 19.2 which shows the appliance used to align the upper labial segment).

Fig. 19.4. Adult with migration of /1 secondary to advanced periodontal disease and a combined perio-endo lesion of /1. Following control of the periodontal disease and root canal therapy, an upper removable appliance in conjunction with a single bracket was used to align /1: (a) prior to orthodontic treatment; (b) appliance used to align /1.

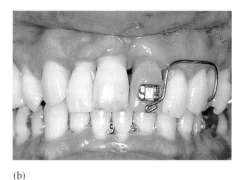

(a)   (b)

Fig. 19.5. Adult patient with migration of the upper incisors secondary to periodontal disease. An upper fixed appliance was used to close the upper labial spacing and to retract the maxillary incisors: (a) pre-treatment: (b) fixed appliance.

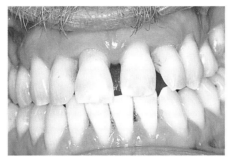 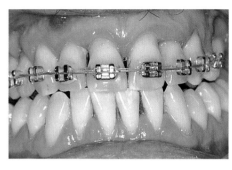

(a)   (b)

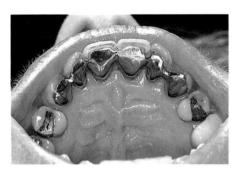

Fig. 19.6. Metal splint to provide retention and support following retraction of periodontally involved incisors.

lead to overbite reduction by extrusion of the molars which will tend to relapse post-treatment. Fixed appliances are required if incisor intrusion is indicated. However, there is a limit to the amount of overbite reduction that can be attempted, and either crown height reduction or surgery may be indicated.

If a forward slide from a premature contact is an aetiological factor, this should be eliminated to allow the patient to attain their true intercuspal position (centric relation). This often necessitates a course of splint therapy, which is best carried out by the restorative member of the team who can then advise on elimination of any premature contacts revealed by this process.

Reduction of the increased overjet is usually relatively straightforward with a fixed appliance in most cases (Fig. 19.5). However, permanent retention is usually necessary following treatment. This can most easily be accomplished with a conventional bonded retainer, although in some cases a metal splint (similar to the retention wings of an acid-etch retained bridge), attached to the palatal aspect of the teeth with composite, may be indicated to provide additional support to periodontally involved teeth (Fig. 19.6).

PRINCIPAL SOURCES AND FURTHER READING

Heasman, P. A. and Millett, D. T. (1996). *The periodontium and orthodontics in health and disease*. Oxford University Press, Oxford.

Howat, A. P. and Warren, K. (1991). A restorative–orthodontic approach in the older patient. *British Journal of Orthodontics*, **18**, 195–201.
● An interesting case report which illustrates the teamwork required in a combined periodontal–orthodontic–restorative treatment for a 60-year-old patient.

Kahl-Nieke, B. (1996). Retention and stability considerations for adult patients. *Dental Clinics of North America*, **40**, 961–94.

Khan, R. S. and Horrocks, E. N. (1991). A study of adult orthodontic patients and their treatment. *British Journal of Orthodontics*, **18**, 183–94.

Melsen, B., Agerbaek, N., Eriksen, J., and Terp, S. (1988). New attachment through periodontal treatment and orthodontic extrusion. *American Journal of Orthodontics and Dentofacial Orthopedics*, **94**, 104–16.

- A thought-provoking article.

Melsen, B., Agerbaek, N., and Markenstam, G. (1989). Intrusion of incisors in adult patients with marginal bone loss. *American Journal of Orthodontics and Dentofacial Orthopedics*, **96**, 232–41.

Nattrass, C. and Sandy, J. R. (1995). Adult Orthodontics — a review. *British Journal of Orthodontics*, 22, 331–7.

Norton, I. A. (1988). The effect of ageing cellular mechanisms on tooth movement. *Dental Clinics of North America*, **32**, 437–46.

20 Orthodontics and orthognathic surgery

Orthognathic surgery is concerned with the correction of dento-facial deformity. In the vast majority of cases a combined surgical and orthodontic approach is required to achieve an optimum result.

20.1. INDICATIONS

Patients with a craniofacial deformity, for example cleft lip and palate, may require orthognathic surgery to correct or mask their underlying abnormality.

Orthognathic surgery may be necessary for those cases with a skeletal discrepancy outside the limits of orthodontic treatment either because of their severity or a lack of growth. Examples include the following:

- severe Class II malocclusions
- severe Class III malocclusions
- vertical discrepancies
- anterior open bite
- markedly increased overbite
- skeletal asymmetry.

20.2. DIAGNOSIS AND TREATMENT PLANNING

An integrated team approach is essential as this allows the surgeon and orthodontist to produce a coordinated treatment plan tailored to an individual patient's needs. This is best achieved by holding joint clinics where treatment can be discussed with the prospective patient. In some centres a psychologist is also a member of the team, helping to identify those patients with unrealistic expectations of treatment. There should also be access to speech and language therapy.

20.2.1. The patient's perception of the problem

Patients seek orthognathic surgery for a number of reasons. The most common are the following:

- appearance
- masticatory difficulties
- speech
- traumatic overbite
- temporomandibular joint dysfunction.

Treatment should always attempt to address the patient's concerns. However, it is important to assess whether an individual's perception of the problem is realistic. A small number of patients project their difficulties in forming relationships or friendships onto a particular facial feature. Their expectations are unrealistic, as they expect surgery to provide an instant solution to their problems and they may react unfavourably post-operatively.

20.2.2. Clinical examination

A systematic approach is required which should include the whole of the patient's face including the forehead and neck. The data given in Table 20.1 can be used as a guide.

Table 20.1 Useful measurements for dentofacial assessment

Mid-facial third	Males 66 mm	Females 60 mm
Lower facial third	Males 66 mm	Females 60 mm
Subnasale to vermilion lower lip	Males 33 mm	Females 30 mm
Vermilion lower lip to menton (ST)	Males 33 mm	Females 30 mm
Intercanthal width	34 ± 4 mm	
Alar base width	34 ± 4 mm	
Interpupillary width	65 ± 4 mm	
Width of mouth	65 ± 4 mm	
Length of upper lip	Males 22 mm	Females 20 mm
Exposure of upper incisor at rest	Males 0 mm	Females 3 mm
Exposure of upper incisor smiling	7–10 mm	
Projection of supra-orbital ridge:	5–10 mm	
Nasolabial angle	110° ± 9°	
Labiomental angle	124° ± 10°	
Neck–chin angle	135°	

Full face

This should include an assessment of the symmetry and balance of the face from the frontal view. Although no face is completely symmetrical, obvious deviations from normal between left and right should be noted. This examination should include the level of the orbits and also the contour of the maxilla and mandible, particularly any deviation of the chin point (Fig. 20.1). In an aesthetically pleasing face the upper, middle, and lower facial thirds are nearly equal in height (Figs. 20.2 and Fig. 20.3), and the face also divides into fifths vertically.

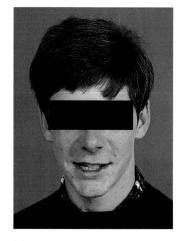

(a)

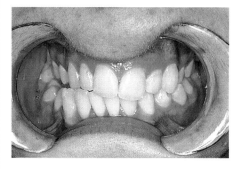

(b)

Fig. 20.1. Patient with mild facial asymmetry: (a) extra-oral; (b) intra-oral.

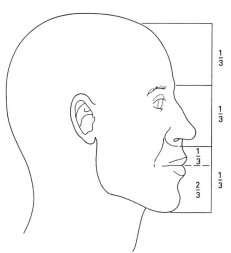

Fig. 20.2. An aesthetic face will divide into thirds vertically. The distance from stomion to menton is two-thirds of the lower facial third.

$\frac{1}{3}$

$\frac{1}{3}$

$\frac{1}{3}$

$\frac{2}{3}$

$\frac{1}{3}$

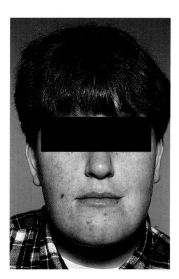

Fig. 20.3. A patient with a long lower third of the face, with a proportionately increased distance between stomion and menton.

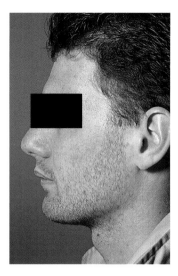

Fig. 20.4. A patient with a Class II division 1 incisor relationship on a Class II skeletal pattern and a good nasolabial angle. Retraction of the upper incisors would lead to a flattening of the upper lip and make the nose appear more prominent.

Fig. 20.5. (a) A patient with a Class II division 1 malocclusion with an excessive amount of upper incisor show; (a) the same patient following segmental surgery in the upper arch and a mandibular advancement. The lips are now competent.

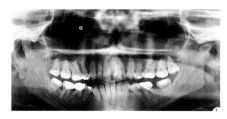

Fig. 20.6. The DPT radiograph of a patient for whom it was decided to avoid presurgical orthodontic alignment in the lower arch.

Profile

The upper, middle, and lower facial thirds should be considered in turn, so that the forehead and the neck–throat angle are assessed as well as the relationship of the maxilla to the mandible. Maxillary retrognathia is more easily diagnosed from this perspective, as the profile appears concave. The shape of the nose and the nasolabial angle are also important, as retraction of the upper incisors will lead to an increase in obliquity of the nasolabial angle, making the nose more prominent (Fig. 20.4). Conversely, proclination of the upper incisors or forward movement of the maxilla will make the angle formed between the nose and the upper lip more acute.

The effect on the profile of surgery to advance the mandible can be judged by asking the patient to posture forwards the desired amount. Advancement of the maxilla can also be evaluated by placing cotton wool rolls under the patient's upper lip.

Soft tissues

The form and tone of the soft tissues should be recorded. The fullness of the lips and the amount of tooth show, particularly the upper incisors, at rest and during function should be assessed (Fig. 20.5). Liposuction and/or platysma plication can sometimes be used to improve the neck–throat angle.

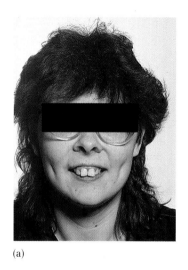
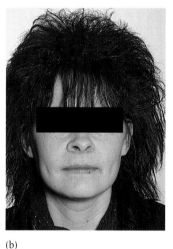

(a) (b)

Temporomandibular joints

The presence of any signs or symptoms of temporomandibular joint dysfunction should be included in the examination of a patient for orthognathic surgery. The role of the occlusion in the aetiology of temporomandibular dysfunction is discussed in more detail in Chapter 1. Ideally, any symptoms should be treated conservatively prior to treatment. However, in patients with grossly deranged occlusions and/or multiple non-working side interferences, it may be necessary to commence treatment which will address these occlusal problems.

Dental health

Good dental health is a prerequisite to a successful outcome. The long-term prognosis of all restored teeth should be taken into consideration when extractions are planned. On occasion this can compromise the treatment plan (Fig. 20.6).

Occlusal assessment

A thorough examination of the occlusion should be carried out by an orthodontist (see Chapter 5). It is important to check whether the centrelines of the upper and lower arches are coincident with each other and the centre of the face, and to note the direction and nature of any discrepancies.

20.2.3. Radiographic examination

This usually includes those radiographs taken as part of the routine orthodontic assessment of a patient with a skeletal discrepancy, namely a panoramic dental view (DPT), a lateral cephalometric radiograph, and, if indicated, a view of the upper incisors. On occasion, other views may be indicated, for example a posteroanterior skull for asymmetry or a submentovertex to assess mandibular flare prior to a mandibular setback.

20.2.4. Cephalometric assessment

In addition to a routine cephalometric analysis (Chapter 6), many surgeons and orthodontists will carry out more specialized analyses to help determine the underlying aetiology of a particular problem. Many such analyses exist, and for details of these the reader is referred to the section on further reading. One commonly used approach is to compare the patient's cephalometric values with the norm by means of a 'standard' tracing. Perhaps the most widely used of these is the Bolton standard (Fig. 20.7). The Bolton standard is a composite tracing derived from the lateral cephalometric radiographs taken every year for a group of individuals followed from birth to maturity. An 'average' tracing is available for each year of age, which can be compared against a patient's tracing to help determine areas of discrepancy. However, care is required, as the discrepancies will alter depending on which structures the tracings are superimposed upon. Also, the Bolton tracings are determined from a relatively small group of individuals of both sexes, and therefore should only be used as a guide and not a treatment goal.

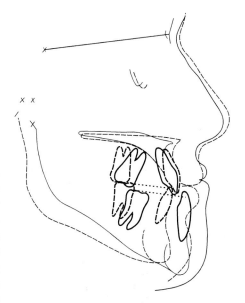

Fig. 20.7. Computer print-out to show superimposition of a Bolton composite for an 18-year-old (bold outline) upon the tracing of a patient with a severe Class III malocclusion on the sella–nasion line at sella.

20.2.5. Planning

The following are essential for the purposes of planning and audit:

1. **Study models** In addition to 'angled' study models, it is often helpful to have at least one set of duplicate models for model surgery, usually mounted on a plane line articulator (Fig. 20.8). However, if it is thought that treatment is likely to involve bimaxillary surgery and/or autorotation of the mandible, a set of models should be mounted on a semi-adjustable articulator.

2. **Photographs** Most orthodontists have a routine set of extra-oral and intra-oral views taken before orthodontic treatment. In addition to these, some surgeons find it helpful to have a negative of the patient's profile enlarged to fit 1:1 to their lateral cephalometric radiograph so that the two are superimposed allowing both soft and bony tissues to be seen. This can then be cut up to help determine the effects of different surgical options upon the patient's profile and can be used to give the patient an idea of his appearance post-surgery. However, care is required not to instill unrealistic expectations, as although some allowance can be made for the responses of the soft tissues to different surgical procedures, there is wide individual variation.

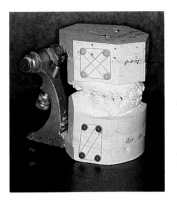

Fig. 20.8. Model surgery.

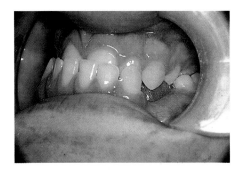

Fig. 20.9.   Dento-alveolar compensation.

Where a skeletal discrepancy exists, the action of the soft tissues can lead to tilting of the teeth which compensates for the underlying skeletal problem to varying degrees. This is known as dento-alveolar compensation. It is most commonly seen in Class III malocclusions where proclination of the upper incisors and retroclination of the lower incisors occurs owing to the action of the lips and tongue striving to form an anterior oral seal (Fig. 20.9). If an orthodontics-only approach is to be undertaken for a skeletal discrepancy, this usually involves a degree of dento-alveolar compensation, whereas if orthognathic surgery is to be carried out, ideally any dento-alveolar compensation needs to be eliminated prior to surgery in order that a full correction of the underlying skeletal discrepancy can be carried out. Obviously, in patients with a marked skeletal discrepancy, consideration should be given to the need for surgery before embarking on orthodontic treatment alone as the tooth movements required are in the opposite direction.

Occasionally it is not feasible or desirable to correct the incisor angulations to their ideal values, for example a narrow mandibular symphysis and/or thin labial periodontal tissues may preclude complete decompensation of retroclined lower incisors in a Class III malocclusion. Therefore it is imperative that the surgeon and orthodontist work closely together at the planning stage to ensure that a co-ordinated approach is employed and the desired skeletal changes can be correlated with the planned occlusion.

A number of methods are used to determine the effect of different treatment plans upon the patient's face and occlusion. There are several manual methods where a 'guesstimate' of the effect of orthodontics and surgery is constructed from the lateral cephalometric tracing. The method described previously, which utilizes a 1:1 photograph superimposed upon a lateral cephalometric radiograph is a variation on this theme. Increasingly, specially designed computer programs (Fig. 20.10) can be utilized to evaluate the effects of different orthodontic and surgical approaches on a particular malocclusion. Use of these sophisticated programs saves considerable time over the manual method, allows the investigation of an almost endless range of treatment permutations, and also provides a database for the subsequent analysis of the results of treatment. However, a degree of

Fig. 20.10.   Print-out of the treatment planned (dashed line) for a patient with a Class III malocclusion using a computer planning program (COGsoft).

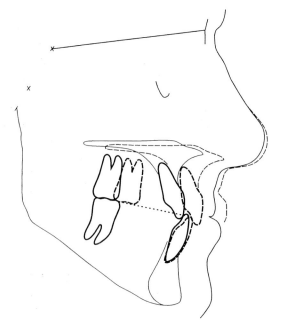

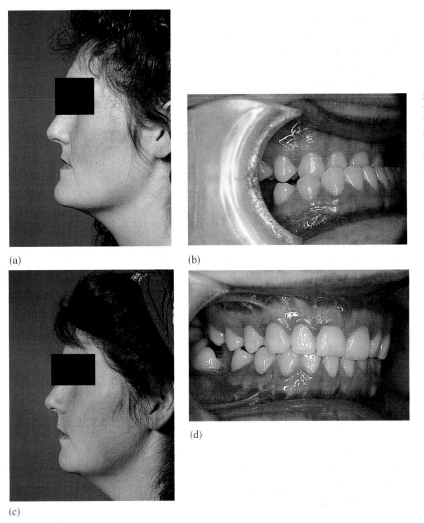

(a)

(b)

(c)

(d)

Fig. 20.11. A patient in her early twenties with a Class III malocclusion who refused to wear orthodontic appliances. She was treated by a maxillary advancement alone, and whilst there is an obvious aesthetic improvement the resulting buccal occlusion is not ideal: (a), (b) pre-operatively; (c), (d) post-operatively.

caution is required when using these programs so that only those approaches that are technically feasible for a particular patient are selected for further consideration.

Following this process it should be possible to determine where the discrepancy lies and whether, and to what degree, it can be corrected. Often, more than one option can be presented to the patient showing varying levels of complexity and final result. Patients often find it helpful to meet a previous (successful!) candidate to discuss the effects of treatment.

A proportion of patients will refuse to consider wearing orthodontic appliances. Rarely, a reasonable occlusion may be possible with surgery alone and perhaps a little judicious occlusal grinding (Fig. 20.11). In the majority a very poor occlusion will result following surgery without orthodontic preparation and if dento-alveolar compensation is not reduced then the facial result may also be prejudiced. In these cases it may be advisable not to proceed unless the patient accepts orthodontic appliances.

20.3. SEQUENCE OF TREATMENT

Except for some of the craniofacial anomalies, orthognathic surgery is usually carried out when the patient has finished growing so that a good result is not spoiled by further growth. However, the presurgical orthodontic preparation can be commenced earlier, so that its conclusion is timed to coincide with the completion of growth.

20.3.1. Extractions

Extractions may be necessary to relieve crowding and to provide space in order to align the teeth over their skeletal bases (i.e. reduce any dento-alveolar decompensation). In addition, it is important for the surgeon to decide whether any impacted third molars should be removed prior to the start of treatment or during surgery itself, particularly if mandibular ramus surgery is planned.

20.3.2. Presurgical orthodontics

A phase of presurgical orthodontics is usually necessary to establish the desired anteroposterior and vertical position of the incisors, and to align and coordinate the arches so that the teeth do not interfere with placing the jaws in their planned relationship. If a segmental procedure is to be carried out, space will need to be created interdentally for the surgical cuts. However, it is inefficient to carry out tooth movements that can be accomplished more readily at or after surgery, for example levelling of the lower arch in a Class II division 2 malocclusion. As with any orthodontic or surgical procedure, some relapse can be anticipated. Therefore it is helpful if the orthodontics can be planned so that the orthodontic relapse is in the opposite direction to the expected surgical relapse, so that they tend to cancel each other out. It is important to forewarn the patient that the presurgical orthodontic phase may make their appearance worse as any dento-alveolar compensation is reduced (Fig. 20.12).

Presurgical orthodontics is carried out using fixed appliances, which are left in place during surgery. The pre-adjusted appliances (see Chapter 17) make this phase of treatment much easier. Rigid rectangular archwires are usually required to complete presurgical alignment. However, it is important that these are passive before surgery is carried out, particularly if inter-occlusal wafers are to be used during surgery. In most cases the rigid archwires are left *in situ* and hooks are added for intermaxillary fixation during surgery. Some orthodontists choose a fixed appliance system with a hook on each bracket for orthognathic cases to save having to place hooks onto the archwire — which can be a fiddly and time-consuming exercise (Fig. 20.13).

Presurgical orthodontics usually takes between 12 and 18 months depending upon the complexity of the case. At this stage new study models, radiographs, and photographs are recorded to check what has been achieved during this phase so that the surgical plan can be modified or confirmed as indicated. Model surgery is often carried out to determine the amount and site of bone removal and to fabricate inter-occlusal wafers (or splints) used to locate the bony segments to the planned position during surgery, prior to fixation.

20.3.3. Surgery

A brief description of the common surgical procedures is given in Section 20.4.

In the past, wires were used to locate and fix the bony segments in their corrected position. This necessitated the use of intermaxillary fixation (i.e. the upper and lower teeth were wired together) for about 6 weeks until bony union had occurred. Apart from being unpleasant for the patient, there was a greater morbidity in the immediate post-operative period, often necessitating admittance to an intensive-care bed for the first 24 hours.

The introduction of small bone plates to fix the position of bony segments semi-rigidly in the maxilla and the use of plates and/or screws in the mandible has completely revolutionized orthognathic surgery. This means that it is not neces-

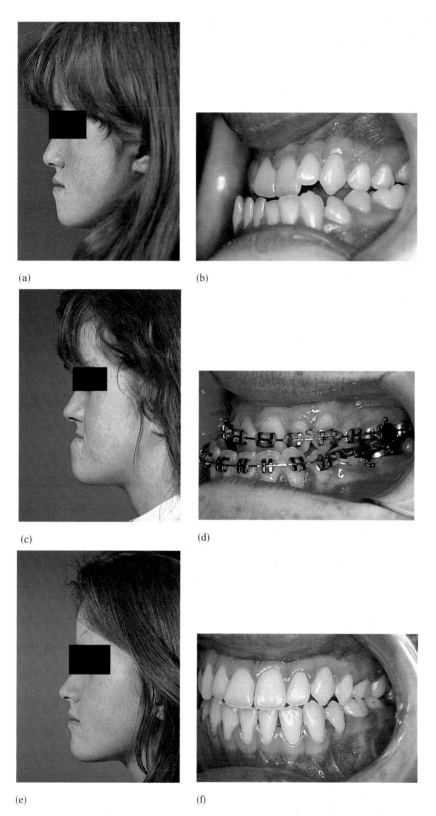

(a)

(b)

(c)

(d)

(e)

(f)

Fig. 20 12. Patient aged 16 years with a Class III malocclusion: SNA = 84°, SNB = 91.5°, ANB = −7.5°, UInc to MxPl = 123°, LInc to MnPl = 76°, MMPA = 21° and FP = 55 per cent. Following the extraction of all four second premolars and presurgical orthodontics, the patient had bimaxillary surgery; (a), (b) pretreatment; (c), (d) at the end of presurgical alignment; (e), (f) at the end of treatment.

Fig. 20.13. (a) Ball hooks crimped onto arch-wire for the application of intermaxillary fixation during surgery. (b) Bracket system with hook incorporated into each bracket.

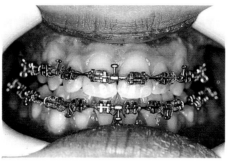
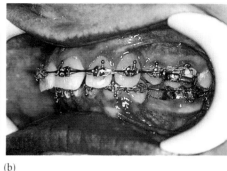

(a)   (b)

sary to rely only on intermaxillary fixation following surgery. This approach, together with advances in the use of steroids to reduce swelling and modern antibiotic regimens, means that patients can often be released from hospital within 2 or 3 days of their operation. More recently, resorbable plates and screws have been introduced.

20.3.4. Post-surgical orthodontics

Although intermaxillary elastic traction can be started immediately post-operatively to help guide the arches into the desired position, active tooth movement is not usually commenced until approximately 4 weeks after surgery. Lighter round wires, and elastic traction are utilized to detail the occlusion into a good interdigitation. This phase of orthodontics should last for about 6 months.

If the bony segments are not correctly positioned during surgery, a limited amount of movement towards the desired position is possible using intermaxillary elastics in the immediate post-operative period. This problem occurs most commonly when the condyles have been displaced from the glenoid fossa during surgery, with the result that when they return to their correct articulation post-operatively the occlusion is wrong.

20.3.5. Retention

This is usually along similar lines as for conventional fixed appliance therapy (see Chapter 17), namely an upper removable retainer and either a lower removable or bonded (lingual to the lower incisors) retainer as indicated.

20.4. COMMON SURGICAL PROCEDURES

Only a brief overview of some of the more popular surgical techniques is included here. Additional information is available in the literature cited in the section on further reading.

As aesthetics are of major importance, where possible an intra-oral approach should be used to avoid unsightly scars. Segmental procedures have an increased morbidity, as damage to the teeth or disruption of the blood supply to a segment is more likely.

20.4.1. Maxillary procedures

Segmental procedures

One or more teeth and their supporting bone can be moved as a segmental procedure. The Wassmund technique involves movement of the upper premaxillary
segment of incisors and canines as a block, either distally to reduce an increased
overjet or upwards to reduce excessive upper incisor show. Nowadays a Le Fort I
procedure is more frequently carried out and the maxilla divided from above into
segments.

Le Fort I (Fig. 20.14)

This is the most widely used technique. The standard approach is a horseshoe
incision of the buccal mucosa and underlying bone, which results in the maxilla
being pedicled on the palatal soft tissues and blood supply. The maxilla can then
be moved upwards (after removal of the intervening bone), downwards (with
interpositional bone graft), or forwards. Movement of the maxilla backwards is
not feasible in practice. Where there is concern regarding the blood supply provided by the palatal vessels, the buccal approach can be made via small vertical
incisions and tunnelling of the mucosa, but this makes plating difficult and may
increase the likelihood of relapse.

A transpalatal approach is favoured in a small number of centres.

Le Fort II

This is employed to achieve mid-face advancement.

Le Fort III

This usually necessitates raising of a bicoronal flap for access and is commonly
used in the management of craniofacial anomalies.

20.4.2. Mandibular procedures

Ramus procedures

The most commonly used ramus techniques are the following.

Vertical subsigmoid osteotomy

This is used for mandibular prognathism and involves a bone cut from the
sigmoid notch to the lower border. This can be performed intra-orally using

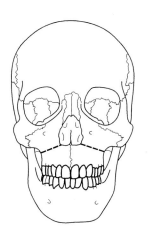 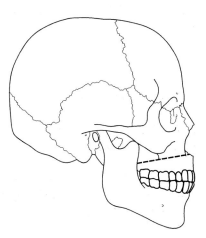

Fig. 20.14. Diagram to show the position of
the surgical cuts (dashed lines) for a Le Fort 1
procedure.

special instruments or extra-orally using standard instruments at the expense of a scar.

Sagittal split osteotomy (Fig. 20.15)

This procedure can be used to advance or push back the mandible or to correct mild asymmetry. The bony cut extends obliquely from above the lingula, across the retromolar region, and vertically down the buccal plate to the lower border. The main complication is damage to the inferior alveolar nerve.

Body osteotomy

This operation is useful if there is a natural gap in the lower arch anterior to the mental foramen in a patient with mandibular prognathism. Now rarely used.

Genioplasty (Fig. 20.16)

The tip of the chin can be moved in almost any direction, limited by sliding bony contact and the muscle pedicle. This technique can sometimes be usefully employed as a masking procedure, thus avoiding more complex treatment (for example, mild asymmetry).

Post-condylar cartilage graft

This technique differs from those discussed previously, as it is usually utilized for the correction of severe mandibular retrognathia in growing children. Insertion of a block of cadaveric or autologous cartilage behind the condylar head can produce results analogous to instantaneous functional appliance treatment in Class II division 1 malocclusions, with remodelling of the condylar fossa and surprisingly few adverse reactions. However, this approach may require multiple interventions to achieve an adequate result and definitive orthognathic surgery may still be required.

20.4.3 Bimaxillary surgery

Many patients require surgery to both jaws to correct the underlying skeletal discrepancy (Fig. 20.17).

20.4.4 Distraction Osteogenesis

One of the difficulties posed by the treatment of congenital craniofacial deformities, is the limitations placed by the soft tissues on the amount of movement that is achievable. Although this problem has been addressed to an extent by the use of tissue expanders, the introduction of 'slow' distraction osteogenesis in the management of limb deformity has opened up a wealth of opportunity for the management of craniofacial anomalies. Basically this process involves the application of incremental traction to osteotomized bone ends. As a result tension arises in the healing callus and new bone is stimulated in the direction of the traction. Thus this technique avoids the problems of harvesting and maintaining a viable bone graft in the treatment of deficiencies and, in addition, the forces also act upon the surrounding soft tissues leading to adaptive changes termed distraction histogenesis. Distraction osteogenesis is useful for the correction of severe deformity in the growing child and it is hoped will help to reduce the number of surgical procedures previously required to treat these children.

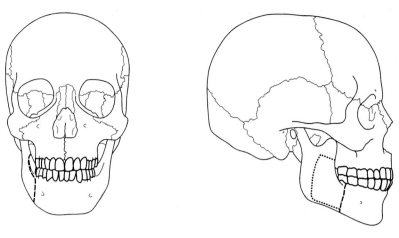

Fig. 20.15. Diagram to show the position of the surgical cuts (dashed/dotted lines) for a sagittal split osteotomy.

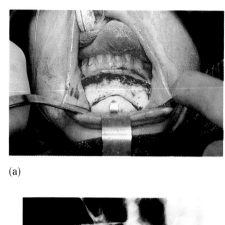

(a)

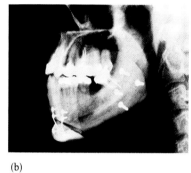

(b)

Fig. 20.16. (a) A genioplasty being carried out; (b) a lateral cephalometric radiograph of a patient who had a genioplasty carried out in addition to a sagittal split ramus procedure (note the plates securing the genioplasty).

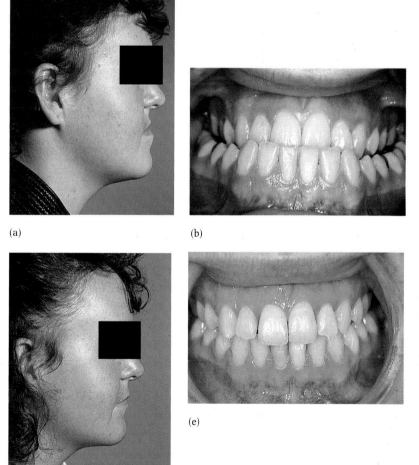

(a)

(b)

(c)

(d)

(e)

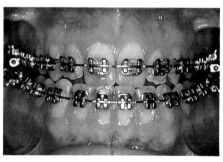

Fig. 20.17. A 16-year-old patient with a Class III malocclusion: SNA = 72.5°, SNB = 79°, ANB = –7.5°, UInc to MxPl = 112.5°, LInc to MnPl = 81°, MMPA = 26.5° and FP = 59 per cent.
Following presurgical orthodontics, the patient had a maxillary advancement and a mandibular set-back: (a), (b) pretreatment; (c) during orthodontic preparation; (d), (e) at the end of treatment.

Whilst this system is still in the process of being developed up to 20 mm of additional mandibular length has been gained by some workers and the technique can also be used for the correction of midface and cranial deformities. Most workers have utilized external fixators, which are manually controlled; however, this approach often leads to significant scarring. Intra-oral mechanisms are now commercially available and future possibilities include implanted telemetrically controlled devices.

20.5. RELAPSE

With biological systems there is always a tendency for any changes to regress. Therefore the potential for relapse should be assessed at the treatment planning stage and if necessary steps should be taken to limit or compensate for it. A number of factors can lead to relapse and these are broadly classified as follows:

1. Surgical factors

   ● Poor planning.
   ● The size of the movement required. Movement of the maxilla by more than 5–6 mm in any direction is more susceptible to relapse, as is movement of the mandible by more than 8 mm.
   ● Direction of movement required (see Table 20.2)
   ● Distraction of the condylar heads out of the glenoid fossa during surgery.
   ● Inadequate fixation.

2. Orthodontic factors

   ● Poor planning.
   ● Movement of the teeth into zones of soft tissue pressure will lead to relapse when appliances are removed. Therefore treatment should be planned to ensure that the teeth will be in a zone of soft tissue balance post-operatively and that the lips will be competent.
   ● Extrusion of the teeth during alignment tends to relapse post-treatment.
   ● Soft tissue habits, for example a tongue thrust, may persist, leading to a recurrence of an anterior open bite.

Table 20.2 Stability of orthognathic surgery

Most stable
Maxillary impaction
Mandibular advancement
Genioplasty (any direction)
Maxillary advancement
Correction of maxillary asymmetry
Maxillary impaction with mandibular advancement
Maxillary advancement with mandibular setback
Correction of mandibular asymmetry
Mandibular setback
Movement of maxilla downwards
Surgical expansion of maxilla
Least stable
Based on the article by Proffit *et al.* (1996).

3. Patient factors

- The nature of the problem; for example, anterior open bites associated with abnormal soft tissue behaviour are notoriously difficult to treat successfully and have a marked potential to relapse, and patients should be warned of this prior to treatment.

- Movements which put the soft tissues under tension, as in the correction of deficiencies, are more susceptible to relapse.

- In patients with cleft lip and palate advancement of the maxilla is difficult and prone to relapse because of the scar tissue of the primary repair.

- Failure to comply with treatment; for example, patient does not wear intermaxillary elastic traction as instructed.

PRINCIPAL SOURCES AND FURTHER READING

Barnard, D. and Birnie, D. (1990). Scope and limitations of orthognathic surgery. *Dental Update*, **17**, 63–9.
- A well-illustrated easy-to-read article introducing the reader to orthognathic surgery.

Cope, J. B., Samchukov, M. D., and Cherkashin, A. M. (1999). Mandibular distraction osteogenesis: A historic perspective and future directions. *American Journal of Orthodontics and Dentofacial Orthopedics*, **115**, 448–60.

Cunningham, S. J. and Feinmann, C. (1998). Psychological assessment of patients requiring orthognathic surgery and the relevance of body dysmorphic disorder. *British Journal of Orthodontics*, **25**, 293–8.

Epker, B. N. and Fish, L. C. (1986). *Dentofacial deformities — integrated orthodontic and surgical correction*. Mosby, St Louis, MO.
- A standard text of its time.

Harris, M. and Reynolds, I. R. (1991). *Fundamentals of orthognathic surgery*. Saunders, London.
- A concise but complete account of the subject for those with little background in the field.

Hunt, N. P. and Rudge, S. J. (1984). Facial profile and orthognathic surgery. *British Journal of Orthodontics*, **11**, 126–36.
- A detailed account of assessment of a patient for orthognathic surgery.

Lee, R. T. (1994). The benefits of post-surgical orthodontic treatment. *British Journal of Orthodontics*, **21**, 265–74.

Proffit, W. R., Turvey, T. A., and Phillips, C. (1996). Orthognathic surgery: a hierarchy of stability. *International Journal of Adult Orthodontics and Orthognathic Surgery*, **11**, 191–204.

Proffit, W. R. and White, R. R. (1991). *Surgical–orthodontic treatment*. Mosby Year Book, St Louis, MO.
- A comprehensive well-written text which is highly recommended.

Tuinzing, D. B., Greebe, R. B., Dorenbos, J., and van der Kwast, W. A. M. (1993). *Surgical orthodontics — diagnosis and treatment*. VU University Press, Amsterdam.
- This book provides a interesting insight into an ingenious method of planning orthognathic management. It also contains a useful section on areas requiring further investigation for those looking for ideas for research projects.

21 Cleft lip and palate and other craniofacial anomalies

21.1. PREVALENCE

Cleft lip and palate is the most common craniofacial malformation, comprising 65 per cent of all anomalies affecting the head and neck. There are two distinct types of cleft anomaly, cleft lip with or without cleft palate and isolated cleft palate, which result from failure of fusion at two different stages of dentofacial development.

21.1.1. Cleft lip and palate

The prevalence of cleft lip and palate varies geographically and between different racial groups. Amongst Caucasians, this anomaly occurs in approximately 1 in every 750 live births. However, the prevalence is increasing. A family history can be found in around 40 per cent of cases of cleft lip with or without cleft palate, and the risk of unaffected parents having another child with this anomaly is 1 in 20. Males are affected more frequently than females, and the left side is involved more commonly than the right. Interestingly, the severity of the cleft is usually more marked when it arises in the less common variant.

21.1.2. Isolated cleft of the secondary palate

Isolated cleft occurs in around 1 in 2000 live births and affects females more often than males. Clefts of the secondary palate have a lesser genetic component, with a family history in around 20 per cent and a reduced risk of further affected offspring to normal parents (1 in 80).

Isolated cleft palate is also found as a feature in a number of syndromes including Down, Treacher–Collins, Pierre–Robin, and Klippel–Fiel syndromes.

21.2. AETIOLOGY

In normal development fusion of the embryological processes that comprise the upper lip occurs around the sixth week of intra-uterine life. 'Flip-up' of the palatal shelves from a vertical to a horizontal position followed by fusion to form the secondary palate occurs around the eighth week. Before fusion can take place the embryological processes must grow until they come into contact. Then breakdown of the overlying epithelium is followed by invasion of mesenchyme. If this process is to take place successfully, a number of different factors need to interact at the right time. An inherited tendency towards short palatal shelves, for example, can be compensated (to a degree) by overdevelopment of other factors. If one of these factors is also affected or an environmental insult occurs at the time that palate formation is taking place, a cleft may result. Therefore cleft lip and palate is described as exhibiting polygenic inheritance with a threshold. Environmental factors (for example anticonvulsant drugs, folic acid deficiency, or steroid therapy) may thus precipitate a susceptible fetus towards the threshold.

It is postulated that isolated cleft palate is more common in females than males because transposition of the palatal shelves occurs later in the female fetus. Thus greater opportunity exists for an environmental insult to affect successful elevation, which is further hampered by widening of the face as a result of growth in the intervening period.

21.3. CLASSIFICATION

A number of classifications exist but, given the wide variation in clinical presentation, in practice it is often preferable to describe the presenting deformity in words (Fig. 21.1). However, in medicine in general, moves to standardize nomenclature have resulted in the introduction of national and international classifications which aim to embrace all medical conditions, thus facilitating epidemiology and management. Of these, the most widely accepted in the UK is the Read coding system. Table 21.1 gives the relevant Read and International Classification of Diseases (ICD) codes for cleft lip and palate anomaly.

Table 21.1   Codes for cleft lip and palate anomalies

Anomaly	Read	ICD
Cleft lip + palate (unspecified)	P9	749
Cleft lip	P91	749.1
Cleft palate	P90	749.0
Cleft lip + palate	P92	749.2
Unilateral complete cleft lip + palate	P921	749.21
Bilateral complete cleft lip + palate	P923	749.23

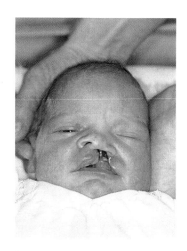

(a)

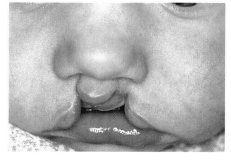

(b)

Fig. 21.1.   (a) Baby with a complete unilateral cleft lip and palate on the left side; (b) baby with a bilateral incomplete cleft lip.

21.4. PROBLEMS IN MANAGEMENT

21.4.1. Congenital anomalies

The disturbances in dental and skeletal development caused by the clefting process itself depend upon the site and severity of the cleft.

Lip only

There is little effect in this type, although notching of the alveolus adjacent to the cleft lip may sometimes be seen.

Lip and alveolus

A unilateral cleft of the lip and alveolus is not usually associated with segmental displacement. However, in bilateral cases the premaxilla may be rotated forwards. The lateral incisor on the side of the cleft may exhibit some of the following dental anomalies:

● congenital absence

● an abnormality of tooth size and/or shape

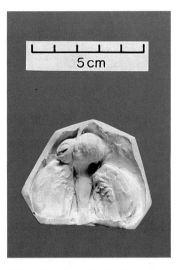

Fig. 21.2. Upper model of a bilateral complete cleft lip and palate showing the inward collapse of the lateral segments behind the premaxillary segment.

- enamel defects
- two conical teeth, one on each side of the cleft.

Lip and palate

In unilateral clefts rotation and collapse of both segments inwards anteriorly is usually seen, although this is usually more marked on the side of the cleft (the lesser segment). In bilateral clefts both lateral segments are often collapsed behind a prominent premaxilla (Fig. 21.2).

Palate only

A widening of the arch posteriorly is usually seen.

It has been shown that individuals with a cleft have a more concave profile, and whilst a degree of this is due to a restriction of growth (see below), research indicates that cleft patients have a tendency towards a more retrognathic maxilla and mandible and also a reduced upper face height compared with the normal population.

21.4.2. Post-surgical distortions

Studies of individuals with unoperated clefts (usually in Third World countries) show that they do not experience a significant restriction of facial growth, although there is a lack of development in the region of the cleft itself, possibly because of tissue hypoplasia. In contrast, individuals who have undergone surgical repair of a cleft lip and palate exhibit marked restriction of mid-face growth anteroposteriorly and transversely (Fig. 21.3). This is attributed to the restraining effect of the scar tissue, which results from surgical intervention. It has been estimated that approximately 40 per cent of cleft patients suffer severe maxillary retrusion. Limitation of vertical growth of the maxilla coupled with a tendency for an increased lower facial height results in an excessive freeway space, and frequently overclosure (Fig. 21.4).

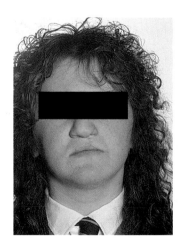

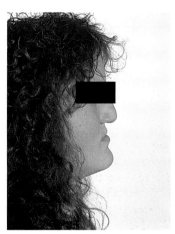

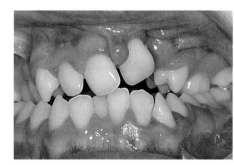

Fig. 21.3. Patient with a repaired unilateral cleft lip and palate of the left side showing mid-face retrusion.

21.4.3. Hearing and speech

Speech development is adversely affected by the presence of fistulae in the palate (Fig. 21.5) and by velopharyngeal insufficiency (where the soft palate is not able to make an adequate contact with the back of the pharynx to close off the nasal airway).

A cleft involving the posterior part of the hard and soft palate will also involve the tensor palati muscles, which act on the Eustachian tube. This predisposes the patient to problems with middle-ear ventilation (known colloquially as 'glue ear'). Obviously, hearing difficulties will also retard a child's speech development. Therefore management of the child with a cleft involving the posterior palate must include audiological assessments and myringotomy with or without grommets as indicated.

21.4.4. Other congenital abnormalities

Around 20 per cent of babies with cleft anomalies, particularly with isolated cleft palate, have associated abnormalities, more frequently of the heart and extremities.

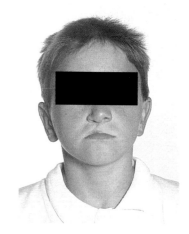

Fig. 21.4. Patient with a repaired cleft lip and palate of the right side who had a degree of overclosure, believed to be due to the restricting effect of the primary repair on vertical growth.

21.4.5. Dental anomalies

In addition to the affects on the teeth in the region of the cleft discussed above, the following anomalies are more prevalent in the remainder of the dentition:

- delayed eruption (delay increases with severity of cleft)
- hypodontia
- general reduction in tooth size
- abnormalities of tooth size and shape (Fig. 21.6)
- enamel defects.

21.5. COORDINATION OF CARE

In order to minimize the number of hospital visits and to ensure integrated inter-disciplinary management, it is essential to employ a team approach with joint clinics. The core members usually include the following:

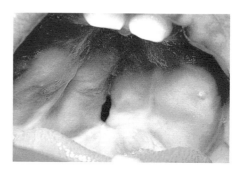

Fig. 21.5. Residual palatal fistula.

- orthodontist
- maxillofacial surgeon
- plastic surgeon
- speech therapist
- ear, nose, and throat (ENT) surgeon.
- health visitor

21.6. MANAGEMENT

21.6.1. At birth

The birth of a child with a cleft anomaly will come as a shock and a disappointment for the parents. It is common for them to experience feelings of guilt and they will need time to grieve for the emotional loss of the 'normal' child that they anticipated. It is important to provide support for the mother at this time to ensure that bonding develops normally and that help with feeding is readily available for those infants with a cleft palate. Because a child with a cleft

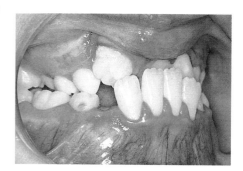

Fig. 21.6. Repaired bilateral cleft lip and palate with absent upper right lateral incisor and hypoplasia of the upper right central incisor.

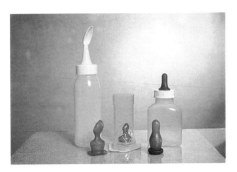

Fig. 21.7. Suitable bottles and teats for feeding cleft babies.

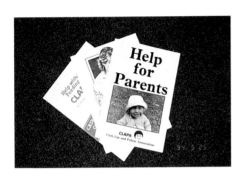

Fig. 21.8. CLAPA leaflets.

will have difficulty in sucking, a bottle and teat which help direct the flow of milk into the mouth is helpful, for example a soft bottle which can be squeezed (Fig. 21.7). Details of a range of useful bottles and teats can be obtained from the support group CLAPA (the Cleft Lip and Palate Association) (Fig. 21.8). This group also provides support and counselling, which is usually greatly appreciated by the parents of a cleft baby. An explanation from a member of the cleft team of probable future management and the possiblities of modern treatment, together with a contact person for advice, is also recommended.

Some centres still advocate the use of acrylic plates designed to help with feeding or to move the displaced cleft segments actively towards a more normal relationship to aid subsequent surgical apposition. This approach, which is known as presurgical orthopaedics, is becoming less fashionable because of a lack of evidence of its efficacy and the good results produced by some cleft teams (for example Oslo) who do not employ presurgical plates.

21.6.2. Lip repair

There is a wide variation in the timing of primary lip repair, depending upon the preference and protocol of the surgeon and cleft team involved. Neonatal repair is still being evaluated. In the UK primary lip repair is, on average, carried out around 3 months of age. A number of different surgical techniques have been described (for example Millard, Delaire, and straight line). The best techniques aim to dissect out and re-oppose the muscles of the lip and alar base in their correct anatomical position. However, there is some controversy as to whether tissue movement should be achieved by subperiosteal dissection or supraperiosteal dissection and skin-lengthening cuts. The degree to which the alar cartlidge is dissected is also contentious, as is the use of a vomer flap.

Most centres repair bilateral cleft lips at the same procedure, but some still carry out two separate operations. Primary bone grafting of the alveolus at the time of lip repair has fallen into disrepute owing to the adverse effects upon subsequent growth.

21.6.3. Palate repair

In many European centres closure of the hard palate is delayed until 5 years of age or older in an effort to reduce the unwanted effects of early surgery upon growth. There is some evidence to suggest that transverse growth of the maxilla is improved. However, the adverse effect upon speech development has been well documented. In the UK hard and soft palate repair is undertaken, on average, between 9 and 12 months of age with the philosophy that any unwanted effects upon growth caused by repair at this stage (which can be compensated for to a degree by orthodontics and surgery) are preferable to fostering the development of poor articulatory habits, which can be extremely difficult to eradicate after the age of 5.

21.6.4. Primary dentition

The first formal speech assessment is usually carried out around 2 years of age, depending upon the needs of the child. Monitoring of a patient's speech should continue throughout childhood, preferably at joint clinics, to pick up any developing problems that may arise with growth. An assessment with an ENT surgeon should also be arranged if this specialty has not been not involved at the time of primary repair.

It is important to minimize surgical interference with the cleft child's life and 'minor' touch-ups should be avoided. Lip revision, prior to the start of schooling, should be performed only if clearly indicated. Closure of any residual palatal fistulae may also be considered to help speech development. In a proportion of cases the repaired cleft palate does not completely seal off the nasopharynx during speech and nasal escape of air may occur, resulting in a nasal intonation to the child's speech. If indicated by evidence from investigations such as speech assessment, videofluroscopy, and nasoendoscopy, a pharyngoplasty may help. These operations, which involve moving mucosal or musculomucosal pharyngeal flaps to augment the shape and function of the soft palate, can reduce velopharngeal incompetence. If indicated, this should be carried out around 4 to 5 years of age.

Orthodontic treatment in the primary dentition is not warranted. However, during this stage it is important to develop good dental care habits, instituting fluoride supplements in non-fluoridated areas.

21.6.5. Mixed dentition

During this stage the restraining effect of surgery upon growth becomes more apparent, initially transversely in the upper arch and then anteroposteriorly as growth in the latter dimension predominates. With the eruption of the permanent incisors, defects in tooth number, formation, and position can be assessed. Often the upper incisors erupt into lingual occlusion and may also be displaced or rotated (Fig. 21.9).

In order to avoid straining patient cooperation, it is better if orthodontic intervention is concentrated into two phases. The first stage is usually carried out during the mixed dentition with the specific aim of preparing the patient for alveolar or secondary bone grafting, and it is preferable, if possible, to delay the correction of the upper incisors until then. The second stage is discussed in Section 21.6.6.

Alveolar (Secondary) bone grafting

This technique has significantly improved the orthodontic care of patients with an alveolar cleft as it involves repairing the defect with cancellous bone which confers the following advantages:

- provision of bone through which the permanent canine (or lateral incisor) can erupt into the arch (Fig. 21.10);
- the possibility of providing the patient with an intact arch;
- improved alar base support;
- aids closure of residual oronasal fistulae;
- stabilization of a mobile premaxilla in a bilateral cleft.

For optimal results this procedure should be timed before the eruption of the permanent canines, at around 8–9 years, particularly as eruption of a tooth through the graft helps to stabilize it.

Before bone grafting is carried out, any transverse collapse of the segments should be corrected to allow complete exposure of the alveolar defect and to improve access for the surgeon. This is most commonly carried out by using the fixed expansion appliance called the quadhelix (see Section 13.4.4). This appliance has the advantage that additional arms or springs can be attached, if indicated, to procline the upper incisors, but in cases with more severe displacement and/or rotation of the incisors a simple fixed appliance can be used concurrently (Fig. 21.11). However, care is required to ensure that the roots of the teeth adjacent to the cleft are not moved out of their bony support, and it may be necessary to defer their complete alignment to the post-grafting stage. The expansion achieved should be retained, for example with a palatal arch, whilst bone grafting is carried

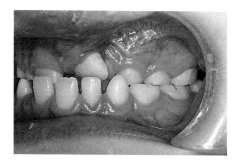

Fig. 21.9. A repaired unilateral cleft lip and palate in the mixed dentition.

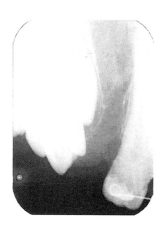

(a)

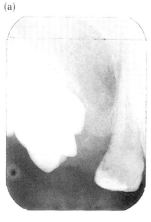

(b)

Fig. 21.10 Radiographs of a patient who had an alveolar bone graft: (a) prior to bone grafting; (b) a month after bone grafting.

Fig. 21.11. Patient with a repaired unilateral cleft of the lip and palate of the left side: (a) pretreatment; (b) following expansion and alignment of the rotated upper left central incisor.

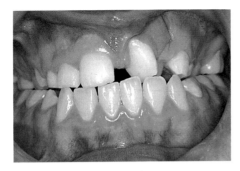
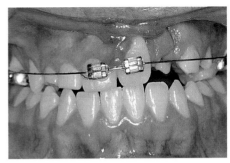

(a)   (b)

Fig. 21.12. The same patient as in Fig. 21.11: (a) palatal arch and sectional archwire to retain position of the upper central incisors, prior to bone grafting; (b) after bone grafting, showing the upper left canine erupting.

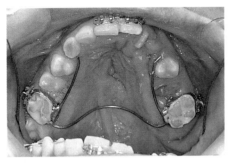
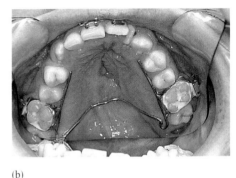

(a)   (b)

out (Fig. 21.12). Removing deciduous teeth and erupted supernumerary teeth in the region of the cleft prior to grafting substantially improves flap quality.

In patients with a bilateral complete cleft lip and palate it may be necessary to stabilize the mobile premaxillary segment after bone grafting in order to ensure that the graft takes. This can be accomplished by placement of a relatively rigid buccal archwire prior to bone grafting, which is left *in situ* for at least 3 months after the operation. If space closure on the side of the cleft is planned, consideration should be given to the need to extract the deciduous molars on that side prior to grafting in order to facilitate forward movement of the first permanent molar. However, any extractions should be carried out at least 3 weeks prior to bone grafting in order to allow healing of the keratinized mucosa.

Cancellous bone is currently used for bone grafting because it assumes the characteristics of the adjacent bone; however, this may change in the future as bone morphogenesis proteins become cheaper and more readily available. Cancellous bone can be harvested from a number of sites, but the iliac crest or the chin are currently most popular. Keratinized flaps should be raised and utilized for closure, as mucosal flaps may interfere with subsequent tooth eruption. Unerupted supernumerary teeth are commonly found in the cleft itself, and these can be removed at the time of operation. There is no substantive evidence to support the contention that simultaneous bone grafting of bilateral alveolar cleft jeopardizes the integrity of the premaxilla.

The complications of this technique include the following:

- granuloma formation in the region of the graft — this often resolves with increased oral hygiene, but surgical removal may be required;
- failure of the graft to take — this usually only occurs to a partial degree;
- root resorption — relatively rare;
- around 15 per cent of canines require exposure.

21.6.6. Permanent dentition

Once the permanent dentition has been established, but before further ortho-dontic treatment is planned, the patient should be assessed as to the need for orthognathic surgery to correct mid-face retrusion (see Chapter 20). The degree of maxillary retrognathia, the magnitude and effect of any future growth, and the patient's wishes should all be taken into consideration. If surgical correction is indicated, this should be deferred until growth is complete (following any presurgical orthodontic alignment).

If orthodontics alone is indicated, this can be commenced once the permanent dentition is established. Usually fixed appliances are necessary (Fig. 21.13). If space closure in the region of the cleft is not feasible, treatment planning should be carried out in collaboration with a restorative opinion regarding the design of the prosthesis required.

At the end of orthodontic treatment, retention will be required. If the maxillary arch has been expanded, this will be particularly prone to relapse, and retention of the arch width with either a removable retainer worn at night or a partial denture (if indicated for prosthetic reasons) is advisable.

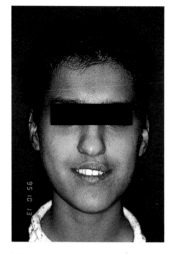

(a)

21.6.7. Completion of growth

A final surgical revision of the nose (rhinoplasty) may be carried out at this stage. However, if orthognathic surgery is planned, this should be carried out first, as movement of the underlying bone will affect the contour of the nose.

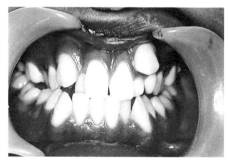

(b)

21.7. AUDIT OF CLEFT PALATE CARE

Audit of cleft palate management is difficult because of the different disciplines involved in providing care and the range of clinical presentations. In order to try to evaluate the effects of treatment, careful records taken before and after any intervention (surgical or orthodontic) must be a priority. These should include study models and photographs of the cleft prior to primary closure, so that the size and morphology of the original cleft can be taken into consideration. In addition, a cleft team should concentrate on a particular treatment protocol in order to gain the necessary expertise and experience to achieve successful results and to collate a meaningful amount of useful data. If the results of one surgical team carrying out a particular treatment protocol are to be compared with another treatment regimen carried out at a different centre, some standardization of these records is required. In the UK the Cranio-facial Society of Great Britain is attempting to standardize record collection with the Cranio-facial Anomalies REgister (CARE).

As in all branches of medicine, concentration of expertise and experience at a centre of excellence produces superior results to those obtained by a lone practitioner carrying out small numbers of a particular procedure each year. Therefore there is pressure to concentrate cleft palate care at regional centres. However, this approach has the disadvantage that the majority of patients will have to travel greater distances to receive their treatment. In other countries this problem is addressed by greater availability of central funding to transport patients and their families to receive treatment; accommodation costs are also included.

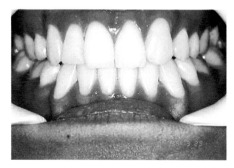

(c)

Fig. 21.13. (a) Patient with a repaired unilateral left cleft lip and palate. The diminutive upper right lateral incisor was extracted and the canine brought forward adjacent to the upper right central incisor: (b) pretreatment; (c) post-treatment.

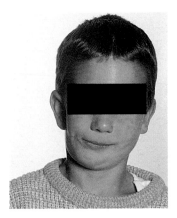

(a)

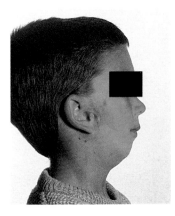

(b)

Fig. 21.14. Patient with hemifacial microsomia.

21.8. OTHER CRANIOFACIAL ANOMALIES

21.8.1. Hemifacial microsomia

This is the second most common craniofacial anomaly, with a prevalence of 1 in 5000 births. It is a congenital defect characterized by a lack of both hard and soft tissue on the affected side of the face, usually in the area of the mandibular ramus and external ear (i.e. in the region of the first and second branchial arches, hence its older name of first arch syndrome). This anomaly usually affects one side of the face (Fig. 21.14), but does present bilaterally in around 20 per cent of cases. A wide spectrum of ear and cranial nerve deformities are found. Goldenhar syndrome or oculo-auriculovertebral dysplasia (the latter name neatly explains the affected sites, but is more difficult to remember — and spell) is a variant of hemifacial microsomia.

Management usually involves a combination of surgery and orthodontic treatment. However, milder cases can sometimes be managed with orthodontic appliances alone. Orthodontic treatment usually involves the use of a specialized type of functional appliance known as a hybrid appliance, so called because components are selected according to the needs of the individual malocclusion, for example encouraging eruption of the buccal segment teeth on the affected side. The degree and type of surgery depends upon the severity of the defect, but three phases are recognized:

- Early reconstruction (5 to 8 years of age), commonly with costochondral rib grafts, is usually reserved for severe cases with no functioning TMJ.
- At the end of the adolescent growth spurt (around 12–15 years of age) — distraction osteogenesis (see section 20.4.4).
- Late teens, to enhance the contour of the skeleton and soft tissues — conventional orthognathic and reconstructive techniques.

21.8.2. Treacher–Collins syndrome

This syndrome is also known as mandibulofacial dysostosis. It is inherited in an autosomal dominant manner and consists of the following features, which are present bilaterally:

- downward sloping (anti-mongoloid slant) palpebral fissures and colobomas (notched iris with a displaced pupil);
- hypoplastic malars;
- mandibular retrognathia;
- deformed ears, including middle and inner ear which can result in deafness;
- hypoplastic air sinuses;
- cleft palate in 30 per cent of cases;
- most have completely normal intellectual function.

The specifics of management depend upon the features of the case, but usually staged craniofacial surgery is required. If a cleft palate is present, this is handled as described above.

21.8.3. Pierre Robin anomaly

This anomaly consists of retrognathia of the mandible, cleft palate, and glossoptosis, which together cause airway problems in the infant. Although originally thought to be due to raised intra-uterine pressure causing the head of the fetus to be compressed against the chest, thus restricting normal development of the mandible, recent research would suggest a metabolic aetiological factor. The first priority at birth is to maintain the airway; in a proportion of cases it is necessary to use an endotracheal tube for the first few days, but once the child is older, or in less severe cases, prone nursing will suffice. Rarely, tracheostomy for medium-term airway protection is required. Subsequent management is as for cleft palate (see above). In a proportion of Pierre Robin children catch-up growth of the mandible does occur, but paediatric distraction osteogenesis (see section 20.4.4) or conventional orthognathic surgery can be planned for those with a markedly retrognathic mandible.

21.8.4. Craniosynostoses

In craniosynostosis and craniofacial synostoses, premature fusion of one or more of the sutures of the bones of the cranial base or vault occurs. The effects depend upon the site and extent of the premature fusion, but all have a marked effect upon growth. In some cases restriction of skull vault growth can lead to an increase in intracranial pressure which, if untreated, can lead to brain damage. If raised intracranial pressure is detected, release of the affected suture(s) before 6 months of age is indicated. This may be the only intervention needed in isolated craniosynostoses. Combined craniofacial synostoses (e.g. Crouzon syndrome, Apert syndrome) require subsequent staged orthodontic and surgical intervention. This may become the prime indication for telemetric distraction osteogenesis.

PRINCIPAL SOURCES AND FURTHER READING

Bergland, O., Semb, G., and Abyholm, F. E. (1986). Elimination of the residual alveolar cleft by secondary bone grafting and subsequent orthodontic treatment. *Cleft Lip and Palate Journal*, **23**, 175–205.

● This paper is now a classic. It describes the pioneering work by the Oslo cleft team on alveolar bone grafting.

Bhatia, S. N. (1972). Genetics of cleft lip and palate. *British Dental Journal*, **132**, 95–103.

● Gives an interesting hypothesis regarding the inheritance of cleft anomalies, but also includes insight on the genetics of other dental anomalies.

Clinical Standards Advisory Group (1998). *Cleft lip and/or palate.* Stationery Office, London.

Cousley, R. R. J. (1993). A comparison of two classification systems for hemifacial microsomia. *British Journal of Oral and Maxillofacial Surgery*, **31**, 78–82.

Edwards, J. R. G. and Newall, D. R. (1985). The Pierre Robin syndrome reassessed in the light of recent research. *British Journal of Plastic Surgery*, **38**, 339–42.

Ranta, R. (1986). A review of tooth formation in children in cleft lip/palate. *American Journal of Orthodontics and Dentofacial Orthopedics*, **90**, 11–18.

Steinberg, M. D. *et al.* (1999). State of the art in oral and maxillofacial surgery: Treatment of maxillary hypoplasia and anterior palatal and alveolar clefts. *Cleft Palate-Craniofacial Journal*, **36**, 283–291.

Thom, A. R. (1990). Modern managment of the cleft lip and palate patient. *Dental Update*, **17**, 402–8.

● An easy-to-read paper emphasizing the integration of preventive care in the overall management of the cleft palate patient.

Definitions

ANCHORAGE The source of resistance to the forces generated in reaction to the active components of an appliance.

ANTERIOR OPEN BITE There is a space vertically between the incisors when the buccal segment teeth are in occlusion.

BALANCING EXTRACTION Extraction of the same (or adjacent) tooth on the opposite side of the arch to preserve symmetry.

BIMAXILLARY PROCLINATION Both upper and lower incisors are proclined relative to their skeletal bases.

BODILY MOVEMENT Equal movement of the root apex and crown of a tooth in the same direction.

BUCCAL CROSSBITE The buccal cusps of the lower premolars and/or molars occlude buccally to the buccal cusps of the upper premolars and/or molars.

CINGULUM PLATEAU The convexity of the cervical third of the lingual/palatal aspect of the incisors and canines.

COMPENSATING EXTRACTION Extraction of the same tooth in the opposing arch.

COMPETENT LIPS Upper and lower lips contact without muscular activity at rest.

COMPLETE OVERBITE The lower incisors occlude with the upper incisors or palatal mucosa.

CROWDING Where there is insufficient space to accommodate the teeth in perfect alignment in an arch, or segment of an arch.

DENTO-ALVEOLAR COMPENSATION The inclination of the teeth compensates for the underlying skeletal pattern, so that the occlusal relationship between the arches is less marked.

HYPODONTIA This term is used when one or more permanent teeth (excluding third molars) are congenitally absent. The equivalent American nomenclature is oligodontia.

IDEAL OCCLUSION Anatomically perfect arrangement of the teeth. Rare.

IMPACTION Impeded tooth eruption–usually because of displacement of the tooth or mechanical obstruction (e.g. a supernumerary tooth).

INCOMPETENT LIPS Some muscular activity is required for the lips to meet together.

INCOMPLETE OVERBITE The lower incisors do not make contact with the opposing upper incisors or palatal mucosa when the buccal segment teeth are in occlusion.

LEEWAY SPACE The difference in diameter between the deciduous canine, first molar, and second molar, and their permanent successors (canine, first premolar, and second premolar).

LINGUAL CROSSBITE The buccal cusps of the lower premolars and/or molars occlude lingually to the lingual cusps of the upper premolars or molars.

MALOCCLUSION Variation from ideal occlusion which has dental health and/or psychosocial implications for the individual. NB The borderline between normal occlusion and malocclusion is contentious (see Chapter 1).

MANDIBULAR DEVIATION The path of closure of the mandible starts from a postured position.

MANDIBULAR DISPLACEMENT When closing from the rest position the mandible displaces (either laterally or anteriorly) to avoid a premature contact.

MIDLINE DIASTEMA A space between the central incisors. Most common in the upper arch.

MIGRATION Physiological (minor) movement of a tooth.

NORMAL OCCLUSION Acceptable variation from ideal occlusion.

OVERBITE Vertical overlap of the upper and lower incisors when viewed anteriorly: one-third to one-half coverage of the lower incisors is normal; where the overbite is greater than one-half it is described as being increased; where the overbite is less than one-third it is described as being reduced.

OVERJET Distance between the upper and lower incisors in the horizontal plane. Normal is 2–4 mm.

RELAPSE The return, following correction, of the features of the original malocclusion.

REVERSE OVERJET The lower incisors lie anterior to the upper incisors. When only one or two incisors are involved the term anterior crossbite is commonly used.

ROTATION A tooth is twisted around its long axis.

SPACING Where the teeth do not touch interproximally and there are gaps between adjacent teeth. Can be localized or generalized.

TILTING MOVEMENT Movement of the root apex and crown of a tooth in opposite directions around a fulcrum.

TORQUE Movement of the root apex buccolingually, either with no or minimal movement of the crown in the same direction.

TRAUMATIC OVERBITE The occlusion of the lower incisors with the palatal mucosa has led to ulceration.

UPRIGHTING Mesial or distal movement of the root apex so that the root and crown of the tooth are at an ideal angulation.

Index